*The Practical Guide to the
Genetic Family History*

The Practical Guide to the Genetic Family History

Second Edition

Robin L. Bennett
Division of Medical Genetics
University of Washington School of Medicine

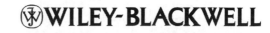
WILEY-BLACKWELL

A JOHN WILEY & SONS, INC., PUBLICATION

Wiley-Blackwell is an imprint of John Wiley & Sons, formed by the merger of Wiley's global Scientific, Technical, and Medical business with Blackwell Publishing.

Published by John Wiley & Sons, Inc., Hoboken, New Jersey.
Published simultaneously in Canada.

For general information on our other products and services or for technical support, please contact our Customer Care Department within the United States at (800) 762-2974, outside the United States at (317) 572-3993 or fax (317) 572-4002.

Wiley also publishes its books in a variety of electronic formats. Some content that appears in print may not be available in electronic formats. For more information about Wiley products, visit our web site at www.wiley.com

Library of Congress Cataloging-in-Publication Data:

Bennett, Robin L., MS, CGC.
    The practical guide to the genetic family history / Robin Bennett. – 2nd ed.
        p.   cm.
    Includes bibliographical references and index.
    ISBN 978-0-470-04072-0 (pbk. : alk. paper)
    1. Genetic counseling.   2. Medical history taking.   3. Genealogy.   I. Title.
    [DNLM: 1. Medical History Taking.   2. Pedigree.   3. Genetic Counseling–methods.
QZ 50 B4722p 2010]
    RB155.7.B46   2010
    616′.042–dc22   2009054241

Printed in the United States of America

10 9 8 7 6 5 4 3 2 1

"I've learned that people will forget what you said, people will forget what you did, but people will never forget how you made them feel."
Maya Angelou

Dedicated to my family–Scott, Maggie and Paul, Colin, Evan, and Maren, Kristin and D. Paul, and auntie Jo; my teacher–Mr. Tougaw; and my friends–Leslie and Nancy.

Contents

Illustrations and Tables

Foreword

The publication of the second edition of Robin Bennett's *The Practical Guide to the Genetic Family History* is an exciting event. This book initially appeared in 1999 with comprehensive coverage of all aspects of the genetic family history and its clinical utility for medical genetics. Bennett is a highly experienced genetic counselor with a deep knowledge of clinical genetics who has worked in the field for 25 years, during a time when medical genetics and its applications have continued growing. From early emphasis on pediatric diseases, medical genetics is now becoming increasingly important for other areas of adult medicine, such as oncology and cardiology. With these developments, our new knowledge of genomics is beginning to be useful in medicine.

The new edition covers practically all conditions encountered by genetic counselors and medical geneticists for diagnosis, reproductive choices, and genetic counseling. Comprehensive listing of diagnostic clues from the family history and patients is particularly useful. The book also deals with many topics requiring genetic knowledge, such as for assisted reproduction in both male and female infertility. The important role of genetic tests by biochemical and molecular methods and their use in patients and family members at genetic risk is covered. There is an extensive chapter about cancer genetics and its practical applications. Many tables allow access to extensive information in an easy manner. Topics such as the current status of adoption provide aid about how to deal with adoptive parents and adoption agencies. Recent developments emphasizing the use of family history by organizations such as the Surgeon General's Office, the Centers for Disease Control and Prevention, and National Institutes for Health reflect current standardization of family histories, an area in which the author's interest and experience has played an important role over the years.

The book is unique not only in accurately and comprehensively covering the medical and genetic aspects of hereditary disease but also in dealing with the many psychological, social, and ethical problems that often arise in such cases. As a medical geneticist who has worked with the author for 25 years, I have admired her approach to patients and their families over a wide range of clinical problems. The new edition of *The Practical Guide to the Genetic Family History* is full of "clinical pearls" for dealing with practical problems posed by patients, their families, and referring health professionals. Bennett provides many insights for dealing sympathetically with the realities and the uncertainties of imperfect knowledge that are often encountered in this area. Specific experiences with patients are often cited to illustrate such problems.

The book is highly recommended for the training of genetic counselors and for MD trainees in medical genetics as well as other professionals such as nurses, social workers, and physician assistants who work with patients who have been diagnosed with a genetic disease. *The Practical Guide to the Genetic Family History* will serve as a most useful reference for all health professionals needing up-to-date advice for practical genetic information.

Arno G. Motulsky, MD, ScD
Professor of Medicine (Division of Medical Genetics)
and Genome Sciences
University of Washington
March 2009

Preface

If there is genetically determined manifest destiny to become a genetic counselor, perhaps mine was set by my maternal great-great-grandfather, Henry Harbaugh who in 1856 wrote in the annals of the Harbaugh family history:[1] "To cherish the memory of our ancestors is a plain dictate of piety. Only those who care not for their destiny, can be careless as to their origin." Although I am not as pious as those Harbaugh and Eyeler ancestors whose descendants still worship in the hollows of mortar that they laid in the hills of the Harbaugh Valley of west-central Maryland, I do have conviction that a medical-family history continues to grow as an essential tool in the armamentarium of clinical diagnosis and client centered care.

The path of my destiny was farther laid by my maternal grandmother, Marjorie Warvelle Harbaugh, who stoked my mind with the art, poems, and images of my ancestors intertwined in elaborate genealogical trees. Her genealogical stories are what I remember best—the guillotined French revolutionary hero Jacques Pierre Brissot de Warville; Leonard Harbaugh, an engineer of the locks of the Potomac canals who was a confidant of George Washington; tales of ancestors voyaging from Denmark, Germany, England, and Ireland during times of persecution and famine; and her artistic sister, Florence, who died in a tuberculosis sanitarium shortly before her marriage. I recall the haunting emotion relayed when she spoke of her brother, Gerald, whom she describes in her memoirs as "the greatest burden of love to his mother as her imbecile son, her only son and greatly wished for child" who at 13 months was "tragically dropped down the stairs" and then never developed normally. The fragments of Gerald's existence are documented with his silver engraved cup in my china cabinet, the half-page of my grandmother's memoirs, and only one picture

---

[1]Henry Harbaugh, Annals of the Harbaugh Family in America from 1736 to 1856. Chambersburg, PA, 1856.

out of thousands of family images: Without question, the photograph of Gerald is of a boy who has Down syndrome (a condition that was just beginning to be recognized in the medical literature a few years after his birth). His short life of 14 years influenced my family for three-quarters of a century.

During my 25-year career as a genetic counselor I have drawn an estimated 20,000 pedigrees from family interviews. The stories documented are beyond a set of neatly drawn symbols. The structure of a medical-family history goes farther than simply assisting the clinician in medical diagnosis; a pedigree can help the clinician identify genetic testing strategies, identify patterns of inheritance, calculate risk of disease, make decisions on medical management and surveillance, develop patient rapport, and serve as a template for patient education. The medical-family history also harbors the stories of a family's beliefs on wellness and disease causality, their tragedies and their dreams. My goal in this book is to provide not only the science of pedigrees but the sensitive approach that must also accompany the gathering and recording of this information.

The Practical Guide to the Genetic Family History provides clinicians not only with the hows of taking a medical-family history and recording a pedigree but also the whys. The utility of taking a family history is reviewed in Chapter 1. In Chapter 2, a brief review of genetics is provided in the context of recognizing patterns of inheritance from a family pedigree and for providing genetic risk assessment and counseling. Standard pedigree nomenclature and the approach to recording a medical-family history are reviewed in Chapter 3. Chapter 4 is similar to a Cliff's Notes version of a basic overview of the directed questions to ask when recording a medical-family history for a specific medical indication (e.g., renal disease, hearing loss, mental illness). This section is greatly expanded on from the first edition. Of course, not every medical system is covered. My choice of disease categories is based on the general categories of disease for which I have had the most inquiries.

Over the past 10 years, cancer genetics has been one of the greatest fields of expansion in medicine and genetics, therefore Chapter 5 is solely devoted to this topic. Medical-family history plays a critical role in identifying families who can benefit from genetic testing and for providing cancer risk assessment so that high-risk families can be offered earlier and more intensive surveillance for cancer.

Pedigree analysis requires that the health facts recorded on individuals be accurate. This requires obtaining medical records on relatives. Although this can be time-consuming, it is often necessary. Chapter 6 details how to assist a patient in obtaining medical records, including death certificates. There is also information about how patients can research their own medical-family history and learn to record their own medical pedigree. It is helpful to the clinician if a patient has done the footwork in obtaining medical-family history information in advance of an appointment.

Adoption and assisted-reproductive technologies using gamete donation provide challenges in taking a medical-family history (see Chapters 7 and 8, respectively). The chapters that focus as these topics have been expanded on from the first edition. There is a growing movement to release closed adoption records and original birth certificates, and for openness in the release of health information about birth parents and gamete donors. A model medical-family history form to be used for adoption is detailed in Appendix 4; it can easily be adapted for use by programs providing assisted-reproductive technology services.

Genetic information carries unique personal, family, and social consequences. If a potential genetic disorder is identified through pedigree analysis, the patient and family members can benefit from referral to a board-certified genetic counselor, a medical geneticist, or genetic nurse specialist. Information on how to find a genetic specialist and what to expect from a genetic consultation is given in Chapter 9.

With the use of electronic health records, there are ethical issues to consider in recording a pedigree; these are detailed in Chapter 10. Researchers and individuals who are considering publishing a pedigree will find valuable information regarding issues to consider when involved in a family study or using a pedigree in publication.

Throughout the book I use clinical examples to illustrate certain themes. The case scenarios and pedigrees are based on hypothetical families. The names, family relationships, and psychosocial issues are fictitious, although the clinical information is often based on facts drawn from several families I have seen in my practice. The genogram of the fictional character Harry Potter (Figure 1.4) is interpreted from the series of four books by J. K. Rowling. The ecomap of soccer legend David Beckham (Figure 1.5), and the pedigrees of the Darwin-Wedgwood family (Figure 3.11) and of actress Elizabeth Taylor's immediate family (Figure 3.6) were drawn from information available in the public domain. I am grateful to the creative energy and genetic experience of Leslie Ciarleglio for the illustrations of the Potter genogram and the Beckham ecomap.

This volume is meant to be a handy reference using a pedigree as a primary tool for making a genetic risk assessment and counseling. Any healthcare provider, including physicians, nurses, medical social workers, and physicians assistants, will benefit from learning this approach to pedigree analysis. To find more information about a specific condition, you will need to turn to one of the many excellent references on genetic disorders, many of which are noted in the references in each chapter. Appendix 5 lists several of the online resources to query for more information about genetic disorders, their inheritance patterns and genetic testing. Appendix 7 is a source for the gene names and symbols associated with most of the disorders mentioned in this book along with the pattern of inheritance.

The pedigree as a tool of practice in health risk assessment and counseling has been available for a century, but the science of the pedigree has really just begun, first with the clarification of standard pedigree nomenclature from the National Society of Genetic Counselor's Task Force and their recommendations published in 1995 and then from national and international efforts of developing tools for decision analysis of pedigree data, such as the efforts of the U.S. Surgeon General's Office, the Centers for Disease Control and Prevention, and the National Institutes of Health State of the Science Conference in 2009. The second edition of the *Practical Guide to the Genetic Family History* continues to expand on earlier work and provide suggestions for future areas of research.

While preparing this edition, I had the privilege of traveling to Saudi Arabia and meeting with genetic counselors and geneticists. I was humbled in recognizing how biased the literature on clinical genetics, family history, and genetic counseling is toward a Western approach to health, disease, and family values. Although I hope that this edition of the *Practical Guide to the Genetic Family History* will reach a worldwide audience, I recognize that my approach is clearly colored from the perspective of a woman of northern European ancestry providing genetic counseling services in the United States. I look forward to hearing from colleagues and families from around the world about different approaches to taking and recording a family history that are more effective from their perspectives.

The foundation of my work lies with my colleagues on the National Society of Genetic Counselors Pedigree Standardization Work Group: Robert Resta, Kathryn Steinhaus French, and Debra Lochner Doyle, and with the assistance of the original task force members who also included Stefanie Uhrich and Corrine O'Sullivan Smith. I am particularly indebted to Robert Resta for his thoughtful edits of my work and his historical perspectives on family history.

I appreciate all I have learned from the opportunity of chairing the Family History Work Group of the National Coalition of Health Professional Education in Genetics (NCHPEG), particularly Joseph McInerney, Chantelle Wolport, Eugene Rich, Maren Scheuner, Siobhan Dolan, and Michael Rackover. I continue to bathe in the primordial soup of genetics with my colleagues at the University of Washington Medical Center, who always support my work including Dr. Arno Motulsky, Dr. Peter Byers, Dr. Virginia Sybert, Dr. Gail Jarvik, Dr. Wylie Burke, Dr. Marshall Horwitz, Dr. Elizabeth Swisher, Dr. Wendy Raskind, and of course my genetic counseling co-workers: Corrie Smith, Mercy Laurino, and Debbie Olson. I was fortunate to have the critical reviews of Heather Hampel, Sara Wyrick, Stephanie Jellison, and Kathleen Delp.

The staff at John Wiley & Sons, including Ian Collins, Kristen Parrish, and Thom Moore, have been generous in their patience and guidance.

I am blessed by a large and close family who continuously inspires me— particularly my sister, Kristin; and brother, Paul (thanks for reminding me to dance the Lucky); my father, Paul; and my cousins Lizz and Tom—and by the support of my husband's family, particularly his sisters Dona, Shelley, and Dale. At the top of my family tree of gratitude are my children, Colin, Evan, and Maren; my aunt Jo, who keeps me plum in family history art quilts; my mother, Maggie, who steers my rudder; and of course, my husband, Scott MacDonald, who is always by my side.

My Mercer Island High School biology teacher, Bill Tougaw, remains the person to whom I dedicate my career and this work. Charles Rice, my uncle and a psychology professor at Kenyon College, provided me with career guidance during my college years.

A pedigree is a map that can help predict disease, but it is not destiny. Knowledge of family history can be used to change the course of family medical history. The families I have worked with continue to impress me with their strength, and they leave imprints on my life. As my gift to them I will end with a long forgotten poem of my maternal grandfather, Marion Dwight Harbaugh, whose life as a geologist was also devoted to maps (and he has left the legacy of geology to his son and grandson):

The Grand Canyon

In a glamorous land on the top of the world
Where the sky is an endless blue
A wedge of heaven has driven deep
And split the earth in two,
And torn its face in a jagged wound
All splotched and stained with blood
That long since poured from its riven veins
In a surging ghastly flood.

I stood one day and gazed in awe
At that gaping, beautiful gash
That stretches from dawn to the setting sun
Like the trail of a dragging lash;
And I looked for miles to its deepest depths
To behold with wondering eyes
The sinuous edge of that mighty wedge
That still presses down from the skies.

Then I trembled to think of the fearful powers
That buffet the world and me,
And I pitied the earth that since its birth
Has suffered so patiently;
But then I began to understand
How a life is shaped and steeled,
And made both rugged and beautiful
By the scars where its wounds have healed.

—*Marion Dwight Harbaugh (1934)*

Chapter *1*

The Language of the Pedigree

Pedigrees are a challenge. With their intricate patterns of geometric symbols, pedigrees are like biological crossword puzzles which dare the clever and creative geneticists to solve them for clues about inheritance, family dynamics, or the localization of a gene.
—Robert G. Resta (1995)

1.1 WHY TAKE TIME TO RECORD A GENETIC FAMILY HISTORY

The field of human genetics has revolutionized the practice of medicine. The cyberspace bible of human genetics—Victor McKusick's *Online Mendelian Inheritance in Man* (better known as OMIM)—lists more than 10,000 hereditary traits and conditions. Identification of genetic mutations through the International Human Genome Project makes genetic testing for most of these conditions a reality. Genetic susceptibility mutations are being identified as part of the causal nexus for complex medical conditions such as cancer, diabetes, heart disease, Alzheimer disease, and mental illness. Human genetics is no longer just a topic for obscure medical journals. Headlines heralding genetic advances are splashed across the fronts of newspapers and popular magazines. The gripping stories of people making heart-wrenching decisions about genetic testing and diagnosis increase the Nielsen ratings of Oprah Winfrey–style talk shows and hospital-based television medical dramas. Patients come to *you* wanting to know if they need to worry about a genetic disease during their pregnancies, in their children, or in relation to their own healthcare.

How can you as a clinician identify individuals at risk for genetic disorders? Often, the first step is to take a genetic family history, recorded in the shorthand form of a pedigree. A pedigree, commonly referred to as a family tree, is a graphic representation of a medical-family history using symbols. A concise pedigree provides both critical medical data and biological relationship information at a glance. In many circumstances, the pedigree is just as important for providing medical services to the patient as any laboratory test. In fact, the pedigree has been described as the "first genetic test." This is both a historical reference to the fact that pedigrees have been used in medicine for over 100 years and also that a pedigree is the first step for genetic evaluation. The pedigree is truly the symbolic language of clinical genetic services and of human genetic research.

Genetic diseases affect all organ systems. Therefore health professionals from all specialties need to learn to think genetic. You need not be a "clever and creative geneticist" (Resta, 1995) to take a genetic family history. The purpose of this book is to provide you with practical screening tools to make an assessment as to whether your client might benefit from more extensive genetic evaluation and/or testing. My goal is provide you with not just the family history questions to ask but the logic behind this questioning. Health professionals working with clients in family practice, internal medicine, pediatrics, neurology, oncology, and obstetrics will find these screening tools particularly useful.

A focus of this book is genetic screening questions for clinical specialists by disease system (see Chapter 4). The emphasis in Chapter 5 and Appendix 3 is family history tools for identifying individuals with an inherited susceptibility to cancer. Researchers in human genetics will find useful information on how to obtain family history information, as well as ethical issues to consider in family studies and the publication of pedigrees (see Chapter 10). For the benefit of professionals involved in adoption, in Chapter 7 I discuss the unique issues surrounding a genetic family history and adoption. In Chapter 8 I delve into some of the challenging aspects of family history in the context of assisted reproductive technologies and the use of donor gametes. Appendix 4 is a medical-family history questionnaire that could be used for a child being placed for adoption, or for health information for an egg or sperm donor, or surrogate mother.

1.2 WHAT DO CRANES HAVE TO DO WITH ANYTHING?

The word *pedigree* comes from the French *pie de grue*, or "crane's foot." The term first appeared in the English language in the 15th century. It described the curved lines resembling a bird's claws that were used to connect an individual with his or her offspring (Resta, 1993). Such vestiges of a bird's talons are obvious in the example of the *sippschaftstafel* drawn by Ernst Rüdin shown in Figure 1.1. The *sippschaftstafel* was a form of depicting family ancestry used by German eugenicists in the early 20th century (Mazumdar, 1992; Resta, 1993).

A pedigree is of limited value if the symbols and abbreviations cannot be easily interpreted. Historically, many different pedigree styles have been used in the

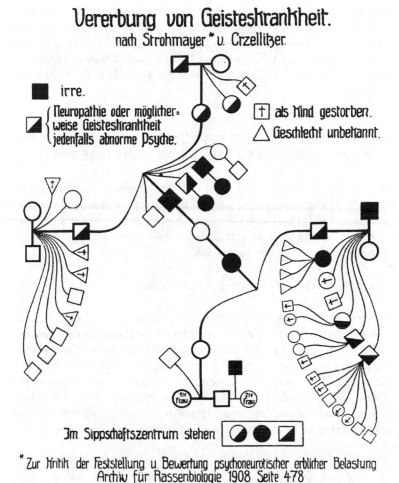

Figure 1.1 *A sippschaftstafel drawn by German eugenicist Ernst Rüdin in 1910. Note the proband (circle with irregular edge) is placed in the center of the pedigree and the maternal and paternal lineages radiate from curved lines drawn to the proband). Here the proband is shown being crushed by the weight of her dysgenic ancestry. (Reprinted with permission from Mazumdar, 1992; and Resta, 1993.)*

published literature and in patient medical records (Bennett et al., 1993; Resta, 1993; Steinhaus et al., 1995). In fact, genetics professionals probably use as many pedigree dialects as there are forms of the human language. As Francis Galton (an early geneticist and cousin to Charles Darwin) observed, "There are many methods of drawing pedigrees and describing kinship, but for my own purposes I still prefer those that I designed myself" (Galton, 1889). By using uniform symbols, it is possible to reduce the chances for incorrect interpretation of patient, family, medical, and genetic information.

Through a peer-reviewed process, the Pedigree Standardization Task Force (PSTF) of the National Society of Genetic Counselors (NSGC) developed standardized nomenclature for symbolizing pedigrees (Bennett et al., 1995). These have become an international standard, and the symbol set has required little revision since the original publication (Bennett et al., 2008). All pedigree symbols in this book conform to these standards.

1.3   THE PEDIGREE IS A COST-EFFECTIVE TOOL FOR GENETIC DIAGNOSIS AND RISK ASSESSMENT FOR MANY DISEASES

"But who has time to take a family pedigree?" is a common lament from the busy practitioner. Most clinicians record some information about a patient's family illnesses in textual form. This can be just as time-consuming as recording a pedigree, and the text may be both lengthier and less informative than a pedigree. For example, consider this excerpt from a medical record:

Linda's grandmother and two aunts died of breast cancer.

Did the cancer occur in Linda's maternal or paternal grandmother? Are the aunts the sisters of Linda's mother or her father? Did they have breast cancer before or after onset of menopause? The exact relationship of these affected relatives to Linda, their ages at diagnosis, and if the breast cancer was unilateral or bilateral can make a critical difference in your clinical assessment of Linda's lifetime risk of developing breast cancer. Instead, using the associative icons of a pedigree, the relevant family and medical information can be recorded quickly and precisely, in an easily interpretable format. A family pedigree has many functions; it is a tool for:

- Making a medical diagnosis.
- Deciding on testing strategies.
- Establishing the pattern of inheritance.
- Identifying at-risk relatives.
- Calculating disease risks.
- Determining reproductive options.
- Distinguishing genetic from other risk factors.
- Making decisions on medical management and surveillance.
- Developing patient rapport.
- Educating the patient.
- Exploring the patient's understanding.

Each of these benefits of collecting a pedigree will be explored further in this chapter.

1.4   JUST DO IT©

The popular advertisement "Just Do It" from the sports company Nike (Center for Applied Research, 2008) is applicable to the attitude that should be assumed by most health professionals regarding documenting a patient's medical-family history. Taking a directed genetic history is a primary step in the evaluation of many medical disorders. Barton Childs (1982) predicts that "to fail to take a good family history is bad medicine and someday will be criminal negligence." Notation of a genetic family history is likely to become an essential component of a patient's electronic medical record (Bennett et al., 2008). The family history that is placed in a newborn's electronic medical record may travel through the health system during that person's life, with the pedigree undergoing various iterations as the individual faces age-related health risks and changing familial risks as diseases develop in relatives.

The ability to elicit a comprehensive medical family history including a family pedigree, is stated as a fundamental skill for all health professionals, according to the National Coalition for Health Provider Education in Genetics (NCHPEG, 2007). Peter Schwartz of Yale University School of Medicine states that for early screening and detection of gynecological malignancies, "Family history is crucial, and it's not a superficial history. You have to go into depth" (Stone, 1998). Both the American College of Obstetrics and Gynecology (ACOG) and the American Society of Clinical Oncologists (ASCO) have had long-standing statements recording the importance of family history in obstetrics evaluations and cancer risk assessment, respectively (ACOG, 1987; ASCO, 1997).

Using a pedigree to symbolize a patient's medical and genetic history is no more time-consuming that dictating a detailed summary for the medical chart. A pedigree is a way to compress pages and pages of medical information on to an $8^1/_2$ by 11-inch piece of paper, or the screen of an electronic medical record. I always keep the patient's pedigree in the front of his or her medical file. This saves me time at subsequent visits because most of the critical information I need is readily accessible and succinctly summarized in one page. The pedigree gives me an immediate image of the family's health and sociological structure without the need to wade through stacks of medical records. Once a pedigree is obtained, the patient's family history can be easily updated on return visits.

1.5   THE PEDIGREE AS A DIAGNOSTIC TOOL

Reviewing a family pedigree can aid the clinician in diagnosis. For example, in making a diagnosis of a familial cancer syndrome, it is imperative to know the cluster of types of cancers; the ages of the individuals diagnosed with cancer; and how closely the individuals with cancer are related to each other (i.e., first-or second-degree relatives) (see Chapter 5). The family history will even influence the kind of genetic diagnostic tests that are ordered.

Take, for example, the family history of Susan, a 30-year-old computer software engineer and the mother of three. She is interested in information about how she can be screened for renal cell cancer because her father, Sam, was recently diagnosed with clear-cell renal carcinoma. Additional family history information is needed to help determine if his cancer was sporadic (the most likely scenario), resulting in a relatively low risk for Susan to develop renal cell cancer, or if Sam has an inherited cancer syndrome for which genetic testing might be available. Some inherited cancer syndromes to consider might include von Hippel-Lindau syndrome, Birt-Hogg Dubé, tuberous sclerosis complex, Lynch syndrome, and Cowden syndrome (see Chapter 5). Many of these inherited cancer syndromes are associated with other tumors besides renal cell carcinoma, thus an accurate diagnosis is important for both Susan and Sam. Taking a multigeneration pedigree (Figure 1.2) can help identify cost-effective approaches to genetic testing for Sam and Susan.

1.6   USING THE PEDIGREE TO DECIDE ON TESTING STRATEGIES AND FOR EVALUATING AT-RISK RELATIVES

Susan's pedigree suggests von Hippel-Lindau (VHL) syndrome, given the history of spinal tumors in her paternal uncle Charlie and the history of a brain tumor in her paternal uncle Adam. Ideally the DNA testing should begin with Sam. If a mutation is identified in Sam, then accurate mutation analysis is available for Susan, her siblings, and other relatives. The pedigree helps you determine the appropriateness of genetic testing, the first person to test, and who else in the family should be tested.

1.7   USING THE PEDIGREE TO ESTABLISH THE PATTERN OF INHERITANCE AND CALCULATE RISKS

John was born with a profound hearing impairment. He and his fiancée are planning a family, and they want to know if they have a high probability of having children who will also have severe congenital hearing impairment. This question is impossible to answer without obtaining a family history. Congenital deafness can have an autosomal recessive, autosomal dominant, X-linked, or mitochondrial inheritance pattern or it could have a maternal teratogenic etiology (see Section 4.3). How to use a pedigree to identify patterns of inheritance is detailed in Chapter 2. Once an inheritance pattern is identified or suspected, John and his fiancée can be given appropriate genetic counseling and possibly genetic testing.

1.8   A PEDIGREE CAN HELP DISTINGUISH GENETIC FROM OTHER RISK FACTORS

A pedigree can be just as useful in determining that a condition is not genetic as in establishing that a condition is inherited in a family. This is particularly true for common complex health conditions such as mental illness, heart disease, and cancer. For example, Jean is a 42-year-old premenopausal woman with unilateral

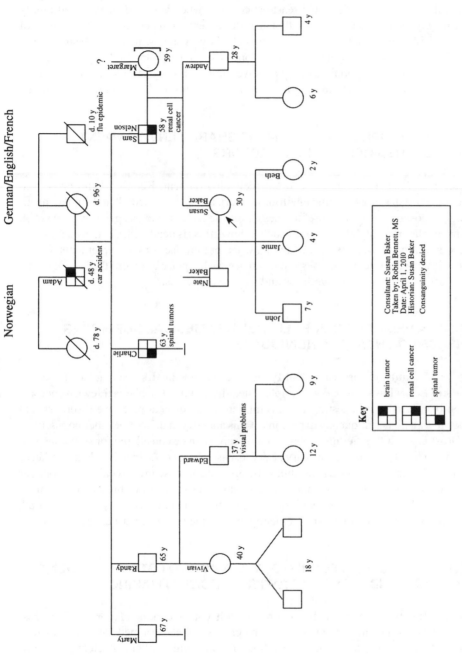

Figure 1.2 *A hypothetical pedigree representative of a family with von Hippel-Lindau syndrome.*

breast cancer. Her mother is healthy at age 65 years, but Jean's maternal grandmother, Pamela, died of breast cancer at age 53. This limited family history may raise your initial suspicion for a familial breast cancer. Yet, when you take an extended family history, you find that Jean's mother has three healthy sisters between the ages of 68 and 72 years. You also find that Pamela had two sisters who died of heart disease in their mid-70s, but they had never developed cancer. For Jean, this "negative" family history is just as important as the "positive" family history of cancer for her cancer risk assessment and determining a strategy for cancer screening and risk reduction.

1.9   A PEDIGREE CAN DOCUMENT SHARED ENVIRONMENT AND SHARED GENETIC RISK FACTORS

Families share their genes and often their environment. Relatives who are raised together often share the same environmental risks (such as secondhand smoke, pesticide exposure, and dietary preferences), lifestyle factors (such as patterns of exercise and alcohol use), styles of coping (such as how stress is dealt with), and even attitudes about health and wellness (for example, whether they use herbal supplements or seek medical care). A pedigree is a simple and accessible place to record these nongenetic factors that can influence wellness and disease processes.

1.10   A PEDIGREE CAN HELP IDENTIFY MEDICAL SCREENING NEEDS FOR HEALTHY INDIVIDUALS

A brief family history can identify genetic and medical screening needs for an otherwise healthy person. For example, a healthy couple of Ashkenazi Jewish ancestry can be offered carrier testing for several genetic autosomal recessive disorders that occur with higher frequency in persons of this ancestry than in some other populations (Gross et al., 2008). Serum cholesterol screening can be considered for someone with a strong family history of coronary artery disease. A person with a first-degree relative with colon cancer before age 50 should be offered colonoscopy screening at a younger age than usual. A young woman with a strong family history of breast cancer might be offered breast cancer screening at an earlier age than is typically recommended, particularly if her relatives are premenopausal at the time of breast cancer diagnosis.

1.11   TAKING A FAMILY HISTORY IS A WAY TO ESTABLISH CLIENT RAPPORT AND FACILITATE PATIENT DECISION MAKING

Your patients are more likely to comply with your recommendations if they trust you and have a relationship with you. The process of taking a medical-family history provides a prime opportunity to establish rapport with a client. A clear picture of family dynamics, family crisis and loss, ethnic and cultural background, and the patient's life experiences usually unfold while taking a patient's medical-family history. These family relationships and life experiences will influence a patient's decisions about medical care and genetic testing.

Querying a patient about his or her family history puts the client in the role of the expert (McCarthy et al., 2003). This can empower a patient who may feel powerless in the healthcare setting or mistrustful of health professionals (Erlanger, 1990). A client may feel more like an active participant in decisions about his or her healthcare. Through the process of taking a family history, a client is likely to feel listened to, and the process may even decrease patient anxiety (Erlanger, 1990; Rogers and Durkin, 1984; Rose et al., 1999).

Compare Amanda, a healthy 37-year-old pregnant woman who has experienced 10 years of infertility, with Beth who is also 37 years old and pregnant but has two healthy children. Both women have the same age-related risk to have a child with a chromosome anomaly, yet each woman may make different choices about genetic testing during her pregnancy. Or consider two 45-year-old women who each have a mother diagnosed with breast cancer at age 38 years; one has a mother who survived her breast cancer, the other has a mother who died 2 years after diagnosis. Their genetic cancer risk assessments (drawn from factual empiric risk models) are similar, but the emotional feelings each woman has about the magnitude of her cancer risk, the effectiveness of breast cancer screening, and usefulness of genetic testing are likely to differ based on each woman's experience with her mother's illness.

The symbols of a pedigree represent more than the "geometric pieces of a biological crossword puzzle," as described by Resta (1993) in the introductory quote to this chapter. I view a pedigree like a quilt, stitching together the intimate and colorful scraps of medical and family information from a person's life (Figure 1.3). Familiar pedigree patterns are the clinician's matrix for providing pedigree risk assessment as well as clinical and diagnostic recommendations. Yet just as the quilter takes artistic liberty with tried-and true patterns to make each quilt a unique work of art, each pedigree has a unique human story behind it. It is from the interwoven fabric of a patient's family, cultural, and life experiences that the patient pieces together his or her decision-making framework.

1.12   A PEDIGREE CAN BE USED FOR PATIENT MEDICAL EDUCATION

"A picture is worth a thousand words," or so the popular saying goes. Reviewing the pedigree with a patient is a vital tool in patient education (Table 1.1). Let us return to Susan's family in Figure 1.2. Susan's pedigree can be used to explain autosomal dominant inheritance: There are people affected in more than one generation, both men and women are affected, and there is male-to-male transmission of the disease. To establish the diagnosis of VHL, you may want to obtain medical records on the people you suspect are affected in the family (such as Susan's father, her uncle Charlie, and her paternal grandfather). By reviewing the pedigree with Susan, it is easy for Susan to see which family members she needs to obtain medical records from and why. The pedigree clearly defines who is at risk to develop VHL syndrome

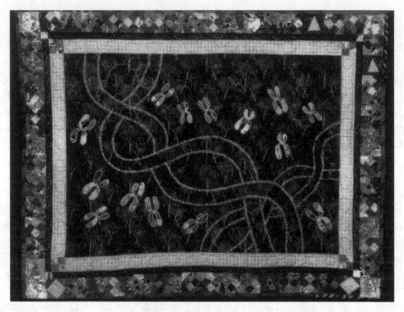

Figure 1.3 *The Family Tree. Designed and stitched in 1997 by Josephine B. Rice of Gambier, Ohio, in celebration of her grandson Brian Alan Forthofer. Brian lived one day before dying from complications of trisomy 13 on March 6, 1997. (Photographed by Ted Rice, reprinted with permission.)*

in Susan's family. You can discuss with Susan a plan for contacting extended family members. Strategies for helping a patient obtain medical records are presented in Chapter 6.

Reviewing a pedigree is a simple tool for showing the variability of disease expression in a family. In Susan's family it is obvious that some people with VHL have lived to an old age with few problems, whereas others are more severely affected. Susan's family history also nicely illustrates the various tumors that can occur together

TABLE 1.1   The Pedigree As a Valuable Tool in Patient Education

The clinician can use a pedigree to:
- Review with the patient the need for obtaining medical documentation on affected family members.
- Help the patient recognize the inheritance pattern of the disorder.
- Provide a visual reminder of who in the family is at risk for the condition and discuss plans for sharing information with relatives.
- Demonstrate variability of disease expression (such as ages of onset).
- Assist the patient in exploring his or her understanding of the condition.
- Discuss shared familial environmental risk factors (such as tobacco).
- Clarify patient misconceptions.

or in isolation in association with VHL. Seeing this visual representation of her family may help motivate Susan to follow your medical screening recommendations because, at a glance, she is reminded of the effect that VHL has had on her extended family.

The visual representation of a pedigree is a stark reminder that a genetic disease is a shared condition; a whole family is influenced. A clinician can use this as a compelling reminder to the patient that it is never any one person's fault that a genetic disease is present in a family.

1.13   USING A PEDIGREE TO EXPLORE A PATIENT'S UNDERSTANDING AND TO CLARIFY MISCONCEPTIONS

Reviewing the pedigree with Susan is an excellent way to explore her feelings about being at risk for VHL as well as her understanding of the disease:

- Should Susan's children have genetic testing and medical screening for VHL?
- How will Susan feel if she finds she is affected with VHL and that her children are at risk for this condition?
- Should Susan's children have genetic testing and medical screening for VHL?
- If Susan has VHL, what type of support does she have from her extended family to deal with her chronic illness?
- How will Susan feel if she is unaffected with VHL, but her sister is affected or vice versa?

Almost invariably a person seeking information about a genetic disease or genetic testing has already reached some of his or her own conclusions about the inheritance of their "family's curse." In fact, considerable family lore may center on complicated theories about the inheritance of the disease in question. For example, Susan might think that she is not a risk for VHL in her family because mostly men are affected. You can point out to Susan that her father did not have any sisters. Or Susan may falsely believe that the eldest sibling is spared from disease. A pedigree can be a wonderful way to clarify patient misconceptions. Table 1.2 lists many of the common misconceptions patients have about the inheritance of a condition in their family.

1.14   OTHER FAMILY DIAGRAMS: GENOGRAMS AND ECOMAPS

Genograms are common tools of therapists and some family practice professionals. They include demographic information (age, dates of birth and death), functional information (data on medical, emotional, and behavioral functioning of different family members) and critical family events (McGoldrick et al., 1999). Nonbiological relationships (such as a housemate or office co-worker) can be included on a genogram.

TABLE 1.2   Common Patient Misconceptions and Beliefs about Inheritance

Ø If no one else in the family is affected, the condition is not inherited.

Ø If several people in the family have the same condition, it must be inherited.

Ø All birth defects are inherited.

Ø The parents (particularly the mother) must have done something before conception or during the pregnancy to cause the condition in their fetus or child.

Ø An external event caused the problem (such as radiation from flying in airplanes, living near a power line or a nuclear reactor, a lunar eclipse).

Ø An evil spirit or an angered ancestor caused the disease.

Ø With a 25% recurrence risk, after one affected child, the next three will be unaffected.

Ø With a 50% recurrence risk, every other child is affected.

Ø The disease skips a generation.

Ø Birth order influences disease status (for example, only the eldest or youngest child can be affected.

Ø If the affected individuals in the family are all women, the condition must be sex-linked.

Ø A person will inherit the genetic condition because he or she looks or acts like the affected relative(s). Or the opposite—a person will not inherit a condition because he or she bears no resemblance to the affected relative(s).

Ø For a condition with sex-influenced expression (such as breast cancer), individuals of the opposite sex cannot transmit the condition (for example, a male cannot pass on a gene alteration for breast cancer).

Source: Modified from Connor and Ferguson-Smith, 1997.

The symbols of a genogram are construed similar to a pedigree (with males as squares and females as circles), with usually three generations pictured. Pertinent relationships are further described by *communication lines* that connect the symbols (McGoldrick et al., 1999):

    ══   Close, open communication with few secrets.

    ≡≡   Very close or fused; open communication without secrets.

    ∧∧∧∧   Poor communication, conflictual, many disagreements and secrets.

    ......   Distant communication (may be from geographic or lifestyle differences).

    ⊣⊢   Estranged or cut off (no communication; may be from conflict or separation such as divorce).

    #### A relationship can be both close and conflictual (a double line with a zigzag through it).

A sample genogram is shown in Figure 1.4 deduced from the fictional families of Harry Potter and Ron Weasley from the acclaimed book series by J. K. Rowling.

Pedigrees also often include information about levels of communication but not in the explicit format of a genogram. For example it may be noted on a pedigree that a person is adopted and has no contact with his or her birth family or that a person is estranged from certain relatives. In general, genograms seem most useful for a

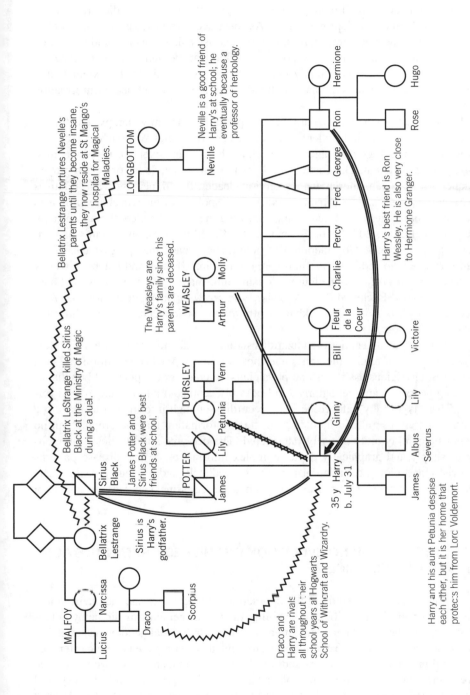

Figure 1.4 Genogram of the fictional families of Harry Potter and Ron Weasley from the J. K. Rowling Harry Potter series. (Illustration courtesy of Leslie Ciarleglio.)

Bellatrix Lestrange tortures Nevelle's parents until they become insane, they now reside at St Mango's hospital for Magical Maladies.

Neville is a good friend of Harry's at school; he eventually because a professor of herbology.

LONGBOTTOM

Neville

Bellatrix LeStrange killed Sirius Black at the Ministry of Magic during a duel.

James Potter and Sirius Black were best friends at school.

The Weasleys are Harry's family since his parents are deceased.

WEASLEY

Arthur   Molly

Hermione

Ron

Rose   Hugo

Fred   George

Percy

Charlie

Harry's best friend is Ron Weasley. He is also very close to Hermione Granger.

Sirius Black

Bellatrix Lestrange

Sirius is Harry's godfather.

DURSLEY

Vern

Petunia

POTTER

James   Lily

35 y Harry
b. July 31

Bill

Fleur de la Coeur

Victoire

Ginny

Lily

James   Albus Severus

MALFOY

Lucius   Narcissa

Draco

Scorpius

Draco and Harry are rivals all throughout their school years at Hogwarts School of Witchcraft and Wizardry.

Harry and his aunt Petunia despise each other, but it is her home that protects him from Lorc Voldemort.

13

therapist's chart or process notes when working with a client in long-term therapy; this documentation is traditionally not part of a patient's common medical record that is shared with other health professionals. As construed currently, a genogram is not as multifunctional as a pedigree, particularly for disease risk assessment and informing strategies for genetic testing. The crisscross effects of the multiple communication lines of a genogram may actually clutter the family graphic to the extent that it becomes difficult for the clinician to attend to the most relevant health information for that office visit.

Ecomaps are also a tool used primarily in personal and family therapy. The format resembles a wheel, with the client in the center, and the social relationships (some of which are also biologic) and agencies (such as church, employer, etc.) are in a circle surrounding the client. The clients "circle of life" may include his or her employer, teacher, sports coach, church and/or religious leader, friend, neighbor, and relatives (partner or spouse, children, parents, etc.). The "spokes" of the wheel are similar to the communication lines of genograms, showing them as close, conflictual, distant, etc. (Rempel et al., 2007). The Ecomap is then used to assess the client's or family's support network. Consideration of how this approach may piggy-back with a traditional genetic pedigree is a future area of research (Kenen and Peters, 2001). A sample ecomap is shown in Figure 1.5 using information on the professional soccer player David Beckham (http://en.wikipedia.org/wiki/David_Beckham; http://en.wikipedia.org/wiki/Victoria_Beckham; http://www.davidbeckham.com/; http://la.galaxy.mlsnet.com).

The professional genetics organizations should coordinate efforts with the professional societies of family therapists and those of family practice practitioners (such as nurses, physicians assistants and physicians) to consider the potential benefits of melding pedigrees and genograms (and possibly ecomaps) into a standardized format. There is a tricky balance between recording enough information to make the family diagram useful and including so much information that the graphic can no longer be quickly and concisely interpreted. The pedigree's utility lies in its ability to simply and graphically depict complex information so that disease patterns and risks, and biological relationships are immediately and obviously visible. The pedigree can already be used as a psychosocial assessment tool as discussed in Section 9.2.

1.15   THE CONTINUING EVOLUTION OF THE PEDIGREE IN THE AGE OF GENOMIC MEDICINE

Genomics describes the study of the interactions among genes and the environment (Guttmacher and Collins, 2002). The ability to practice genomic medicine by potentially viewing the molecular status of each patient's individual genome has an effect on all medical disciplines. Yet it is absurd to think that a complete genomic reference map will then lead to the understanding of all that is human or that we are all the direct and inevitable consequence of our genome. The genetic family history will continue to play an essential role in the medicine of the 21st century. As Reed Pyeritz

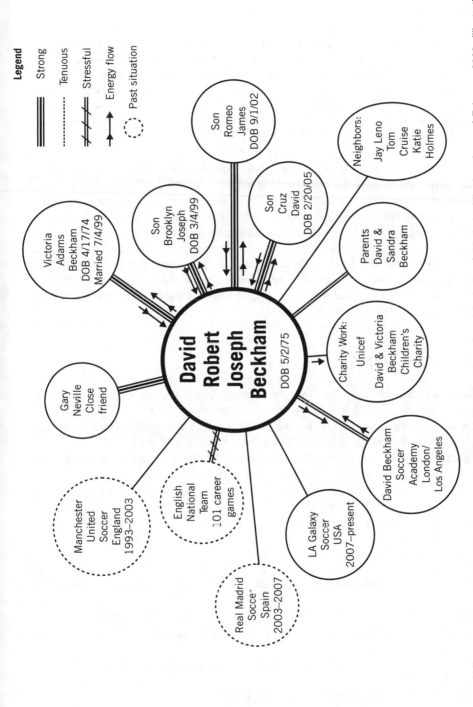

Legend

Strong

Tenuous

Stressful

Energy flow

Past situation

Neighbors: Jay Leno Tom Cruise Katie Holmes

Son Romeo James DOB 9/1/02

Son Cruz David DOB 2/20/05

Son Brooklyn Joseph DOB 3/4/99

Victoria Adams Beckham DOB 4/17/74 Married 7/4/99

Parents David & Sandra Beckham

David Robert Joseph Beckham DOB 5/2/75

Charity Work: Unicef David & Victoria Beckham Children's Charity

Gary Neville Close friend

David Beckham Soccer Academy London/ Los Angeles

Manchester United Soccer England 1993–2003

English National Team 101 career games

Real Madrid Soccer Spain 2003–2007

LA Galaxy Soccer USA 2007–present

Figure 1.5 *Ecomap of professional soccer player David Beckham, based on information from the public domain as of February 2009. (Illustration courtesy of Leslie Cia:leglio.)*

15

(1997), former president of the American College of Medical Genetics succinctly summarized:

> The importance of the family history will only be enhanced in the future. Even when an individual's genome can be displayed on a personal microchip, interpreting that information will depend in large part on the biological and environmental context in which the genome is expressed, and the family milieu is as good a guide as any. Physicians can help define those contexts through careful family and social histories. How those histories can be obtained and interpreted, when the average time for patient interaction with a physician continues to diminish, are crucial areas for research.

Variation is the hallmark of humans—even within well-established diseases with known patterns of inheritance, there is remarkable disease variability. Pedigree assessment will continue to play a critical role in our understanding of gene expression. A patient who has a genetic disorder or one who carries a genetic susceptibility mutation cannot be viewed in isolation from the background of his or her family history. How is it that five relatives with the same gene mutation can all have different ages of disease onset and varying clinical manifestations of the same genetic disorder? The patient and his or her genotype must be examined in the context of his or her genetic and environmental exposures. The clues from buried ancestors can reach out to the present to provide solutions for the future.

1.16 REFERENCES

American College of Obstetricians and Gynecologists. (1987). Antenatal Diagnosis of Genetic Disorders. *ACOG Technical Bulletin* 108. Washington, DC: ACOG.

American Society of Clinical Oncologists. (1997). Resource document for curriculum developing in cancer genetics education. *J Clin Oncol* 15:2157–2169.

Bennett RL, Steinhaus KA, Uhrich SB, O'Sullivan C. (1993). The need for developing standardized family pedigree nomenclature. *J Genet Couns* 2:261–273.

Bennett RL, Steinhaus KA, Uhrich SB, et al. (1995). Recommendations for standardized human pedigree nomenclature. *Am J Hum Genet* 56 (3):745–752.

Bennett RL, Steinhaus French K, Resta RG, Lochner Doyle D. (2008). Standardized pedigree nomenclature: Update and assessment of the recommendations of the National Society of Genetic Counselors. *J Genet Couns* 17(5):424–433.

Center for Applied Research. (2008). Mini case study: Nike's "Just Do It" Advertising Campaign: RES3:990108. Available at www.cfar.com/Documents/nikecmp.pdf. Accessed July 5, 2008.

Childs B. (1982). Genetics in the medical curriculum. *Am J Med Genet* 13:319–324.

Connor M, Ferguson-Smith M. (1997). *Essential Medical Genetics*. 5th ed. Oxford: Blackwell Science.

Erlanger MA. (1990). Using the genogram with the older client. *J Mental Health Couns* 12:321–331.

Galton F. (1889). *Natural Inheritance*. London: Macmillan.

Gross SJ, Pletcher BA, Monaghan KG, Professional Practice and Guidelines Committee. (2008). Carrier screening individuals of Ashkenazi Jewish descent. *Genet Med* 10(1):54–56.

Guttmacher AE, Collins FS. (2002). Genomic medicine—A primer. *N Engl J Med* 347(19): 1512–1520.

Kenen R, Peters J. (2001). The colored, eco-genetic relationship map (CEGRM): A conceptual approach and tool for genetic counseling research. *J Genet Couns* 10(4):289–301.

Mazumdar PMH. (1992). *Eugenics, Human Genetics and Human Failings*. London and New York: Routledge.

McCarthy Veach P, LeRoy B, Bartels D. (2003). *Facilitating the Genetic Counseling Process: A Practice Manual*. New York: Springer.

McGoldrick M, Gerson R, Shellenberger S. (1999). *Genograms: assessment and intervention*, 2nd ed. New York: Norton.

NCHPEG: National Coalition for Health Care Professional Education in Genetics. (2007). *Core Competencies in Genetics for Health Professionals*, 3rd ed. Available at www.nchpeg.org/core/core_comp_English_2007.pdf. Accessed July 5, 2008.

Online Mendelian Inheritance in Man, OMIM. Available at www.ncbi.nlm.nih.gov/omim. Accessed July 5, 2008.

Pyeritz RE. (1997). Family history and genetic risk factors. Forward to the future. *JAMA* 278(15):1284–1285.

Rempel GR, Neufeld A, Kushner KE. (2007). Interactive use of genograms and ecomaps in family caregiving research. *J Fam Nurs* 13:403–419.

Resta RG. (1993). The crane's foot: The rise of the pedigree in human genetics. *J Genet Couns* 2(4):1284–1285.

Resta RG. (1995). Whispered hints. *Am J Med Genet* 59:131–133.

Rogers J, Durkin M. (1984). The semi-structured genogram interview: I. Protocol, II. Evaluation. *Fam Systems Med* 2:176–187.

Rose R, Humm E, Hey K, et al. (1999). Family history taking and genetic counseling. *Fam Practice* 16:78–83.

Steinhaus KA, Bennett RL, Uhrich SB, et al. (1995). Inconsistencies in pedigree nomenclature in human genetics publications: A need for standardization. *Am J Med Genet* 56(3):291–295.

Stone Ml, ed. (1998). *Screening and Early Detection of Gynecologic Malignancies*. Update Vol. 23. Washington, DC. American College of Obstetricians and Gynecologists.

Chapter 2

Practical Inheritance

No genetic factor works in a void, but in an environment which may help or hinder its expression.
—Eliot Slater (1936)

2.1 A TRIBUTE(ARY) TO MENDEL

In some far-off recess of the human mind hides the Mendelian rules of inheritance that we learned in our early school education. While Mendelian patterns of inheritance remain a foundation for understanding many genetic principles, like many ideas of the 1860s, the principles of Gregor Mendel do not reflect the changing times. Should we be surprised that inheritance patterns in humans are more complex than those in garden peas or that an Augustinian monk is an unlikely resource in matters of human reproduction?

Mendel's laws work under the simple assumption that genetic factors are transmitted from each parent as discrete units that are inherited independently from one another and passed, unaltered, from one generation to the next. Thus begin the tributaries from Mendelian principles. We now know that genes do not function in isolation, but interact with each other and the environment (for example, modifying genes and regulating elements of genes). Genes that are in close proximity to each other may be inherited as a unit rather than independently (such as *contiguous gene syndromes*). Some genes are indeed altered from one generation to the next, as is evidenced by *dynamic mutations* (seen in *trinucleotide repeat disorders*), *new mutations*, and *parental imprinting*. Chemical markers on our genomes' DNA sequences actually change as we age without changing the actual sequence (*epigenetics*). Mendelian principles really do not apply when applied to *mitochondrial inheritance* because, in

The Practical Guide to the Genetic Family History, Second Edition, by Robin L. Bennett
Copyright © 2010 John Wiley & Sons, Inc.

this instance, there is virtually no paternal genetic contribution, and in *uniparental disomy* where only one parent contributes the homologous chromosomes (or segment of chromosomal material).

Despite these caveats, it is still useful to divide hereditary conditions into three classic inheritance patterns: single gene (classic Mendelian), multifactorial and polygenic, and chromosomal. Single-gene disorders are classified by whether they are dominant or recessive and by their locations on the chromosomes. Genes for autosomal disorders are on one of the 22 pairs of non-sex chromosomes (*autosomes*). Genes for sex-linked disorders are on the X and Y chromosomes. Sporadic inheritance usually refers to the one-time occurrence of a condition. In these instances, unaffected siblings usually do not have affected children but the parents of the affected child may have a risk of recurrence due to factors such as *gonadal moscaicism* and parental imprinting.

Clues for identifying the standard and not-so-standard patterns of inheritance are reviewed in Table 2.1. This chapter includes representative pedigrees for the primary inheritance patterns as well as tables with a sampling of common genetic conditions and their estimated incidences (Tables 2.2–2.4).

2.2 A BRIEF GENETICS PRIMER

This is a cursory review of some principles of human genetics. I have chosen points that may be useful to recall when one is interpreting family history information and genetic test results.

Humans carry an estimated 30,000 expressed genes. Genes are the basic chemical unit of heredity. They are packaged in rows (like beads on a string) on rod-like structures called chromosomes in the cell nucleus. Each gene has a specific place or *locus* on the chromosome. Every person inherits one copy of a gene from his (or her) mother and one from the father. Alternative copies of the same gene are called *alleles*. Although any single person has only two alleles of a gene (one from each parent), there may be many different types in the population. For example, in the genes for hereditary breast-ovarian cancer syndrome (*BRCA1* or *BRCA2*) there are over 1,000 different gene mutations that can occur in each gene. The *genotype* is an individual's genetic constitution. The *phenotype* is the observed expression (physical, biochemical, and physiological) of an individual's genotype.

Humans have 23 pairs of chromosomes in each cell of the body, except the egg and sperm, which have only one copy of each chromosome. There are 22 pairs of non-sex chromosomes called autosomes. The 23rd pair of chromosomes, the sex chromosomes, are called X and Y. Females have two X chromosomes. Males have an X and a Y chromosome. The centromeres are the sites of attachment of the spindle fibers during cell division. A centromere divides a chromosome into a short (upper) arm called the p arm and a long (lower) arm called the q arm. The telomeres are hot spots for mutation and are the section of DNA or "caps" located at each end of the chromosome.

A gene is as a molecule of DNA (deoxyribonuclei acid). Four letters (representing nitrogenous bases) in the DNA alphabet: A (adenine), C (cytosine), G (guanine), and

TABLE 2.1   Pedigree Clues for Distinguishing the Primary Patterns of Human Inheritance

Inheritance Pattern	Pedigree Clues	Confounding Variables
Autosomal dominant (AD)	Males and females affected Condition seen in multiple successive generations Both males and females transmit (male-to-male transmission observed) Often see variability of clinical disease expression Homozygotes may be more severely affected than heterozygotes Homozygous state may be embryonic lethal	Sex-limited expression (e.g., if individual has primarily male relatives this makes it difficult to recognize an inherited breast cancer or ovarian cancer syndrome) Small family size may mask inheritance Limited information about the health of prior generations may mask inheritance Mild expression and/or late onset of disease symptoms may cause disease to be unrecognized New dominant mutation may mask inheritance Gonadal mosaicism may cause disease to be mistaken for AR inheritance because parents are unaffected but sibling are affected
Autosomal recessive (AR)	Males and females affected Affected individuals usually in just one generation Symptoms often seen in newborn, infancy, or early childhood Often inborn errors of metabolism Disease may be more common in certain ethnic groups Sometimes see parental consanguinity	Small family size—may be mistaken for sporadic occurrence
X-linked (XL)	Males affected, may occur over multiple generations Females often express condition but have milder manifestations or later onset of symptoms Male-to-male transmission not observed Some conditions have embryonic male lethality so might see many miscarriages or paucity of males in pedigree	Small family size may mask inheritance Limited knowledge about prior generations may mask inheritance May be missed if paucity of males in family Disorder may have high new mutation rate Gonadal mosaicism (in females)

TABLE 2.1 (*Continued*)

Inheritance Pattern	Pedigree Clues	Confounding Variables
Chromosomal	Males and females affected Suspect in a person with two or more major birth anomalies, or one major and two minor birth anomalies, or three minor birth anomalies Suspect in a fetus with a major structural defect Unexplained intellectual disability (static, nonprogressive), especially if associated with dysmorphic features or birth anomaly Unexplained psychomotor delays Ambiguous genitalia Lymphadema or cystic hygroma in newborn Multiple pregnancy losses Family history of intellectual disability Family history of multiple congenital anomalies Unexplained infertility (male or female)	
Contiguous gene (segmental aneusomy)	Males and females affected Intellectual disability with other recognized genetic or medical conditions Recognized single-gene condition with uncharacteristic dysmorphic features Family history usually unremarkable	
Mitochondrial	Males and females affected, often in multiple generations Father does not transmit condition, only mother does Highly variable clinical expressivity Often nervous system disorders May be degenerative	
Multifactorial	Males and females affected No clear pattern May skip generations Few affected family members	

T (thymine). Nucleotides are composed of a nitrogenous base, a sugar molecule, and a phosphate molecule. The nitrogenous bases pair together—A with T, and G with C—like rungs on a ladder, with the sugar and phosphates serving as the backbone. The DNA ladder is shaped in a twisted helix. The DNA helix unzips and free nucleotides join the single-stranded DNA to form a matching ribonucleic acid molecule called messenger RNA (mRNA) in a process called transcription. The initial mRNA *sense strand* matches the complementary *anti-sense DNA template* with the exception that thymine (T) is replaced by uracil (U).

The DNA sequence has coding regions called *exons* that are interrupted by *intervening sequences* (IVSs), or *introns*. The DNA molecule also has regulatory regions (such as those for starting and stopping transcription and translation) and specialized sequences related to tissue-specific expression. The initial mRNA (or primary transcript) is modified before diffusing to the cytoplasm so that the final mRNA is composed of only exons (the IVSs are spliced out during the mRNA processing).

The mRNA molecule diffuses to the cytoplasm, where it is translated into a polypeptide chain by the ribosomes. Each mRNA codon is recognized by a matching complementary tRNA anticodon that is attached to a corresponding amnio acid. For example, the DNA sequence GCT is transcribed into the mRNA sequence CGU. The mRNA sequence CGU is read on the ribosomes by the tRNA anticodon GCA, which attaches the amino acid arginine to the growing polypeptide chain. The sequence of the 20 amino acids determines the form and function of the resulting protein (e.g., structural protein, enzyme, carrier molecule, receptor molecule, hormone). Proteins usually undergo further modification after ribosomal translation (e.g., phosphorylation, proteolytic cleavage, glycosolation).

Each cell contains hundreds of mitochondria in the cytoplasm. Mitochondria are the powerhouses of the cells and are essential for energy metabolism. Each mitochondrion has about 10 single copies of small, circular chromosomes. These chromosomes consist of double-stranded helices of DNA (mtDNA). Human mtDNA has only exons, and both strands of DNA are transcribed and translated. The mitochondria behave as semi-autonomous organisms within the cell cytoplasm with their own self-replicating genome and replication, transcription, and translation systems.

All mitochondria are maternally inherited. The mitochondria in each cell are derived at the time of fertilization from the mitochondria in the cytoplasm of the ovum. There are about 100,000 mitochondria and mtDNA in the ovum and about 100 mtDNA in the sperm. The sperm mtDNA are degraded on entrance into the oocyte (Wallace et al., 2007).

2.3   TYPES OF MUTATIONS

Understanding the ways genes can be changed is helpful in interpreting a test result for your patient or when interpreting medical records on relatives. There are many ways the genetic code can be altered. Part of the code for a gene can be deleted or a change can be inserted. Pieces of the gene can be swapped between chromosomes (a translocation).

Point mutations alter the genetic code by changing the letters in the codons; this change can mean the protein is not made or too much or not enough protein is made. *Frameshift mutations* cause the DNA message to start in the wrong place. For example, if the normal instruction to code for the amnio acid and thus the protein is CAT EAT THE RAT, a frameshift mutation might be CAE ATT HER ATS. A mutation at the end of the gene in the stop codon prevents the protein from being made: CAT EAT THE. If the mutation affects the mRNA splicing, a portion of the message is missing, leading to a shortened protein: CAT THE RAT.

A *missense mutation* causes an amino acid substitution: CAT EAT THE HAM. Missense mutations do not always affect the function of the gene. When the gene alteration is of unclear significance (termed a VUS or *variant of unknown significance*), this is often a frustrating result for the patient and the clinician. Sometimes a family *tracking study* can be done to determine if the variant is present in relatives with the same condition. For example, if a woman with premenopausal breast cancer has a variant identified in the *BRCA1* gene associated with hereditary breast-ovarian cancer syndrome, then a close relative with premenopausal breast cancer (such as her sister, aunt or mother) could be tested to see if she also had the variant. If the affected relative does not have the gene variant, the gene alteration is unlikely to be the direct cause of the disease.

2.4 SINGLE-GENE DISORDERS

Single-gene disorders arise as a result of a mutation in one or both alleles of a gene located in an autosome, a sex chromosome, or a mitochondrial gene. A person who has identical alleles for a gene is *homozygous*, and an individual in whom the alleles are not identical is *heterozygous*. Because the X and Y chromosomes do not have homologous (matching) genes, males are said to be *hemizygous* for genes on the X and Y chromosomes.

Single-gene disorders generally refer to conditions inherited in patterns that follow the rules originally described by Gregor Mendel. These traditional Mendelian patterns are autosomal dominant (AD), autosomal recessive (AR), X-linked (XL) (both recessive and dominant), and Y-linked. Chromosomal disorders are present if there is a visible alteration in the number or structure of the chromosomes.

2.5 MULTI-ALLELIC INHERITANCE

Multifactorial inheritance refers to the complex interplay of multiple genes and environmental factors that assumes an additive effect leading to a phenotype. *Polygenic inheritance* describes the effects of three or more genes that are involved in the expression of a trait. *Digenic inheritance* refers to a phenotype being expressed when the individual is heterozygous for two different genes at unlinked loci. This is distinguished from *biallelic,* which pertains to inheritance of both alternative forms of a gene.

As we recognize more readily the contributions of genes interacting with the environment and with each other, the boundary between single- gene disorders and the complex expression of multiple genes continues to blur.

2.6 CONFOUNDING FACTORS IN RECOGNIZING PATTERNS OF INHERITANCE

Failure to obtain complete medical-family history information from a patient may compromise the clinician's ability to recognize an inheritance pattern. Sometimes the lack of pertinent information is actually voluntarily withheld by the patient for various reasons such as feelings of guilt about the cause of a disease or fear of stigma. Ideally, the pedigree should extend at least three generations to include the patient's parents, siblings and half-siblings, children, aunt and uncles, and grandparents; it can be helpful to include nieces and nephews, cousins, and grandchildren (see Chapter 3).

Remember to record the ages, gender, and health information of both affected and unaffected relatives. *Information on unaffected relatives is just as important as information on affected relatives.* For example, if you obtain a history of a 50-year-old woman recently diagnosed with breast cancer, and she has sisters cancer-free in their 60s, and her mother lived to be elderly without developing cancer, you are more likely to consider this cancer a sporadic occurrence than to suspect an autosomal dominant inheritance pattern (Section 2.7.2).

A person with only mild clinical symptoms may be missed as being affected in a pedigree. *Variable expressivity* means that the clinical severity of a disorder differs from one individual to another. For example, two siblings with cystic fibrosis (an autosomal recessive condition characterized by pancreatic insufficiency and progressive accumulation of mucus in the lungs) may each have very different manifestations of the disease. It is not uncommon for the seemingly healthy sibling of a child with cystic fibrosis to be diagnosed serendipitously through molecular genetic testing rather than by clinical symptoms.

Recognizing that individuals within a family have the same genetic syndrome is also confounded by *clinical* or *genetic heterogeneity*. This means that individuals with similar phenotypes can have entirely different genetic causes. For example, ovarian cancer is often not due to mutations in a single gene, but of the estimated 10–14% cases that are familial, mutations in multiple cancer susceptibility genes associated with ovarian cancer have been identified (such as *BRCA1* and *BRCA2* with hereditary breast-ovarian cancer syndrome, and *MLH1*, *MSH2*, *TACSTD1*, *MSH6* and *PMS2* with Lynch syndrome).

The expression of a syndrome may be influenced by the sex of an individual even when the gene is located on an autosome (a non-sex-linked chromosome). This is called *sex-influenced* or *sex-limited gene expression*. For example, it may be difficult to recognize a family with an inherited breast cancer susceptibility if most of the relatives are men, because men rarely develop breast cancer. The breast cancer mutation can be inherited through healthy men in the family.

I came across a 6-year-old who described love as, "One of the people has freckles and so he finds someone else who has freckles too." This could be the definition of *assortative mating*. Humans do not choose a mating partner randomly. We tend to have children with people with similar cultural and ethnic backgrounds. It is not unusual for people with comparable medical conditions to have children together (such as a couple who both have deafness or short stature). Because there are multiple etiologies for each of these conditions, it may be challenging to determine an inheritance pattern and disease risk assessment.

Misattributed paternity is a common explanation for confusion in pedigree interpretation (i.e., the stated father in the pedigree is not the biological father). The rate of misattributed paternity in the United States is estimated to be in the range of 2–4%. Misattribution of paternity crosses all racial and socioeconomic groups. In some circumstances, it may be important for the clinician to verify paternity with DNA testing—for example, if there is a suspicion of a child conceived through incest and thus a high risk of social and genetic pathology (Bennett et al., 2002) or if there is an autosomal recessive condition and testing of the parents for carrier status identifies the carrier state in only one parent (but could be uniparental disomy, see Section 2.8.6).

Small family size is a common problem that limits the ability to recognize patterns of inheritance from a pedigree. In a family of an affected person in which both healthy parents have no siblings and the affected person does not have siblings either, it may be impossible to distinguish a pattern of inheritance from pedigree analysis.

Other potential explanations for a seemingly "negative" family history are listed in Table 3.4.

2.7 RECOGNIZING PATTERNS OF INHERITANCE

2.7.1 Dominant and Recessive Inheritance Patterns: A Shifting Paradigm

Historically, *dominant inheritance* is the term used when only one copy (heterozygosity) of a gene mutation or alteration is needed for clinical (phenotypic) expression. Recessive inheritance traditionally pertains to individuals who are clinically affected when they have a double dose (homozygosity) of a gene alteration. The ability to examine gene action at the biochemical and molecular levels demonstrates that gene expression is not strictly dominant or recessive; each allele usually has distinct phenotypic expression. Thus there can be phenotypic expression of both alleles in the heterozygous state. This can be described as *co-dominant inheritance*, *semi-dominant inheritance*, or *intermediate expression* (Strachan and Read, 1996; Vogel and Motulsky, 1996). Although the expression of any trait or character requires the expression of multiple genes and environmental factors, if a particular genotype is sufficient for the trait to be expressed, the trait is considered to be inherited in a Mendelian pattern.

2.7.2 Autosomal Dominant Inheritance

Conditions inherited in an AD pattern account for approximately half of all single gene disorders (Nussbaum et al., 2007). Table 2.2 lists some conditions with AD inheritance. Figure 2.1 is a representative pedigree of AD inheritance. In AD inheritance, an affected individual has a 50:50 chance to pass the gene mutation to each son or daughter. Multiple relatives of both sexes are usually affected in more than one generation. A key feature that identifies AD inheritance in a pedigree is observation of transmission of the trait from a father to his son (male-to-male transmission),

TABLE 2.2   Examples of Autosomal Dominant Conditions

Condition	Approximate Prevalence
Familial hypercholesterolemia	1/500
Breast-ovarian cancer syndrome (*BRCA1* and *BRCA2*)	1/300-1/500
Adult polycystic kidney disease	1/1,000
Von Willebrand disease	1/1,000
Lynch syndrome (multiple genes)	1/660-1/2,000
Long-QT syndrome (multiple genes)	1/2,500
Polydactyly (postaxial)	1/3,000 (Caucasians)
Neurofibromatosis 1	1/3,500
22q.11.2 deletion syndrome (velocardiofacial syndrome, DiGeorge syndrome)	1/5,000
Oculo-auriculo-vertebral spectrum (hemifacial microsomia)	1/5,600
Charcot-Marie-Tooth type I/hereditary motor sensor neuropathy (heterogeneous)	1/6,600
Myotonic muscular dystrophy	1/7,500
Familial adenomatous polyposis (FAP)	1/8,000
Tuberous sclerosis complex (types I and II)	1/10,000
Dominant blindness	1/10,000
Dominant congenital deafness	1/10,000
Achondroplasia	1/10,000-1/15,00
Marfan syndrome	1/16,000-1/25,000
Osteogenesis imperfecta (all types)	1/20,000
Huntington disease	1/20,00
Li-Fraumeni syndrome	1/20,000
Waardenburg syndrome	1/33,000-1/50,000
Van der Woude syndrome	1/35,000
Von Hippel-Lindau syndrome	1/36,000

Sources: Connor and Ferguson-Smith, 1997; Rimoin et al., 2007; Schwartz et al., 2009.
Refer to Appendix A.7 for gene symbols and names.

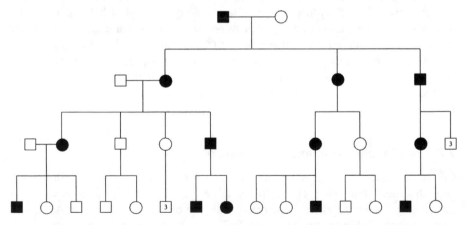

Figure 2.1 *Representative pedigree of autosomal dominant (AD) inheritance. Note that male-to-male disease transmission can occur, and affected individuals of both sexes are observed in successive generations.*

although women can also transmit the trait. Many AD conditions have variable expression. *Because a parent and other extended relatives may have only minor features of the condition, it is crucial to examine both parents for subtle clinical symptoms of the disease in question.*

The recognition of an AD pattern in a pedigree can be complicated by the *penetrance* of the condition. Penetrance refers to the percentage likelihood that a person who has inherited a gene mutation will actually show the disease manifestations in his or her lifetime. Some conditions are fully penetrant at birth, while others may have age-related penetrance. For example, an AD cleft lip and palate syndrome may have a penetrance of 40%. Thus an unaffected person in such a family could carry a "hidden" mutation that could be passed to offspring who may or may not be affected with cleft lip and palate. In contrast, familial adenomatous polyposis (FAP) is an AD colon cancer syndrome that approaches 100% penetrance by the age of 40. Anyone with a gene mutation in the FAP gene (called *APC*) should have multiple adenomatous (precancerous) colonic polyps by age 40 years, but a 5-year-old child with the *APC* gene mutation may have no observable manifestations. Persons with classic FAP often have a carpet of hundreds of polyps in the colon by their early 20s. It is now recognized that individuals with an attenuated form of FAP often have fewer adenomatous polyps and later age of onset of polyposis, although the lifetime disease penetrance still approaches 100%.

When a couple with the same AD condition has children together there is a 75% chance with each conception that they will have an affected son or daughter. There is a 25% chance that they will have a child who has a double dose of the mutation (referred to as *homozygosity* if it is the same gene mutation and *compound heterozygosity* or *biallelic* if there are two different mutations in the same gene). In some instances, the child with homozygous dominant or compound heterozygous dominant mutations may be severely affected by the condition. The homozygous or compound heterozygous state may even be lethal to a fetus or embryo (for example, *FGFR3* mutations and achondroplasia—a disproportionate short state syndrome, or *BRCA1* mutations associated with hereditary breast-ovarian cancer syndrome).

Many conditions with AD inheritance have a high frequency of observed *new mutations* in individuals with the condition (i.e., neither parent is affected with the condition). For example, estimates of the occurrence of persons with a new mutation for neurofibromatosis 1 is 50%, for bilateral retinoblastoma is 30%, and for Marfan syndrome is 25% (OMIM). This means that the mutation occurred in the egg or sperm from which the person was conceived, and that the parents are not affected. Thus an individual can be the first person in the family with the condition. The person who has the condition has a 50:50 chance to pass the mutation causing the condition on to each of his or her children, but the person's brothers and sisters are usually not at risk for the condition. The exception is if one of the parents is mosaic for the mutation in the testes or ovaries. This phenomenon of *gonadal mosaicism* is discussed in more detail near the end of this chapter (see Section 2.9.2)

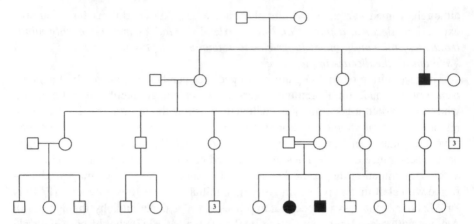

Figure 2.2 *Representative pedigree of autosomal recessive (AR) inheritance. Although consanguinity is a clue suggesting AR inheritance, most individuals with an AR condition are born to unrelated parents.*

2.7.3   Autosomal Recessive Inheritance

Figure 2.2 is a representative pedigree of autosomal recessive inheritance. Parents who each carry an AR gene mutation have a 25% chance, with each conception, to have an affected son or daughter. All humans carry several "hidden" AR gene mutations. Many inborn errors of metabolism are inherited in an AR pattern. A pedigree in which a condition is autosomal recessive will usually show only affected relatives in a sibship. *Consanguinity* in a pedigree can be a clue to an AR pattern, because couples who are closely related (such as first cousins) are more likely to have inherited the same AR gene mutation from a common ancestor. A person who has two mutations in the same gene traced to a common ancestor is *autozygous* for the mutation.

Some AR conditions are common in certain ethnic groups because individuals of the same ethnic and cultural background are more likely to have children together (see Table 3.2). For example, Tay-Sachs disease has a 1/30 carrier frequency in the Ashkenazi population (Jews from eastern and central Europe) as compared to a 1/300 carrier frequency in individuals of non-Ashkenazi northern European ancestry. Cystic fibrosis has a frequency of 1/3,300 in individuals of northern European ancestry, 1/15,300 in individuals of African American ancestry (a carrier frequency of approximately 1/60–65), and about 1/50,000 in Native Americans (NIH Consensus, 1997). Table 2.3 lists some common conditions that are inherited in an AR pattern.

The sibling of a parent with a child with a known autosomal recessive condition has a one in two (50%) chance to be a carrier of the mutation for the condition. The unaffected sibling of a person with an AR condition has a two in three (66%) chance to be a mutation carrier (the reason this is not 50% is because the chance of being homozygous affected has already been ruled out so there remains two of three possibilities: One chance to be homozygous unaffected and two chances to be heterozygous gene mutation carrier).

TABLE 2.3   Examples of Autosomal Recessive Conditions

Condition	Approximate Prevalence[a]
Hemochromatosis	1/300–1/500 (Caucasians)
Sickle cell anemia	1/400–1/600 (African Americans)
β-thalassemia	1/800–1/2,000 (Italians or Greek Americans)
Cystic fibrosis	1/2,500 (northern Europeans)
	1/8,000 (Hispanic Americans)
	1/15,300 (African Americans)
	1/32,100 (Asian Americans)
Nonsyndromic neurosensory deafness (DFNB1)	1/5,000
Medium-chain-acyl-dehydrogenase (MCAD)	1/6,000
α-1 antitrypsin deficiency	1/4,400–1/8,000
Spinal muscular atrophy I (Werdnig-Hoffman)	1/10,000
Phenylketonuria (PKU)	1/19,000
21-Hydroxylase deficiency	1/8,000–1/26,000
Albinism (all types)	1/20,000
Smith-Lemli-Opitz syndrome	1/20,000–1/40,000
Infantile polycystic kidney disease	1/20,800
Usher syndrome (type)	1/23,000–1/33,000
Glutaric aciduria	1/30,000–1/50,000
Galactosemia	1/40,0000
Homocystinuria	1/6,000–1/83,000
Tay-Sachs disease	1/3,600 (Ashkenazi Jews)
	1/300,000 (non-Ashkenazi)
Tyrosinemia type 1	1/100,000 (northern European)
	1/12,500 (Quebec)
	1/1,800 (Saguenay Lac Saint-Jean, Quebec)

[a]The frequency of these diseases may vary widely among ethnic groups. Most figures are from U.S. populations. Table 3.2 lists some autosomal recessive conditions that have a high frequency in certain population groups.
Sources: Clarke, 2006; Connor and Ferguson-Smith, 1997; Rimoin et al., 2007; Watson et al., 2006.
Refer to Appendix A.7 for gene symbols and names.

The chance a mutation carrier for an AR condition will have an affected child depends on the chance that his or her partner carries an AR gene mutation for the same disorder. This possibility will be higher if the partner is a blood relative (e.g., a cousin), or if he or she is from a population group in which the carrier frequency for the disease is high.

For most rare AR conditions, the chance that healthy siblings of the person with the AR condition will have children with the condition is low (in the range of 1% or less). Likewise, individuals with AR conditions usually do not have children who are affected with the disease, although all their children are obligate carriers of the gene mutation (the person homozygous for the gene mutation can pass on only the mutation to each child because the person has no non-mutated copy). Depending on the carrier frequency of the gene alteration, the chance that the children will be affected usually is in the range of 0.5–3%; a higher chance of having an affected child would be associated with a higher population carrier frequency of the mutation. For example if the carrier frequency of the condition is 1 in 100, a person homozygous for the mutation (thus usually affected) would have a 1 in 200 (0.5%) chance of having a child with the condition:

1 (chance person with condition carries the mutation) × 1/100 (chance partner carries the mutation) × 1 (chance person with the condition passes mutation their child) × 1/2 (chance partner passes the mutation to their offspring) = 1/200.

With the same general population carrier frequency, for a person who is a known mutation carrier (heterozygous), the chance to have an affected child would be 1 in 400 (0.25%):

1 (chance of heterozygous carrier being a mutation carrier) × 1/100 (chance partner carries the mutation) × 1/2 (chance known heterozygous carrier passes the mutation to their offspring) × 1/2 (chance partner passes the mutation to their offspring) = 1/400.

Alternatively, if the population carrier frequency is 1 in 25, the chance of having an affected child becomes 2% (1 × 1/25 × 1 × 1/2 = 1/50) for the person who is the homozygous carrier, and 1% (1 × 1/25 × 1/2 × 1/2 = 1/100) for the person who is a known heterozygous carrier.

2.7.4 X-Linked Inheritance

Women who carry an X-chromosome gene mutation have a 50:50 chance, with each pregnancy, to have an affected son. Also, there is a 50:50 chance with each pregnancy to have a daughter who carries the mutation. Often daughters are unaffected. A pedigree in which only males are affected, often in more than one generation, suggests a traditional X-linked inheritance pattern. The family history of an X-linked disorder may show few affected family members, particularly if most of the relatives are female. Figure 2.3 is a representative pedigree of a condition inherited in an X-linked

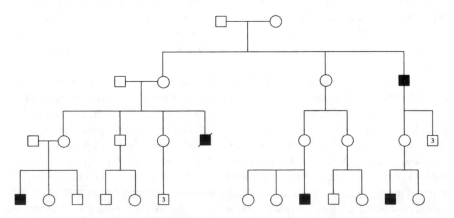

Figure 2.3   Representative pedigree of an X-linked condition.

TABLE 2.4   Examples of X-Linked Conditions

Condition	Approximate Prevalence (Males)
Red-green colorblindness (Europeans)	8/100
Fragile X syndrome (full mutation)	1/2,500–1/4,000 (1/8,000 females)
Duchenne muscular dystrophy	1/3,000–1/5,000
Hemophilia A (factor VIII)	1/2,500–1/4,000
Hemophilia B (Christmas disease, factor IX)	1/4,000–1/7,000
Vitamin D–resistant rickets (X-linked hypophosphatemia)	1/25,000
Fabry disease	1/40,000[b]
Hunter syndrome (MPSII)	1/144,000
Spinobulbar muscular atrophy	1/50,000
Orofacial digital syndrome I[a]	1/50,000
Ornithine transcarbamylase deficiency (males usually die in first few years of life)[a]	1/20,000–1/30,000
Rett syndrome (lethal in males)[a]	1/10,000 (females)
Nephrogenic diabetes insipidus[a]	1/30,000–1/50,000[b] (about 10% are autosomal recessive)
Incontinentia pigmenti (lethal in males)[a]	rare

[a]Disorders that are traditionally considered X-linked dominant.
[b]Females also frequently have manifestations but are not included in this prevalence figure.
Sources: Connor and Ferguson-Smith, 1997; Rimoin et al., 2007.
Refer to Appendix A.7 for gene symbols and names.

pattern. Examples of X-linked conditions and their approximate prevalence in males are shown in Table 2.4.

The concept of dominant and recessive inheritance blurs when applied to X-linked inheritance. Heterozygous women can be affected with an X-linked condition, but usually they are more mildly affected than their male relatives. The main explanation for this is *lyonization* or *X-inactivation*. Soon after fertilization when the embryo contains several hundred to several thousand cells, the genes on one of the X chromosomes in each cell is inactivated. A single X chromosome remains active per cell. This inactivation is a random process. If the clones of these original cells carry the inactive X with the normally working gene, then the woman may have symptoms of the condition. For example, females who carry the X-linked Duchenne muscular dystrophy (DMD) mutation may have subtle symptoms of DMD (such as large calves and high blood levels of the contractile muscle enzyme creatine kinase, and dilated cardiomyopathy). Affected males, in contrast, will have highly elevated creatine kinase levels at birth and progressive muscle weakness, such that they usually require wheelchair assistance by the age of 10–12 years and have a shortened life expectancy (Emery, 2007).

There are some X-linked conditions, particularly those involving enzyme deficiencies, in which it is common for heterozygous female carriers to show mild symptoms (*intermediate expression*) because women have some level of enzyme activity. A female can also be as severely affected as a male with the condition. For example, girls and women who are carriers for a rare condition called nephrogenic diabetes insipidus I (NDI, hereditary renal tubular insensitivity to antidiuretic hormone and mutations in *AVPR2*) often show symptoms of increased thirst for water and dilute urine but often do not need extensive treatment. In contrast, boys and men affected with NDI are treated with free access to water, diuretics, and a low sodium diet to prevent repeated bouts of hypernatremia (a form of dehydration) that can cause damage to the kidneys and, in infants, seizures, failure to thrive, mental retardation, and even death (Knoers, 2007). Ornithine transcarbamylase deficiency (OTCD; a urea cycle defect leading to hyperammonemia with mutations in *OTC*) is usually lethal in males in the first few years of life, even with strict protein restriction and dietary arginine. The female carriers may have protein intolerance but may not require treatment beyond dietary modifications (Summar, 2005). Fabry disease (an enzyme defect of α-galactosidase A with mutations in the *GLA* gene) is another example of an X-linked condition in which the men are usually more severely affected but women also can have severe symptoms, though the age that complications manifest in women may be at least 10 years later and sometimes less severe then men (Deegan et al., 2006; Hughes, 2008). Classic symptoms in men include episodes of burning pain in the in the hands and feet, difficulty sweating, hearing loss, stroke, kidney failure, and hypertrophic cardiomyopathy.

X-linked dominant inheritance traditionally describes conditions in which the heterozygous female manifest disease symptoms, and the condition is usually lethal (in utero or in infancy) for the male who is hemizygous. In this instance, the pedigree clues include only females being affected and multiple miscarriages (representing in utero death of a male fetus) (Figure 2.4). These conditions are rare. Incontinentia pigmenti (IP) is an example of an X-linked lethal (dominant) condition. Female infants with this condition have blisters that spontaneously resolve, leaving marbled brown or slate gray pigmentation that fades into hypopigmented macules in an adult. Other features may include hypodontia (congenital absence of primary or secondary teeth), partial hair loss (alopecia), mental delay, and ocular problems. The condition is lethal in males (Sybert, 2010).

A family history of an X-linked condition in which the women express the condition is distinguishable from AD inheritance by the absence of male-to-male

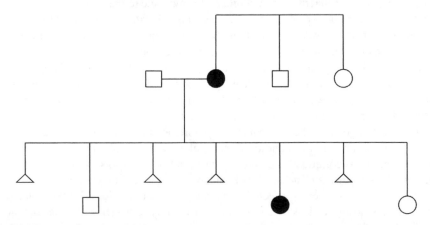

Figure 2.4   *Pedigree suggestive of an X-linked mutation that is lethal in males. Note the absence of affected males and the multiple pregnancy losses.*

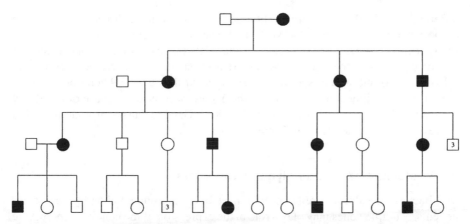

Figure 2.5 *Representative pedigree of X-linked dominant inheritance. Note that males and females are affected and that males have affected daughters but no affected sons. Females may have less severe manifestations or later onset of symptoms that their male relatives.*

transmission (Figure 2.5). Male-to-male transmission can be mimicked in pedigrees where there is consanguinity (a union between relatives) because an affected father may have children with a female relative who is a carrier for the same condition; thus sons can inherit the gene alteration from the mother. Another feature that distinguishes an X-linked pedigree from an autosomal dominant pedigree is that in X-linked conditions the females are generally more mildly affected than the males, whereas in AD conditions, both males and females may have variable expression of the disease.

Because men pass the X chromosome only to their daughters, the daughters of a man with an X-linked condition are always mutation carriers (and rarely affected), and their sons are never affected. The carrier daughters each have a 50:50 chance to have an affected son. Thus the grandsons of these males who carry the mutation are at risk to be affected.

Similar to AD conditions, many X-linked conditions are associated with a high incidence of persons with new mutations. For those X-linked conditions causing severe physical impairment in which it is unusual for affected men to father children, the new mutation rates are often 20–30% (Nussbaum et al., 2007). For example, if a woman has a son with Duchenne muscular dystrophy and she has no affected relatives, the chance that her affected son has a new mutation in the dystrophin gene is approximately $\frac{1}{3}$.

2.7.5 Y-Inheritance (Holandric)

The Y chromosome is small. It contains only a short segment of functional genes that are largely responsible for determining maleness (autosomal genes are also associated with sex determination). A gene on the short arm of the Y chromosome called the *SRY* (sex-determining region of Y) mediates the male-determining effect of the Y chromosome. Genetic alterations in this segment can affect human sex differentiation, leading to such conditions as XY females and XX males. The long arm of the Y chromosome carries the MSY (male specific Y) region, which is responsible for spermatogenesis. Microdeletions in the AZF (azoospermia factor) regions of the long (q) arm of the Y chromosome are associated with decreased sperm count (oligospermia) and absent sperm (azoospermia) in the semen. Alterations in these regions and possibly other gene loci on the Y chromosome are a cause of hereditary infertility (Disteche, 2007; Lissens et al., 2007). Genetic causes of male infertility are reviewed in greater detail in Section 4.18.3.

2.7.6 Multifactorial and Polygenic Disorders

Multifactorial conditions are believed to have both environmental and genetic components. Multiple genes may play a role in the expression of the condition (polygenic inheritance). Height and skin color are examples of conditions in which multiple genes and their environment are involved in phenotypic expression. Many isolated birth defects, such as pyloric stenosis, clubfoot, scoliosis, and neural tube defects, are believed to have a multifactorial etiology. Common illnesses in adults, such as diabetes, asthma, hypertension, epilepsy, and mental disorders are thought to have multiple genetic and environmental factors at the root of their expression.

Pedigrees documenting conditions that have a multifactorial or polygenic etiology usually have no other, or few, affected relatives (Figure 2.6). Males and females may be affected. The risk of recurrence is based on empirical data tables, derived from population studies. The more closely related a person is to the affected individual, the higher the chance of being affected. For these conditions, "chance has a memory," meaning that the recurrence risks rises as the number of affected individuals within the family increases. If a family has multiple instances of a condition that is traditionally considered multifactorial, it is important to investigate the possibility of a single gene disorder.

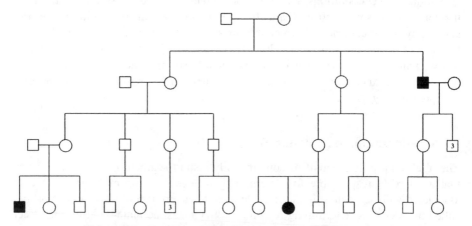

Figure 2.6 Representative pedigree of multifactorial inheritance.

2.7.7 Chromosomal Inheritance

A chromosome problem involves a missing or added segment of either a partial chromosome (such as a duplication or deletion) or a whole chromosome. Because the functions of multiple genes are disrupted, the affected individual usually has multiple problems, including varying degrees of intellectual disability. Hundreds of chromosomal syndromes have been described (Shashidhar et al., 2003).

There are several family and medical history clues that suggest a chromosomal problem (Table 2.1). Always "think chromosomes" any time a child is born with three or more minor birth anomalies (such as protuberant ears, unusually shaped hands, and wide-spaced eyes). Minor anomalies are generally defined as characteristics that are of no serious cosmetic or functional consequence to the patient (Jones, 2006). A chromosome aberration should also be considered in an individual with two major birth anomalies (such as cleft lip and palate and a heart defect) or with one major anomaly and two minor anomalies, particularly if there are accompanying dysmorphic features. Consider requesting a chromosome study in any person with intellectual disability, particularly if there are accompanying dysmorphic features or birth anomalies. A history of multiple miscarriages (three or more) suggests a parental chromosomal rearrangement. This is particularly true if there is a history of multiple miscarriages and intellectual disability with or without multiple birth anomalies. Figure 2.7 is a representative pedigree of a family with an inherited chromosome translocation.

A karyotype to search for a sex chromosome anomaly should be considered in:

- An individual with ambiguous genitalia.
- A fetus with cystic hygroma(s) (also common in trisomies 21 and 18).

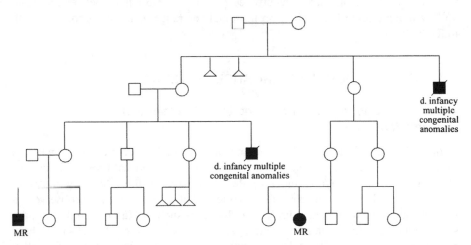

Figure 2.7 *Representative pedigree of an inherited chromosome translocation. Note the history of multiple miscarriages and individuals with intellectual disability (MR) and multiple congenital anomalies.*

- A newborn with lymphedema (females associated with Turner syndrome, males and females with trisomy 21).
- A female with an inguinal hernia.
- A female with primary amenorrhea.
- A female with short stature and/or delayed or arrested puberty.
- A male or female with failure to develop secondary sexual characteristics.
- A male with hypogonadism and/or significant gynecomastia.

The intellectual delay associated with chromosome problems is not regressive. Although a child with a chromosome anomaly may be born with serious medical problems, including severe cognitive delay, usually he or she slowly advances to some ultimate level of functioning (albeit this level is often below the average).

Changes in chromosome number are attributable to errors in meiosis (non-disjunction), resulting in trisomy (such as trisomy 18 or trisomy 21) or monosomy (such as the single X in Turner syndrome). These numerical chromosome errors are much more common than structural chromosomal changes (translocations). Most individuals with a chromosome anomaly will have an unremarkable family history.

The recurrence risk to have another child with a chromosome anomaly depends on the etiology of the chromosome anomaly. For example, the risk for a couple to have another child with a non-disjunctional chromosome anomaly is 1% or the maternal age-related risk (whichever is higher). If a parent is a carrier for a structural chromosome translocation, the recurrence risk depends on the size of the rearrangement, the chromosomes involved, and which parent is a carrier. The chance to have a child with an unbalanced chromosome rearrangement when the mother carries the chromosome rearrangement is often higher than when the father is the carrier. Large unbalanced chromosome rearrangements may be lethal early in pregnancy. Most hereditary chromosome translocations have a recurrence risk for the parents of between 1% and 15%, although some hereditary chromosomal rearrangements are associated with much higher risks.

2.8 NONTRADITIONAL INHERITANCE PATTERNS

2.8.1 Triplet Repeat Disorders and the Inheritance of Dynamic Mutations.

Anticipation describes the clinical phenomenon in which a genetic condition seems to worsen over successive generations. For example, a child with myotonic dystrophy may have severe hypotonia and failure to thrive, yet the affected grandfather has only early balding and presenile cataracts. Anticipation has been observed in several autosomal dominant neurological disorders such as Huntington disease, the spinocerebellar ataxias, and myotonic dystrophy (La Spada et al., 1994). In these conditions, nucleotide runs of three are excessively repeated in the DNA. Thus they are called *trinucleotide repeat disorders*. Spinobulbar muscular atrophy and fragile X syndrome are X-linked neurological trinucleotide repeat disorders.

Most genes are transmitted unaltered through each generation of a family. In triplet repeat disorders, the triplet repeat is unstable once it reaches a critical size threshold, and the size can increase in successive generations. These unstable mutations are called *dynamic mutations* (Sutherland and Richards, 1994). It is normal to have fewer than a certain number of these trinucleotide repeats. The instability of the trinucleotide repeats tends to be related to their size (with longer repeats being more unstable and more likely to increase in size). Rarely, contractions in size occur, and the contractions are usually small (LaSpada, 1994). Often repeats are transmitted unchanged with neither expansion nor contraction.

A *premutation* describes an intermediate size range between trinucleotide repeats with sizes in the normal (stable) range and larger repeats in the range associated with disease. Individuals who carry a permutation often have no symptoms of disease, mild symptoms of disease, or a later onset of disease than individuals with larger trinucleotide repeat expansions. Premutations are unstable and may expand into the full mutation range during meiosis.

For some trinucleotide repeat disorders, the stability of the mutation is influenced by the sex of the parent transmitting the mutation. Congenital myotonic dystrophy seems to be inherited primarily from the mother whereas childhood-onset Huntington disease occurs more often from the father. The risk for severe childhood presentation is also correlated with the affected parent having a large trinucleotide repeat expansion. In fragile X syndrome, premutation carrier males cannot transmit a full mutation to their daughters, though all their daughters inherit the premutation. However, when the unstable fragile X mutation is transmitted by females, it often increases in size (with larger CGG repeats having a much higher risk of expansion in the offspring) (McConkie-Rosell et al., 2005).

A large trinucleotide repeat expansion is often associated with a more severe presentation of the disease (LaSpada, 1994; Nance, 1997). For example, in myotonic dystrophy, it is normal to have 37 or fewer CTG repeats. In the premutation range between 38 and 49 repeats, the individual does not have symptoms of myotonic dystrophy. However, an expansion can occur in the egg or sperm of an unaffected premutation carrier; thus the person's offspring are at risk to be affected (with milder symptoms often occurring with CTG repeats in the range of 50–80, and more severe symptoms associated with CTG repeats over 200). An individual with 1,000 or more CTG repeats usually displays the severe congenital form of myotonic dystrophy (Harper, 2002).

Huntington disease (HD) is an example of an autosomal dominant trinucleotide repeat disorder showing variable expressivity, age-related penetrance, anticipation, and parental bias in the stability of the trinucleotide repeat. Huntington disease is a progressive neurological condition characterized by uncontrolled movements (chorea) and problems with thinking, coordination, and judgment. The penetrance is believed to approach 100% by the age of 90, with an average age of symptom onset between 40 and 45 years (Firth and Hurst, 2005). The gene alteration in HD is a CAG repeat located on the tip of the short arm of chromosome 4. An affected individual has 40 or more CAG repeats; an unaffected individual has 35 or fewer CAG repeats. Alleles between 36 and 39 CAG repeats are considered intermediate, and this range is considered an area of reduced penetrance. In the premutation range between 27 and 35 repeats, the individual will not be affected but an expansion can occur in the sperm (Brinkman et al., 1997). Juvenile Huntington disease is associated with CAG repeat expansions over 80 repeats (persons with 60 or more CAG repeats may have symptoms in the teenage years) (Nance and Myers, 2001). The majority of children with juvenile Huntington disease have an affected father, although mothers with a large CAG repeat expansion also are at risk to have offspring with childhood onset Huntington disease.

2.8.2 Mitochondrial Inheritance

When P. D. Eastman penned the classic children's book *Are You My Mother?* (1960), little did he realize that he had discovered the mantra of mitochondrial geneticists. Disorders caused by mitochondrial mutations have an unusual pedigree pattern—both males and females are affected, but the disease is transmitted exclusively through females (Figure 2.8). There appears to be a random distribution of affected children. The expression of the disease is quite variable, both between families and within a family.

Within each cell the number of mtDNA that carry the mutation vary. All the mtDNA within the mitochondrion may carry the mutation (*homoplasmy*) or only a fraction of the cellular mtDNA may be mutated (*heteroplasmy*). There is a threshold effect at which a certain proportion of mutant mitochondria within a cell are tolerated (no disease). Severe disease is manifested when the proportion of mutant mitochondria is very high. Thus recurrence risk for the condition ranges from 0 to 100%.

It is easy to confuse mitochondrial diseases and mitochondrial mutations. Genes within the nucleus (nuclear DNA) code for the majority of mitochondrial proteins, including the subunits of protein involved in electron transport (oxidative phosphorylation). Mutations in these nuclear genes can be inherited in classic Mendelian

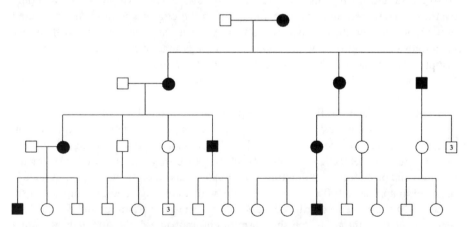

Figure 2.8 *Representative pedigree of mitochondrial inheritance. Note that males and females are affected and that the condition is passed only through females. Usually there is wide variability in the disease manifestations.*

patterns (autosomal recessive, autosomal dominant, or X-linked). Many mitochondrial disorders controlled by mutations in nuclear DNA have been identified. The mtDNA contains genes that code for the production of ribosomal RNA and various tRNAs necessary for mitochondrial electron transport.

Mitochondria are important for energy production, specifically in their role in oxidative phosphorylation. Certain tissues and body organs depend more on the mitochondrial energy metabolism than others. Mitochondrial diseases are most often associated with disorders of organs and tissues with high-energy demands such as the central nervous system, the heart, skeletal muscles, endocrine glands, and kidneys (Wallace et al., 2007). They generally have a delayed onset with a degenerative course. Some of the clinical features of mitochondrial diseases are listed in Table 2.5. When taking a family history where a mitochondrial disorder is suspected, it is important to note all medical problems in family members. Because so many organ systems can be involved, even a seemingly minor medical problem may connect to a diagnosis of a mitochondrial disorder. Examples of common conditions caused by mitochondrial mutations are shown in Table 2.6.

TABLE 2.5 Medical and Family History Features Suggesting Conditions Caused by Mitochondrial Inheritance[a]

Frequent Features
Persistent lactic acidosis
Progressive or intermittent muscle weakness
Hypotonia
Failure to thrive
Psychomotor retardation/regression
Seizures
Ptosis

Other Suggestive Features
Oculomotor abnormalities
Retinal degeneration
Optic atrophy
Cataract
Sudden loss of vision
Deafness (sensorineural, including aminoglycoside induced)
Slurred speech
Short stature
Apnea or tachypena (periodic)
Cardiomyopathy (hypertrophic)
Cardiac rhythm disturbances
Renal tubular dysfunction
Diabetes mellitus
Stroke (at a young age)
Myoclonus
Ataxia (progressive or intermittent)
Sideroblastic anemia/pancytopenia

[a]Any of these features with lactic acidosis or combinations of the features strongly suggest mitochondrial disorders.
Source: Adapted with permission from Clarke, 2006.

TABLE 2.6   Examples of Conditions with Mitochondrial Inheritance

Syndrome	Features
Kearns-Sayre syndrome	Ophthalmoplegia (paralysis of the extraocular eye muscles) and retinal degeneration (usually before age 20 years), cerebellar dysfunction, psychomotor regression, ataxia, seizures, sensorineural deafness, cardiac conduction defects, short stature, lactic acidosis
MERRF (mitochondrial encephalomyopathy with ragged-red fibers)	Ataxia, spasticity, psychomotor regression, myoclonic seizures, sensorineural hearing loss, short stature, diabetes, lactic acidosis, lipomas (neck)
MELAS (mitochondrial encephalomyopathy, lactic acidosis, and strokes)	Bilateral cataracts, cortical blindness, ataxia, intermittent migraine headaches, seizures, myoclonus, sensorineural deafness, stroke-like episodes, myopathy, renal tubular dysfunction, cardiac conduction defects, short stature, diabetes mellitus, lactic acidosis
NARP (neuropathy with ataxia and retinitis pigmentosa)	Retinitis pigmentosa, ataxia, sensory neuropathy, proximal muscle weakness, developmental delay, seizures, dementia, diabetes mellitus (occasional), lactic acidosis (occasional)
LHON (Leber hereditary optic neuropathy)	Midlife onset of optic atrophy (sudden central vision loss), cerebellar dysfunction (dystonic), and cardiac conduction defects
CPEO (chronic progressive external ophthalmoplegia)	Progressive ophthalmoplegia, ptosis (droopy eyelids)
Diabetes mellitus type II and sensorineural hearing loss	Several families have been described with mitochondrial mutations

Sources: Clarke, 2006; Firth and Hurst, 2005; Wallace et al., 2007.

Our understanding of mitochondrial diseases and mitochondrial inheritance has greatly expanded since their first description in the 1980s. More than 50 diseases have been linked to mitochondrial inheritance (Wallace et al., 2007). Mitochondrial inheritance has been implicated for some manifestations of common diseases such as nonsyndromic hearing loss, stroke, epilepsy, and diabetes mellitus (Wallace et al., 2007). The recognition of mitochondrial inheritance patterns will undoubtedly play an increasingly important role in the evolving clinical realm of genomic medicine.

2.8.3   Contiguous Gene Syndromes or Segmental Aneusomy

If the affected individual has multiple systems or organs involved (*pleiotropy*), this may be a *contiguous gene syndrome* (CGS). This terminology is somewhat archaic now that technology such as FISH (fluorescence in situ hybridization; a technique of using molecular probes to visual minute chromosomal changes) and array CGH (comparative genomic hybridization) allow more precise definition of the segment of genetic material that varies from normal. Historically a contiguous gene syndrome described a loss of chromosomal material resulting in disruption of function in several genes located in a row. Such conditions are now often referred to as microdeletion syndromes, referring to submicrosopic deletions or duplications of multiple unrelated genes that are located next to each other at a specific choromosome locus that in the hemizygous state may each independently contribute to the phenotype. Not all of the genes that map to the segment of the chromosome are likely to contribute to the phenotype. For example, neurofibromatosis is an autosomal dominant syndrome characterized by multiple café au lait spots and neurofibromas. Rarely this syndrome is also associated with intellectual delay and dysmorphic features. It is now known that this association represents a large deletion that includes the *NF1* gene (Jenne et al., 2000). Not all the contiguous genes that map to the segment of the chromosome are likely to contribute to the phenotype. The term *segmental aneusomy* has been used to refer to the affect of multiple contiguous genes on abnormal dosage as a result of a cytogenetic abnormality or imprinting effect (Spinner et al., 2007).

The recognition and description of contiguous gene syndromes have played an important role in the isolation and localization of disease genes. For example, in 1985 Francke and colleagues described a boy with Duchenne muscular dystrophy, chronic granulomatous disease, retinitis pigmentosa, and McLeod syndrome, who was missing a segment of chromosomal material at Xp21. This finding led to the discovery of gene alterations for all the aforementioned syndromes. The study of such syndromes is helping researchers define genetic loci and phenotypic expression in the hemizygous state (loss-of-function of dominant genes).

2.8.4 Genomic Imprinting

Imprinting refers to the modification of a gene (or a chromosomal region) such that it is expressed differently if it is inherited from one parent as compared to the other parent. The imprinted copy of the gene is inactivated; therefore, it is not expressed. The imprint is reversible because a man passes on his genes with his own paternal imprint if those genes were inherited with a maternal imprint from his mother (Strachan and Read, 1996). The mechanism of imprinting appears to involve DNA methylation (the modification of DNA by the addition of a methyl group) and/or histone modification (histones are the protein-spools around which DNA winds), but the details are complex and not well understood. Usually the nonmethylated allele is expressed and the methylated gene is repressed. Imprinting appears to occur at the level of transcription, most likely in the germline. It is unclear whether imprinting is a critical process in embryonic development and the expression of genetic disease or a property of a limited number of genes (or small chromosomal regions). Most genes are not subject to imprinting, or we would not so readily recognize simple Mendelian inheritance patterns. Over 50 genes are known to be imprinted in humans, and many of these genes play a role in growth regulatory pathways and/or behavioral/neurological expression (Weksberg et al., 2007). The imprinted genes tend to cluster together in "imprinted chromosomal domains." Duke University has a fascinating website about advances in gene imprinting (human and other species), visit www.geneimprint.com.

Classic examples of imprinting disorders are Prader-Willi syndrome (PWS) and Angelman syndrome. Both of these distinctly different genetic conditions involve altered genetic expression of the same genetic region—a tiny segment of the long (q) arm of chromosome 15 (15q11-q13). If the altered region is inherited from the father, the child (son or daughter) has PWS. The hallmark features of PWS are hypotonia in childhood, almond-shaped eyes, small hands and feet, behavioral difficulties, and a mean IQ of 56. Early feeding difficulties are replaced by overeating and morbid obesity in childhood. If the same altered region is inherited from the mother, the child (son or daughter) has Angelman syndrome. Severe developmental delay, limited speech, jerky movements, ataxia, excitable personality with hysterical laughter, and an unusual facial appearance characterize Angelman syndrome.

Providing genetic counseling and risk assessment for families with Angelman syndrome or Prader-Willi syndrome is complicated and requires a careful family history and sophisticated genetic testing. Multiple genetic mechanisms of inheritance of PWS and Angelman syndrome have been identified (Firth and Hurst, 2005):

- *Deletions.* Between 70% and 75% of people with Prader-Willi have large deletions of the paternal 15q11-q13 region, and a similar proportion of persons with Angelman syndrome have the deletion of this region of chromosome 15 that is maternally derived. These may be detectable through standard karyotype or require FISH.
- *Uniparental disomy* (UPD). Another 25% of persons with PWS have maternal uniparental disomy or UPD (inheritance of two maternal chromosome 15s and no paternal contribution) with the opposite pattern for Angelman syndrome.
- *Imprinting defect.* About 5% of those with PWS inherit a copy of chromosome 15 from each parent, but they have abnormal DNA methylation and gene expression of the Prader-Willi/Angelman syndrome critical region (FISH studies will be normal).
- *Chromosome translocation.* A small percentage of persons with Angelman syndrome or Prader-Willi syndrome have a chromosome translocation.
- *UBE3A (E3 ubiquitin-protein ligase) mutation.* For about 20% of individuals with Angelman syndrome the mother carries a mutation in this gene.

The chance of having another affected child varies, depending on the origin of the problem. The risk of recurrence if the affected child has a deletion or uniparental disomy is less than 1%. The risk is 50% if there is a mutation of the imprinting critical region and up to 25% if there is a parental chromosome translocation. Women carrying a *UBE3A* mutation have a 50% risk of having a child with Angeleman syndrome with each pregnancy. When a *UBE3A* mutation is transmitted by a father, development is normal because the gene is silenced. All patients with an interstitial deletion, UPD, or an imprinting defect will have a SNRPN (small nuclear ribonuclear protein-associated polypeptide N) methylation abnormality and have only unmethylated alleles (normally there would be one methylated and one unmethylated paternal allele). A person with Angelman syndrome due to *UBE3A* mutations would have a normal SNRPN methylation assay (Firth and Hurst, 2005).

2.8.5 Uniparental Disomy

Uniparental disomy refers to the phenomenon whereby an individual receives both pairs of a specific chromosome (or portion of a pair) from one parent and no copy from the other parent. If the two homologues are identical (replica copies of the same homolog) and from the same parent this is referred to as *uniparental isodisomy*. Such errors occur during meiosis II or postzygotic duplication. If the two homologues are different (heterozygous) but from the same parent, this is referred to is *uniparental heterodisomy* (this indicates an error in meiosis I). Thus far UPD has been documented for more than 18 of the 22 autosomes, both X chromosomes, and the XY pair (Engel and Antonarakis, 2001). The most common mechanism is through *trisomy rescue* (the loss of a chromosome from an initial trisomy). This involves the original meiotic error leading to trisomy and then the mitotic error in which the normal diploid state is returned through non-disjunction or anaphase lag. This has mostly been observed in maternally derived isodisomy occurring during oogenesis (Engel and Antonarakis, 2001). Engel and Antonarakis (2001) provide a fascinating discussion of uniparental disomy, the diseases identified to date, and the complex genetic counseling issues.

Several genetic conditions have been described in which UPD has been observed. For example, a few individuals with classic autosomal recessive cystic fibrosis have inherited both chromosomes from the cystic fibrosis mutation from one parent (the other parent has two normal alleles) (Cutting, 2007). Uniparental disomy has been observed in 2–3% of individuals with Angelman syndrome in which the child inherits two critical regions of chromosome 15 from the father. The opposite has also occurred, in which a child inherits two chromosome 15s from the mother and thus has Prader-Willi syndrome (Section 2.8.4).

For some chromosomes, uniparental disomy may produce no effect, and for other chromosomes it may be lethal (Strachan Read, 1996, Engel 1998; Spinner et al., 2007). Uniparental disomy can cause morbidity or lethality by altering imprinting processes, mimicking disease deletions or duplications, generating recessive disorders when only one parent is a carrier, or prompting malignant tumor development (Engel, 1995). Although misattribution of paternity is the most likely explanation if a child with a classic autosomal recessive condition has only one parent identified as a mutation carrier, uniparental disomy should be a consideration.

2.9 OTHER FACTORS TO CONSIDER

2.9.1 New Hereditary Mutations

Many autosomal dominant, X-linked, and mitochondrially inherited conditions have a high new mutation rate. This means that the affected person is the first person in the family to have the condition. The mutation occurred in the egg or sperm that "created" that person. All of the daughter cells from the fertilized egg carry the alteration, including the gonads. The affected individual has a chance to pass the mutation on to his or her children. The siblings and parents of the affected individual do not have an increased chance to have a child with the same condition.

2.9.2 Mosaicism

Mosaicism describes the phenomenon when some cells in an organ or tissue have a different genetic constitution from the other cells. Chromosomal mosaicism refers to a chromosome abnormality that occurs after fertilization during mitosis at an early cell stage. For example, a child who has mosaic trisomy 21 (Down syndrome) has some cells that are normal (diploid), and some cells that have the extra chromosome 21 (trisomy).

If the cells in the gonads (testes and ovaries) are mosaic, this is called gonadal mosaicism. The risk to have an affected child depends on the percentage of gonadal involvement. Recurrence risk ranges from 0% to 50%. In somatic mosaicism there is no increased risk for affected offspring because the mutation is not in the gonads. Somatic mosaicism occurs in tumor cells—some cells in the body contain an altered chromosome or single gene mutation, whereas others do not. It is interesting to note that somatic mitochondrial mutations accumulate in all cells with age. It is hypothesized that these mitochondrial mutations play a central role in late-onset degenerative diseases, cancer, and aging (Wallace et al., 2007).

2.9.3 Sporadic Conditions

Inheritance of a condition is described as "sporadic" when the parents' chance to have another child with the condition is considered negligible (in the range of less than 1%). These conditions are often severe, and the affected child does not reproduce. As we learn more about genetic mechanisms, some of these conditions are now known to be a result of contiguous gene syndromes, gonadal mosaicism in one of the parents, or new autosomal dominant or X-linked mutations. In these instances, the parents of the affected child may have a risk for recurrence. The affected individual may have as much as a 50:50 chance to have an affected son or daughter if he or she carries a new dominant mutation. Usually the healthy siblings of the affected individual have a low risk of having affected children.

2.10 ENVIRONMENTAL FACTORS

In taking a genetic family history, it is important to remember the role that the environment plays in gene expression. For example, a history of two sisters dying of lung cancer is much more worrisome if the sisters never smoked cigarettes than if they each smoked a pack of cigarettes a day for 20 years. The contribution of environmental factors to gene expression will continue to be elucidated as more genes are identified for common genetic disorders.

2.11 SUMMARY

The patterns of Mendelian inheritance have been genetic dogma since the turn of the 20th century. Health professionals must be receptive to new ways of thinking about human inheritance. Sixty years ago genetic doctrine was rocked by the recognition that a human cell has 46 chromosomes, not 48. The past 20 years mark the discovery and increased understanding of entirely new genetic inheritance patterns and their mechanisms, such as mitochondrial inheritance, imprinting, and dynamic mutations. The family pedigree will undoubtedly serve as a template for new discoveries in gene action and interaction as the practice of genomic medicine unfolds.

It seems appropriate to end this chapter with a poem by the late-19th-century author and poet Thomas Hardy (1917):

Heredity

I am the family face;
Flesh perishes, I live on,
Projecting trait and trace
Through time to times anon,
And leaping from place to place
Over oblivion.

The years-heired feature that can
In curve and voice and eye
Despise the human span
Of durance—that is I;
The eternal thing in man,
That heeds no call to die.

2.12 REFERENCES

Bennett RL, Motulsky AG, Bittles AH, et al. (2002). Genetic counseling and screening of consanguineous couples and their offspring: Recommendations of the National Society of Genetic Counselors. *J Genet Couns* 11(2):97–119.

Brinkman RR, Mezei MM, Theilmann J, et al. (1997). The likelihood of being affected with Huntington disease by a particular age, for a specific CAG size. *Am J Hum Genet* 60(5):1202–1210.

Clarke JTR. (2006). *A Clinical Guide to Metabolic Diseases*, 3rd ed. Cambridge: Cambridge University Press.

Connnor M, Ferguson-Smith M. (1997). *Essential Medical Genetics*, 5th ed. Oxford: Blackwell Scientific.

Cutting GR. (2007). Cystic fibrosis. In: Rimoin DL, Connor JM, Pyeritz RE, Korf BR, eds., *Emery & Rimoin's Principles and Practice of Medical Genetics*, 5th ed. Philadelphia: Elsivier, pp. 1354–1394.

Deegan PB, Baehner AF, Barba Romero MA, et al. (2006). Natural history of Fabry disease in females in the Fabry outcome survey. *J Med Genet* 43(4):347–352.

Disteche CM. (2007). Y chromosome infertility. March 19, 2007. Available at www.genereviews.org. Accessed February 7, 2009.

Eastman PD. (1960). *Are You My Mother?* New York: Random House.

Emery AEH. (2007). Duchenne and other X-linked muscular dystrophies. In: Rimoin DL, Connor JM, Pyeritz RE, Korf BR, eds., *Emery & Rimoin's Principles and Practice of Medical Genetics*, 5th ed. Philadelphia: Elsevier, pp. 2911–2927.

Engel E. (1995). Uniparental disomy: A review of causes and clinical sequelae. *Ann Genet* 38(3):113–136.

Engel E. (1998). Uniparental disomies in unselected populations. *Am J Hum Genet* 63:962–966.

Engel E, Antonarakis SE. (2001). *Genomic Imprinting and Uniparental Disomy in Medicine: Clinical and Molecular Aspects*. New York: Wiley-Liss.

Firth HV, Hurst JA. (2005). *Oxford Desk Reference Clinical Genetics*. Oxford, New York: Oxford University Press.

Francke U, Ochs HD, De Martinville B et al. (1985). Minor Xp21 chromosome deletion in a male associated with expression of Duchenne muscular dystrophy, chronic granulomatous disease, retinitis pigmentosa, and McLeod syndrome. *Am J Hum Genet* 37(2):250–267.

Hardy T. (1917). Moments of vision. The Literature Network. Available at www.online-literature.com/hardy/moments-of-vision/12. Accessed September 20, 2008.

Harper PS. (2002). *Myotonic Dystrophy—The Facts*. Oxford: Oxford University Press.

Huges DA. (2008). Early therapeutic intervention in females with Fabry disease? *Acta Paediatr Suppl* 97(457):41–47.

Jenne DE, Tinschert S, Stemann E, et al. (2000). A common set of at least 11 functional genes is lost in the majority of NF1 patients with gross deletions. *Genomics* 66(1): 93–97.

Jones, KL. (2006) *Smith's Recognizable Patterns of Human Malformation*, 6th ed. Philadelphia: Saunders.

Knoers N. (2007). Nephrogenic diabetes insipidus. June 8, 2007. Available at www.genereviews.org. Accessed February 7, 2009.

LaSpada AR, Paulson HL, Fishbeck KH. (1994). Trinucleotide repeat expansions in neurological disease. *Ann Neurol* 36: 814–822.

Lissens W, Liebaers I, Van Steirteghem. (2007). Male infertility. In: Rimoin DL, Connor JM, Pyeritz RE, Korf BR, eds. *Emery & Rimoin's Principles and Practice of Medical Genetics*, 5th ed. Philadelphia: Elsevier, pp. 856–874.

McConkie-Rosell A, Finucane B, Cronister A, et al. (2005). Genetic counseling for fragile X syndrome: Updated recommendations of the National Society of Genetic Counselors. *J Genet Couns* 14: 249–270.

Nance MA (1997). Clinical aspects of CAG repeat disorders. *Brain Pathol* 7(3):881–900.

Nance MA, Myers RH. (2001). Juvenile onset Huntington's disease–clinical and research perspectives. *Ment Retard Dev Disabil Res Rev* 7:153–157.

Nussbaum RL, McInnes RR, Willard HF. (2007). *Thompson and Thompson: Genetics in Medicine*, 7th ed. Philadelphia: Elsevier.

OMIM (2009). Online Mendelian Inheritance in Man. Available at www.ncbi.nlm.nih.gov/omim/. Accessed November 17, 2009.

Reeves WB, Andreioli TE. (1995). Nephrogenic diabetes. In: Scriver CR, Beaudet AL, Sly WS, Valle D, eds, *The Metabolic and Molecular Bases of Inherited Disease*. New York: McGraw-Hill, pp. 3045–3071.

Rimoin, DL, Connor JM, Pyeritz RE, Korf BR, eds. (2007). *Emery and Rimoin's Principles and Practice of Medical Genetics*, 5th ed. Philadelphia: Elsevier.

Riva P, Coorado L, Natacci F, et al. (2000). NF1 microdeletion syndrome: Refined FISH characterization of sporadic and familial deletions with locus-specific probes. *Am J Hum Genet* 66: 100–109.

Sinnreich M, Karpati G. (2006). Inclusion body myopathy 2. May 24, 2006. Available at www.genereviews.org. Accessed February 15, 2009.

Shashidhar P, Lewandowski RC, Borgaonkar D. (2003). *Handbook of Chromosomal Syndromes*. New York: Wiley.

Spinner NB, Saitta S, Emanuel BS. (2007). Deletions and other structural abnormalities of the autosomes. In: Rimoin DL, Connor JM, Pyeritz RE, Korf BR, eds., *Emery and Rimoin's Principles and Practice of Medical Genetics*, 5th ed. Philadelphia: Elsevier, pp. 1058–1081.

Strachan T, Read. (1996). *Human Molecular Genetics*. New York: Wiley-Liss.

Summar ML. (2005). Urea cycle disorders overview. August 11, 2005. Available at http://genereviews.org. Accessed February 7, 2009.

Sutherland GR, Richards RI. (1994). Dynamic mutations. *Am Scientist* 82: 157–163.

Sybert VP. (2010). *Genetic Skin Disorders*, 2nd ed. New York: Oxford University Press.

Vogel F, Motulsky AG. (1996). *Human Genetics: Problems and Approaches*, 3rd ed. Berlin: Springer.

Wallace DC, Lott MT, Procaccio V. (2007). Mitochondrial genes in degenerative diseases, cancer, and aging. In: Rimoin DL, Connor JM, Pyeritz RE, Korf BR, eds., *Emery & Rimoin's Principles and Practice of Medical Genetics*, 5th ed. Philadelphia: Elsevier, pp. 194–298.

Watson MS, Lloyd-Puryear MA, Mann MY, et al. (2006). Newborn screening: Toward a uniform panel and system. *Genet Med* 8(5)Suppl:12S–252S.

Weksberg R, Sadowski P, Smith AC, Tycko B. (2007). Epigenetics. In: Rimoin DL, Connor JM, Pyeritz RE, Korf BR, eds., *Emery & Rimoin's Principles and Practice of Medical Genetics*, 5th ed., Philadelphia: Elsevier, pp. 81–100.

Chapter 3

Getting to the Roots: Recording the Family Tree

A complete pedigree is often a work of great labour, and in its finished form is frequently a work of art.
—Karl Pearson, 1912 (From Resta, 1993)

3.1 CREATING A MEDICAL PEDIGREE: GETTING STARTED

The basic medical pedigree is a graphic depiction or map of how family members are biologically related to one another, from one generation to the next; social and legal relationships can also be shown (e.g., adoption and divorce). Each family member is represented by a square (male), or circle (female), and they are connected to each other by lines that form the trunks and branches of the family tree (Figure 3.1). This family map is meaningless if the symbols cannot be interpreted from clinician to clinician. The symbols outlined here are from the National Society of Genetic Counselors Pedigree Standardization Work Group (Bennett et al., 1995; Bennett et al., 2008); this nomenclature is now the international standard (Bennett et al., 2008). Appendix A.1 is a convenient cheat sheet for the common pedigree symbols, the basic information to include on a pedigree, and a prototype fictional pedigree demonstrating all the standardized symbols. The pedigree icons in isolation provide scant information; the power of a pedigree lies with the associative network of symbols.

Generally, the pedigree is taken in a face-to-face interview with the patient, before any physical examination. A patient is usually more comfortable sharing the intimate details of his or her personal and family life while fully clothed rather than wearing one of the highly fashionable rear-exposure gowns that are available in most examination

The Practical Guide to the Genetic Family History, Second Edition, by Robin L. Bennett
Copyright © 2010 John Wiley & Sons, Inc.

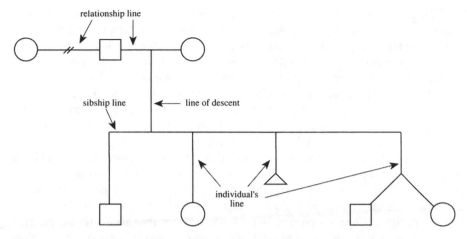

Figure 3.1 *Pedigree line definitions.*

rooms. A pedigree may also be drawn from family history questionnaires that are mailed in advance of the appointment.

There are a growing number of web-based family history programs for recording a medical family history. These programs and computer software programs for drawing pedigrees are reviewed in Appendix A.5. Most of the currently available software programs are cumbersome for drawing a quick pedigree in a clinical setting, and they often lack flexibility to reflect the nuances of a pedigree (such as multiple partners, including more than three generations, and tracking multiple diseases). These drawing programs are efficacious for clinics that will be seeing the same patient for multiple visits, for large research pedigrees, for patient registries, and for preparing a pedigree for professional publication. Such electronic versions may replace the old-fashioned pen-and-paper way, particularly when the patient is providing the pedigree and the content of the family history information is considered reliable. The pedigree drawing tool "My Family Health Portrait" developed through the U.S. Surgeon General's Office is a free web-based tool that is a useful, consumer-friendly method of recording a family history (https://familyhistory.hhs.gov).

I find it helpful to take a preliminary pedigree on the telephone. Many patients have limited knowledge of the health of their extended relatives. By asking medical-family history questions in advance of the appointment, the patient can do the homework of contacting the relevant family members to get more accurate details. The patient can also help arrange to obtain medical records (see Chapter 6). At the appointment, the pedigree that was obtained in advance can be verified with the patient. Medical-family history questionnaires can be a useful tool to collect pertinent information before the patient's appointment. However, a questionnaire is rarely a substitute for an actual pedigree. Appendix A.4 is a sample family history questionnaire designed for use when a child is being placed for adoption; this form has also been used for sperm and egg donor programs. A questionnaire for a family history of cancer is included in Appendix A.3.

The *consultand* is the individual seeking genetic counseling. This person is identified on the pedigree by an arrow, so that he or she can be easily identified when referring to the pedigree. If more than one person (consultands) come to the appointment (such as two sisters), identify each person with an arrow on the pedigree. The consultand can be a healthy person or a person with a medical condition.

The *proband* is the affected individual that brings the family to medical attention (Marazita, 1995). Identifying the proband is important in genetic mapping studies and research. Some researchers use the term *propositus* (plural is propositi) interchangeably with proband(s). The *index case* is a term used in genetic research to describe the first affected person to be studied in the family. Sometimes an individual is both a proband and the consultand. In addition, there can be two probands in a family if each independently brings that branch of the family to medical attention.

Even with the use of standardized pedigree symbols, a *key* or *legend* is essential for any pedigree. The main purpose of the key is to define the shading (or hatching) of symbols that indicate who is affected on the pedigree. The key is also used to explain any less frequently used symbols (such as adoption or donor gametes) or uncommon abbreviations.

Table 3.1 serves as a quick reference to the information essential to record on a pedigree. Remember to document on the pedigree your name and credentials (such as R.N., M.D., D.O., P.A., M.S.), and the name of the consultand. It is also helpful to record the name of the historian (the person giving the information), who may

TABLE 3.1   Essential Information on Family Members to Record in a Pedigree

Age (year of birth)
Age at death (year if known)
Cause of death
Full sibs distinguished from half sibs
Relevant health information[a]
    Significant health problems
    Significant surgeries
Age at diagnosis
Affected/unaffected status (define shading of symbol in key/legend)
Pregnancies with gestational age noted
    (LMP = last menstrual period or EDD = estimated date of delivery)
Pregnancy complications with gestational age noted (e.g., 6 wk, 34 wk): miscarriage
    (SAB), stillbirth (SB), pregnancy termination (TOP), ectopic (ECT)
Infertility or no children by choice
Personally evaluated or medically documented[a]
Ethnic background /country of origin, for each grandparent
Use a "?" if family history is unknown/unavailable
Consanguinity (noted degree of relationship if not implicit in pedigree)
First names (if appropriate, be cautious of privacy)
Date pedigree taken or updated
Reason pedigree taken
Name of person who took pedigree, and credentials (M.D., R.N., M.S., C.G.C., P.A.)
Key/legend

[a]Height and weight of first-degree relatives may be useful if specific to condition (such as condition with short stature, and obesity and disease risk.)

be different from the consultand. For example, an aunt in the family may be the "kin-keeper" or custodian of the family's medical information; a foster or adoptive parent may have access to only limited information about the biological relatives of the child.

Remember to date the pedigree. This is particularly important if ages rather than year of birth are recorded for family members on the pedigree. Was the pedigree taken yesterday or 10 years ago?

Use abbreviations sparingly and define them in the key. For example, CP may be short for cleft palate or cerebral palsy; MVA may mean motor vehicle accident or multiple vascular accidents; SB may be interpreted as stillbirth, spina bifida, or even shortness of breath.

Because the pedigree is part of the patient's medical record, it should be drawn with permanent ink. Using a black pen is best because blue ink may be faint if the record is scanned. It is acceptable to draft a pedigree in pencil; just be wary of errors in transcription. My favorite pedigree drawing tool is a corrective pen or tape that obliterates my frequent drawing errors. Some medical centers may not allow the use of corrective ink or tape in the patient's permanent record because of medical-legal concerns.

Draw the pedigree on your institution's medical progress notepaper (if available). A sample pedigree form is included in Appendix A.2. A standardized pedigree form has the advantage that you can include common pedigree symbols as a reference on the form. This fill-in-the-blanks approach serves as a reminder to document easily overlooked family history information (such as family ethnicity and whether there is consanguinity). These forms are limited in that pedigrees of large families may be difficult to squeeze onto the page.

Plastic drawing templates of various-size circles, squares, triangles, diamonds, and arrows are helpful for keeping the pedigree symbols neat and of uniform size. Such templates are available at most art and office supply stores.

3.2 LAYING THE FOUNDATION—PEDIGREE LINE DEFINITIONS

Pedigree can become quite complicated when they include multiple generations. Add to this the common occurrence of a person having children with multiple partners, and a pedigree soon looks a football play book. There are four main line definitions that form the trunk and branches of a medical family tree (Figure 3.1). Here are some rules to remember:

- A *relationship line* is a horizontal line between two partners; a slash or break in this line documents a separation or divorce.
- When possible, a male partner should be to the left of the female partner.
- A couple who is consanguineous (meaning they are biological relatives such as cousins) should be connected by a double relationship line (Figures 3.10 and 3.11).
- The *sibship line* is a horizontal line connecting brothers and sisters (siblings).

- Each sibling has a vertical *individual's line* attached to the horizontal sibship line (always above the individual's symbol).
- The *line of descent* is a vertical bridge connecting the horizontal sibship line to the horizontal relationship line (either below the individual's symbol or beneath the relationship line).

The application of these line definitions is important in the pedigree symbolization of adoption (Figure 3.7), and in symbolizing assisted reproductive technologies (ART) (see Chapter 8 and Figure 8.1).

3.3   KEEPING TRACK OF WHO IS WHO ON THE PEDIGREE

Begin by explaining to the consultand (or parent if the consultand is a child) that you will be taking a family health history by asking questions about his or her health and that of his or her family, and drawing a family tree. You may prefer to use the terminology of a *family health portrait* as advocated by the office of the U.S. Surgeon General (U.S. Department of Health and Human Services, 2009). To explain why family medical history information is important, I usually say, "Your family-health history is one of the best tools we have to provide you with information about the diseases in your family, what we can do to diagnose and even prevent disease, and what genetic tests, if any, may be appropriate."

Begin with simple, factual questions:

Do you have a partner, are you married, or were you married in the past?

How many children do you have? Are they with the same partner?

Have you had any miscarriages or babies who died, or other pregnancies?

How many biological brothers and sisters do you have?

Do your siblings share the same mother and father as you?

The answers to these questions will give you an idea of how much room you will need on your paper. If you are interviewing an elderly person, you may be taking a five-generation pedigree (e.g., grandparents, parents, aunts and uncles, cousins, siblings, nieces and nephews, children, and grandchildren). If you begin your pedigree in the middle of the page, it is easy to extend your pedigree up and down. If the consultand is a child or a pregnant woman, usually it is easier to start the pedigree toward the bottom of the page and extend your pedigree up toward the top of the paper as you inquire about prior generations. Large pedigrees are often easier to record with the paper in a landscape, or lengthwise, orientation as compared to a portrait, or up-and-down, orientation.

When possible, draw siblings in birth order, from left to right. Record the age, or year of birth, of each sibling. Always ask if siblings share the same mother and father—people often do not distinguish an adopted sibling or a step-sibling from biological kin. Figure 3.6 shows how to demarcate half-siblings. It is not necessary to draw each sibling's partner or spouse on the pedigree, particularly if the couple does

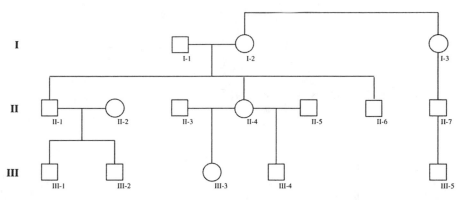

Figure 3.2 *Numbering generations and individuals on a pedigree. The numbering system allows for easy reference to individuals on a pedigree when names are not recorded.*

not have children. It may be important to record the partner of a sibling if there is a significant medical history in their offspring. This is particularly important when a family history of a common medical condition (such as cancer) is identified. Remind the historian that you are also interested in deceased relatives and pregnancy losses. An adult may forget to tell you about a sibling who died 25 years ago or in childhood.

Each generation in a pedigree should be on the same horizontal plane. For example, a person's siblings and cousins are drawn on the same horizontal axis; the parents, aunts and uncles are drawn on the same horizontal line. In pedigrees used for publication or research, usually each generation is defined by a Roman numeral (e.g., I, II, III), and each person in the generation is given an Arabic number, from left to right (e.g., I-3, I-4, II-3). This makes it easy to refer to family members in the pedigree by number, and thus protects family confidentiality (Figure 3.2). In clinical pedigrees, names are usually recorded on the pedigree (parallel or next to the individual's line). The family surname is placed above the sibship line, or above the relationship line. Of course, if names are recorded on the pedigree, care must be taken to preserve the confidentiality of the pedigree. First names or initials would meet most privacy compliance standards (Bennett et al., 2008).

3.4 HOW MANY GENERATIONS ARE INCLUDED IN A PEDIGREE?

A basic pedigree usually includes a minimum of three generations—the consultand's *first-degree relatives* (parents, children, siblings) and *second-degree relatives* (half siblings, grandparents, aunts and uncles, grandchildren). *Third-degree relatives*, particularly cousins are often included, even if only to note that they "exist." For example, one can place a diamond with a *3* inside to show that an aunt or uncle has three children. Figure 3.3 shows the pedigree framework for denoting a relative's relationship to the consultand (for example, a first cousin is a third-degree relative to the consultand).

If a health problem of significance is identified, the pedigree is extended back as far as possible (refer to Table 4.1 for clues to family history features suggestive of a

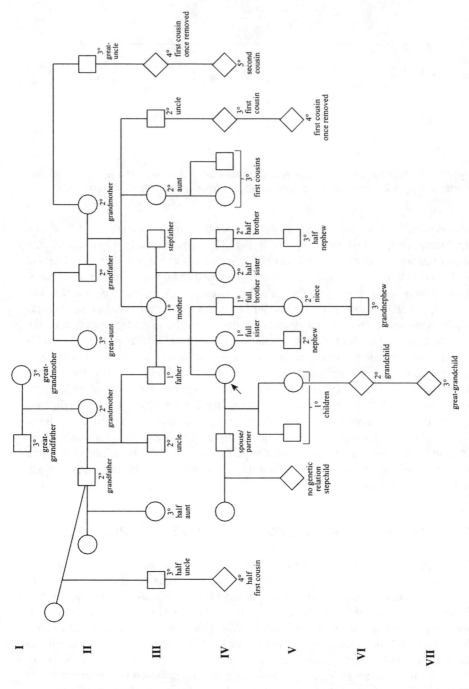

Figure 3.3 The pedigree framework for denoting a relative's relationship to the consultand (i.e., first-degree, second-degree, and third-degree relatives).

genetic condition). For example, if a 60-year-old woman with breast cancer is interested in genetic risk assessment for the benefit of her two daughters, you would ask her
about any cancer in her parents, grandparents, uncles and aunts, cousins, children, and
grandchildren. If a positive family history for a medical condition is identified, you
would inquire about great-aunts and great-uncles, and great-grandparents. A pedigree
may be quite extensive for a person with a family history of genetic condition with a
late age of symptom onset.

3.5 THE BASIC PEDIGREE SYMBOLS

The most common pedigree symbols are shown in Figures 3.4 and 3.5. The gender of
an individual is assigned by the outward phenotype. Males are denoted with squares
and females with circles. A pregnancy is represented with a diamond with a *P* inside.
A diamond can be used when it is not important to specify the gender or if the
information is unknown. For example, if the consultand is aware that a grandparent
had one or more siblings but does not know their gender, a diamond can be used with
an *n* placed inside. A diamond can also represent persons with congenital disorders
of sex development in which chromosomal, gonadal, or anatomic sex is atypical. The
karyotype is noted below the symbol (such as 46, XY). The diamond can also be
used for a transgendered individual or for a person who self-identifies as somewhere
on the spectrum between the opposites of male and female (Bennett et al., 2008).

Information about each person can be written in the space below and to the lower
right of each symbol. The age or year of birth is noted. The birth date is considered
protected health information and should be avoided unless necessary for correlating
family medical records with pedigree information (Bennett et al., 2008). Record the
cause of death and age at death for all individuals on the pedigree. Noting the year
of death is useful because this can provide you with clues as to the diagnostic tools
available during that medical era. For example, DNA diagnostic testing did not exist
before the mid-1980s. The identification of a structural brain anomaly may have been
made with the aid of a pneumonencephalogram in the 1960s and 1970s as compared
to the modern brain imaging technique of brain MRI.

Relevant health information such as height (h.) and weight (w.) is placed below
the pedigree symbol. The recommended order of this information is: (1) age or year
of birth, (2) age at death and cause, (3) relevant health information, (4) pedigree
number.

It is the rare historian who knows the precise details of such information as current
ages, ages at death, and the heights of his or her extended relatives. A tilde ($\sim$) can
be used when approximations are given.

3.6 YOURS, MINE, AND OURS—THE BLENDED FAMILY

Correct documentation of how individuals are biologically related to each other is
essential for accurate pedigree assessment. It is almost inevitable when taking a family
history that at least one person in the family will have more than one partner. For each

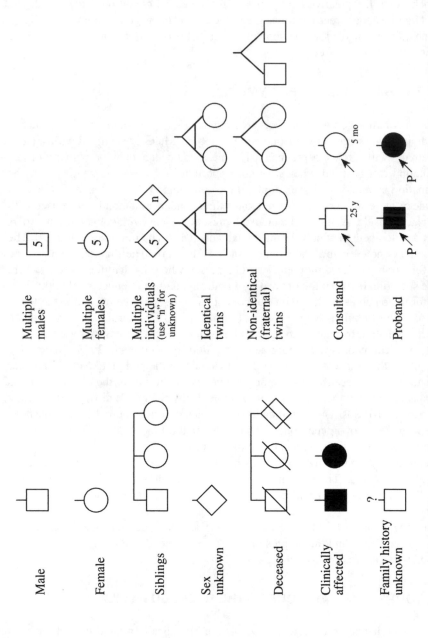

Figure 3.4 The most common pedigree symbols. Pregnancy-related symbols are shown in Figure 3.5.

Male

Female

Siblings

Sex unknown

Deceased

Clinically affected

Family history unknown

Multiple males

Multiple females

Multiple individuals (use "n" for unknown)

Identical twins

Non-identical (fraternal) twins

Consultand

Proband

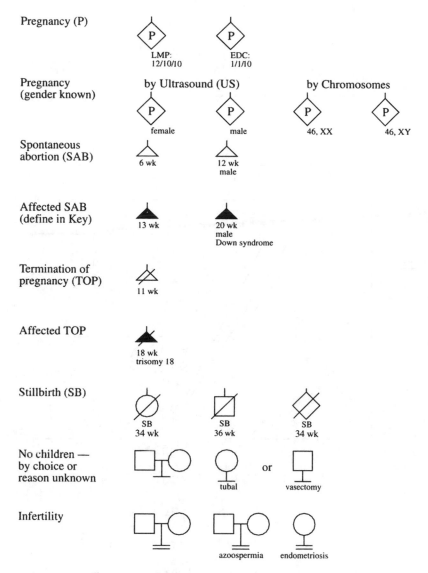

Figure 3.5 *Pedigree symbols related to pregnancy.*

sibling group on the pedigree, ask if they share the same mother and father. If the answer is no, ask "Which of your brothers and sisters share the same mother and which share the same father?" Not uncommonly patients confuse half-sibs from step-sibs.

If there is a big gap in age between siblings, this is a clue that they may be half-siblings. The gap may also be an indication of a period of infertility.

It is not necessary to include each partner of an individual on a pedigree—doing so can make a pedigree quite complicated as is illustrated in actress Elizabeth Taylor's marriage history shown in Figure 3.6.

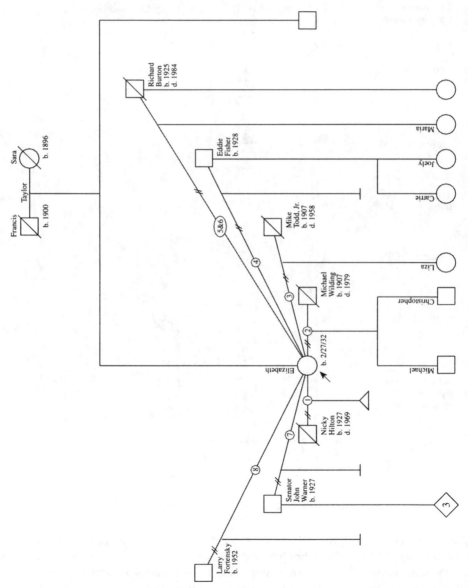

Figure 3.6 A pedigree of actress Elizabeth Taylor demonstrating how to illustrate multiple marriage partners, step-children, and half siblings. (Source: www.celebsite.com.)

3.7 PEDIGREE SYMBOLS RELATED TO PREGNANCY AND REPRODUCTION

The various pedigree symbols related to pregnancy, spontaneous abortion, termination of pregnancy, stillbirth, and infertility are shown in Figure 3.5. If the gestational age is known, place the gestational age in weeks (wk.) below the symbol. An approximation of dates can be shown such as "~12 wk." Usually the gestational age is stated as the date from the first date of the last menstrual period (LMP) or the estimated date of delivery (EDD). The older terminology of estimated date of confinement (EDC) is considered archaic. Pregnancy dating by ultrasound can be noted as "US 12 wk."

A stillbirth (SB) is defined as "the birth of a dead child with gestational age noted" (Bennett et al., 1995).

If the gender of the fetus is known then one can write "male" or "female" under the symbol. This is preferable to making the symbol a square or a circle. If a chromosome study has confirmed the sex of the fetus, this can be noted under the symbol as "46,XX" or "46,XY."

3.8 ASSISTED REPRODUCTIVE TECHNOLOGIES (ART) AND USE OF DONOR GAMETES

The importance of recording family history for persons conceived through ART, including information on the family history of egg or sperm donors is detailed in Chapter 8. The symbols to use in recording this information are noted in the tables to Chapter 8. Some birth defects may be related to assisted reproductive technologies (e.g., in vitro fertilization, frozen embryos), and therefore the method of ART should be recorded on the pedigree.

3.9 ADOPTION

It is important to distinguish a person who is adopted *in* to a family (a nonbiological relative) from a person who is adopted *out* (a biological relative). To symbolize adoption, brackets are placed around the symbol for male (square) or female (circle) or unknown (diamond). If a person or couple adopts an individual, the individual's line is dotted (indicating a nonbiological relationship). A person who is placed for adoption has a solid individual's line to the birth parents.

It is not uncommon for a family member to adopt a relative—for example, a sibling adopting a niece or nephew, or grandparents adopting a grandchild. The method of recording this situation on a pedigree is shown in Figure 3.7.

When a person or couple adopts a child it is useful to inquire if there was a medical reason; perhaps an adoptive parent had a genetic condition or the couple who adopted the child experienced infertility. The reason can be noted below the line of descent.

When a child is placed for adoption, information about the child's medical heritage is usually given to the adoptive parents (see Chapter 7). A sample adoptive medical-family history form can be found in Appendix A.4.

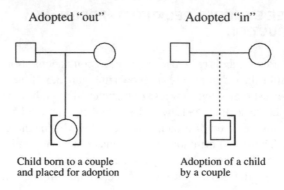

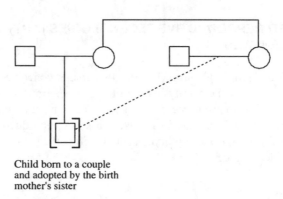

Figure 3.7 Pedigree symbolization of adoption.

3.10 INFERTILITY AND NO CHILDREN BY CHOICE

If a person or couple is of reproductive age and has no children, inquire if this is by choice or for a biological reason. The cause of infertility should be noted below the individual's line (e.g., azoospermia, endometriosis, etc.).

3.11 AFFECTED STATUS: SHADING THE PEDIGREE SYMBOLS

Accurately documenting who is affected and unaffected on a pedigree is critical for pedigree analysis. A symbol should only be shaded if the person, pregnancy, miscarriage, or abortion is clinically affected. Of course, whether a person is considered affected may be a function of the sensitivity of the clinical tool that is used to define affected status. For example, the 2-year old sister of a 5-year old boy with classic symptoms of cystic fibrosis may have no obvious symptoms, yet she can have elevated sweat chloride levels. Methods of documenting this information are described in Figure 3.9.

Most families will have more than one genetic or potentially heritable medical condition. Different shading can be used to define separate diseases on the pedigree. For example, when documenting a family history of cancer, shading in the various quadrants of each square (male) or circle (female) is a way to symbolize multiple cancers (Figure 3.8).

3.12   A & W

A & W is a simple method of showing on the pedigree that a relative is "alive and well." By noting "A & W" under each healthy person on the pedigree, you demonstrate that you have inquired about the health of each family member on the pedigree. If the health status of a relative is unknown, this can be demarcated below the pedigree symbol with a question mark (?).

3.13   "HE DIED OF A BROKEN HEART"—FAMILY HEARSAY

Family members often use non-medical terms to describe medical illnesses in a family. If Uncle Billy "died of a broken heart," the clinician should not automatically assume that the person died of a heart attack. Family lore can be recorded on the pedigree in "quotes," using the words that the relative used to describe the ailment. Asking questions such as, "Was this a long-standing illness?" and "Was the death unexpected?" might help clarify the nature of a family member's illness." The clinician should never assume a diagnosis based on a family member's description; any presumed diagnosis should be noted as unconfirmed on the pedigree.

3.14   FAMILY HISTORY UNKNOWN

Sometimes little information is known about a parent, grandparent, or other family member. Placing a question mark above the pedigree symbol shows that you inquired about that person's medical history and that the information is unknown or unavailable. Another way to note that there is limited information available is "ø contact" (no contact) (Figure 3.4).

3.15   DOCUMENTING MEDICAL EXAMINATIONS AND EVALUATIONS

Genetic counseling requires accurate medical and health history information. An asterisk (*) is placed near the lower right edge of the pedigree symbol for anyone who

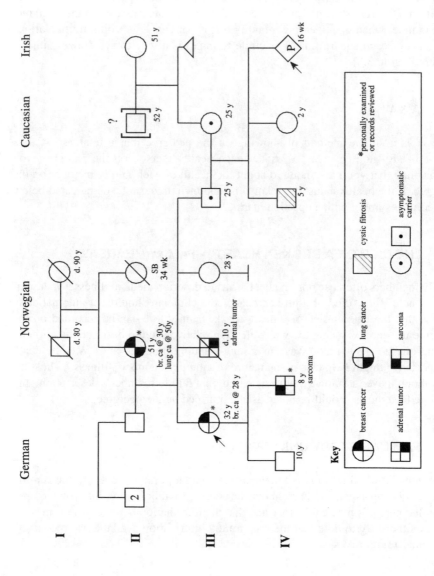

Figure 3.8 *Hypothetical pedigree demonstrating how to shade affected individuals when more than one condition is segregating in a family.*

Instructions:
— E is used for evaluation to represent clinical and/or test information on the pedigree
  a. E is to be defined in key/legend
  b. If more than one evaluation, use subscript (E_1, E_2, E_3) and define in key
  c. Test results should be put in parentheses or defined in key/legend
— A symbol is shaded only when an individual is clinically symptomatic
— For linkage studies, haplotype information is written below the individual. The haplotype of interest should be on left and appropriately highlighted
— Repetitive sequences, trinucleotides and expansion numbers are written with affected allele first and placed in parentheses
— If mutation known, identify in parentheses

Definition	Symbol	Scenario
1. Documented evaluation (*) Use only if examined/evaluated by you or your research/clinical team or if the outside evaluation has been reviewed and verified.		Woman with negative echocardiogram.
2. Carrier—not likely to manifest disease regardless of inheritance pattern		Male carrier of Tay-Sachs disease by patient report (* not used because results not verified).
3. Asymptomatic/presymptomatic carrier—clinically unaffected at this time but could later exhibit symptoms		Woman age 25 with negative mammogram and positive BRCA1 DNA test.
4. Uninformative study (u)	Eu	Man age 25 with normal physical exam and uninformative DNA test for Huntington disease (E_2).
5. Affected individual with positive evaluation (E+)	E+	Individual with cystic fibrosis and positive mutation study; only one mutation has currently been identified.
		10 week male fetus with a trisomy 18 karyotype.

Scenario column annotations:
- E– (echo)
- E_1– (mammogram) / E_2+ (5385insC BRCA1); 25 y
- E_1– (physical exam) / E_2u (36n/18n); 25 y
- E+(ΔF508) ... Eu / E+(ΔF508/u)
- 10wk / E+(CVS) / 47, XY,+18

Figure 3.9 *How to document results of medical evaluations and genetic testing on a pedigree (including presymptomatic testing and obligate carrier status). (Reprinted with permission from Bennett et. al, 1995; Bennett et al., 2008.)*

has been personally examined by you or you have verified information with medical records (Figure 3.9). See Chapter 6 for specific information on how to help families obtain medical records on relatives.

Medical evaluations on relatives can be recorded on the pedigree. Each clinical evaluation or test can be represented by an "E" and defined in the key. An evaluation may represent information obtained by clinical examination, medical testing (e.g., brain imaging, biopsy, nerve conduction studies), or laboratory results. If a test or examination result is considered abnormal it is considered a "+" (positive) result, and a normal result is documented "−." If the test is uninformative, a "u" follows the "E." For example, there are over 1,000 mutations in the cystic fibrosis gene. A child with known cystic fibrosis may have only 1 gene mutation identified. Such a result could be noted on the pedigree as E = ΔF08/u (Figure 3.9).

3.16   A NOTE ON GENETIC TESTING

Genetic testing can be confusing to patients and even to many health professionals. Some patients falsely assume that any genetic test is a chromosome test. Others assume that all genetic testing involves direct analysis of the DNA (as compared to enzyme analysis or tumor marker studies). A patient may assume that a genetic test was "positive" when in fact the result is inconclusive or a gene variation of uncertain significance was detected. It is important to clarify how the term *positive result* is being used because to a patient this may be "good news" but the health professional may be referring to an abnormal result. It is always important to obtain documentation of the patient's or family member's actual laboratory result.

3.17   THE HEALTHY PERSON WITH AN ABNORMAL GENETIC TEST RESULT: THE DIFFERENCE BETWEEN A PRESYMPTOMATIC OR ASYMPTOMATIC CARRIER AND AN OBLIGATE CARRIER

Advances in genetic testing now allow a healthy person to be tested for a genetic condition that he or she may or will develop in the future. Many geneticists reserve the description *presymptomatic carrier* for a healthy person who is likely to develop the disease in his or her lifetime (Bennett et al., 1995). For example, a person who is predicted to develop Huntington disease in his or her lifetime has a segment of genetic material called a CAG trinucleotide repeat that is repeated too many times. A person with 40 or more CAG repeats is likely to have symptoms of Huntington disease by the time he or she reaches the age of 70.

In contrast, a woman who has a mutation in *BRCA1* or *BRCA2* (the genes associated with two hereditary breast-ovarian cancer syndromes) has up to an 85% lifetime chance of developing breast cancer to age 70, but the development of cancer is not inevitable. This is usually referred to as *predisposition* or *susceptibility genetic testing*. The description *asymptomatic carrier* is sometimes used for a person who carries a susceptibility or predisposition mutation. Some geneticists take exception to the use of the terminology *predictive testing* because no genetic test provides and absolute gaze into a person's medical future.

A person who carries a gene mutation but will not develop clinical symptoms is referred to as an *obligate carrier* (Bennett et al., 1995). For example, the parents of children affected with a classic autosomal recessive disorder are obligate carriers. A healthy mother of two boys with an X-linked recessive condition (such as Duchenne muscular dystrophy) is an obligate carrier. A problem with this terminology is that the spectrum of recognizing disease expression has broadened for many diseases.

For example, women with a fragile X premutation have been traditionally thought of as healthy obligate carriers, but it is now known that some of these women experience premature ovarian insufficiency as an expression of the disease (McConkie-Rosell et al., 2005).

Figure 3.9 demonstrates how to document genetic test results and asymptomatic or presymptomatic and obligate carrier status. Individuals who are obligate carriers are represented on the pedigree with a dot in the middle of the male (square) or female (circle) symbol. Persons who are asymptomatic or presymptomatic carriers are represented with a line down the middle of the pedigree symbol. If the person later develops the disease, the symbol is shaded.

3.18 PEDIGREE ETIQUETTE

3.18.1 The Skeletons in the Closet

For many reasons, people tend to keep genetic information private. There is often a sense of stigma, even embarrassment about "bad blood" or a "curse" in the family. As Francis Galton observed, "Most men and women shrink from having their hereditary worth recorded. There may be family diseases of which they hardly dare to speak, and then in whispered hints or hushed phrases as if timidity of utterance could hush thoughts..." (Resta, 1995). People may be reluctant to share medical and genetic information because of fear they will be blamed for the family imperfections.

3.18.2 Choose Your Words Wisely

The difference between the right word and the almost right word is the difference between lightening and the lightning bug.

—Mark Twain

When you take a medical-family history, you are inquiring about the very essence of an individual. You are asking not only about the individual's personal health but also about intimate relationships and the health of family members (with whom he or she may have little contact). Before you begin taking a genetic family history, it is helpful to warn the client: "I need to ask you some personal questions about your health and the health of people in your family. Your answers to these questions are an important part of providing you with appropriate medical care."

The clinician should be careful not to perpetuate feelings of guilt or fears of stigmatization. Use words such as *altered*, *changed*, or *not working properly* to describe genes, instead of *mutation*, *bad*, or *faulty*. Emphasize to the patient that relatives have no choice in the genetic conditions that are passed in a family; the diseases are nobody's fault.

Be sensitive to terms like an *uneventful pregnancy*. Although a healthy pregnancy may be uneventful to the clinician, it is very eventful to the proud parents! I often hear clinicians refer to a family history without apparent genetic problems as a "negative" family history, as compared to "positive." A positive family history is usually experienced as negative by the patient and family (Fisher, 1996). I usually describe health problems in the family history as being *contributory* or *remarkable* as compared to *noncontributory* or *unremarkable* in reference to the medical problems in question.

Questioning should focus on "people-first-language" (www.disabilityisnatural. com), with inquires about the diagnosis not the label (e.g., a person with Down syndrome not a Down's person, or a person with autism not an autistic). It is a challenge in taking a family history not to focus solely on health problems, but it is important not to use words with negative connotations such as *abnormal, crippled, retarded* (intellectual disability is appropriate), *birth defect* (congenital disability is preferred), or *wheelchair bound* (as compared to saying the person uses a wheelchair or mobility devise). Avoid phrases that ask if relatives "suffer" or "struggle" from a disease.

Ask questions one at a time. Do not jump from one topic to another. Begin with general questions, and then move to more specific questions that may be more complex or threatening (McCarthy Veach et al., 2003). Do not interrogate.

The ultimate test of the appropriateness of a question is "Will this information be helpful to my patient" (Hill and O'Brien, 1999). If the patient asked you, "Why do you need to know this information?" what would be your reply (McCarthy Veach et al., 2003)?

3.18.3 Use Common Language

You are more likely to be successful in obtaining an accurate family history if you use terms that are familiar to people. For example, rather than asking about myopathies in the family, inquire if individuals have muscle weakness or if anyone uses a cane or wheelchair.

3.18.4 Beware the Leading Question

If you say, "So, your brothers and sisters are healthy, right? No health problems in your parents?" you will most likely receive a reply of "Un-huh," regardless of whether this is a true statement. Instead, try to be specific with your questioning by asking open-ended questions: "Do your brothers and sisters have any health problems?"

3.18.5 Listen

Let your client tell his or her story. If the client's dialogue is heading down a path that is not leading to information relevant for your evaluation, gently lead the questioning back on task. For example interject with, "That is interesting information. Now let me ask you more about . . ."

Respect a client's belief system of causality of a problem. Be aware of the emotional and cognitive effect that your history gathering is having on your client, and slow your pace of questioning or pause as needed (Stanion et al., 1997).

3.18.6 Acknowledge Significant Life Events

Common courtesy should be the rule in taking a family history. If a woman tells you that she recently miscarried or that her mother died of breast cancer a few months ago, it is appropriate to acknowledge this with "I am sorry to hear of your loss," or "This must be a difficult time for you." Conversely, the news of a recent birth, marriage, or desired pregnancy can be greeted with "Congratulations."

Each family history tells a story. Sometimes that story leaps from the page and must be acknowledged. A person may be the only survivor from a house fire or a car accident that took the lives of several relatives. A family may have perished in the Holocaust or from a similar criminal act against humanity. Your comments such as "That must have been hard for you," or "I cannot imagine what that must have been like for you," in acknowledgment of such obviously life-changing events up-rooted in the family tree, will be appreciated by your client and assist in cementing rapport, respect and trust with your patient.

3.18.7 Be Sensitive to Cultural Issues and Differences

If your patient does not speak English, get an interpreter. Do not rely on a family member to provide interpretation. The family member may be tempted to interject his or her opinions, particularly about family matters, as part of the translation or omit or censor information. Using an interpreter can be problematic if the interpreter is from the same social community as the patient; in this circumstance the patient may be reluctant to share confidential information.

Culture consists of shared patterns, knowledge, meaning, and behaviors of a social group (Fisher, 1996). Individuals have different customs and beliefs based on their race, socioeconomic status, gender, religious beliefs, sexual orientation, education, or health status. When taking a family history, it is important to acknowledge belief systems that are different from one's own. For example, a traditional Latino woman may believe that her child's cleft lip and palate is the result of supernatural forces during a lunar eclipse, "susto" (Cohen et al., 1998). Individuals from a traditional Southeast Asian culture may have strong belief in karma and fate. Several cultures believe in the evil eye as a cause of family illness and woes (Abboud, 1998; Kalofissudis, 2003). Traditional Chinese views may relate genetics to Buddhist ideas of retribution in this life for wrong-doings committed in a previous life. Accepted Chinese beliefs are in patrilineal descent (through the male lines) and thus the male blood line is genetically stronger and diseases can be passed through the male line more readily than the female line (Barlow-Stewart et al., 2006). Persons from certain religious and cultural groups may believe bad thoughts or sins cause a birth defect or genetic disorder (Cohen et al., 1998). References to "bad illnesses" in the family may disturb the "good aura" of the family or ancestors (Fisher and Lew, 1996).

An individual's belief system is likely to influence the type of health information he or she shares with the healthcare provider. A vivid example of this is the description of a Hopi woman with severely disabling congenital kyphoscoliosis who was described by her sister as being small and having pain in her legs and back that kept her from her normal activities. The woman's sister was not portrayed as disabled, because she had high status in the community due to her ability to make piki, a thin wafer bread (Hauck and Knoki-Wilson, 1996). While it is important to listen to and respect a person's cultural health beliefs, it is just as essential to avoid stereotypes by assuming that all persons from that cultural share the same views of health and disease causation.

Exceptional references on providing healthcare for diverse populations are *Cultural and Ethnic Diversity: A Guide for Genetics Professionals* (Fisher, 1996), *Developing Cross-Cultural Competence: A Guide for Working with Young Children and Their Families*, (Lynch and Hanson, 2004), *Cultural Awareness in the Human Services: A Multi-Ethnic Approach* (Green, 1999), and *Counselling the Cultural Diverse: Theory and Practice* (Wing Sue and Sue, 2002).

3.19   RECORDING A BASIC PEDIGREE: THE QUESTIONS TO ASK

Obtaining an extended medical-family history is really no different from obtaining a person's medical history. I usually inform the consultand, "I will now ask you questions about you and your relatives. I am interested in your family members who are both living and dead." Then I ask general questions, reviewing medical systems from head to toe. If a positive history is found, I ask directed questions based on that system, and the genetic diseases that are associated with it. For additional directed family history questions focused on a positive family history for several common medical conditions (e.g., heart disease, hearing loss), see Chapter 4.

3.19.1   Medical-Family History Queries by Systems Review

3.19.1.1   Head, Face, and Neck.   Begin by asking, *Does anyone have anything unusual about the way he or she looks?* If yes, have the historian describe the unusual facial features. In particular inquire about unusual placement or shape of the eyes and ears.

Anyone with an unusually large or small head?

Are there problems with vision, blindness, cataracts, or glaucoma? (If so, inquire as to the age the problems began, the severity, and any treatment.)

Anyone with unusual eye coloring (e.g., eyes that are different colors, or whites of the eyes that are blue)?

Do any family members have cleft lip or opening in the lip, with or without cleft palate?

Anyone with unusual problems with his or her teeth (e.g., missing, extra, misshapen, fragile, early teeth loss)?

Any problems with hearing or speech?

Anyone with a short or webbed neck?

Anything unusual about the hair (e.g., coarse, fine, early balding, white patch)?

3.19.1.2 Skeletal System.

Is any family member unusually tall or short? (If so, record the heights of the person, the parents, and siblings. If someone is short, is he or she in proportion?)

Anyone with curvature of the spine? (If so, did this require surgery or bracing?)

Anyone with multiple fractures? (If yes, inquire as to how many fractures, how the breaks occurred, the bones that were broken, and the age the fractures occurred.)

Anyone with an unusual shape to his or her chest?

Anyone with unusually formed bones?

Anyone with unusually shaped hands or feet, such as extremely long or short fingers or toes, missing fingers or toes? Have the historian describe these anomalies.

Anyone with joint problems, such that they are unusually stiff or flexible, or dislocate frequently?

3.19.1.3 Skin.

Anyone with unusual lumps, bumps, or birthmarks? (If so, have the patient describe them, their location, their coloration, and number.) Were these skin changes ever biopsied or treated?

Any problems with healing, scarring, or excessive bruising?

Anyone with unusual problems with their fingernails, or toenails, such as absent nails, or growths under the nails?

3.19.1.4 Respiratory System.

Any family members with any lung diseases? (If so, were they smokers? Were they treated for the lung condition, and how?)

3.19.1.5 Cardiac System.

Anyone with heart disease? (If so, at what age, and how were they treated?)

Was anyone born with a heart defect? (If so, did they have birth anomalies or intellectual delay?)

Anyone with heart murmurs?

Anyone with high blood pressure?

Were there any heart surgeries? (If so, what was done, and at what age?)

3.19.1.6 Gastrointestinal System.

Anyone with stomach or intestinal tract problems? (If so, were they treated for the problem, and how? How old were they at the age of symptom onset?)

3.19.1.7 Renal System.

Anyone with kidney disease? (If so, were they treated for the problem, and how? What was their age of onset and their symptoms?)

3.19.1.8 Hematological System.

Anyone with bleeding, clotting, or healing problems?
Have any relatives been told they are anemic?
Have there been relatives who needed transfusions?

3.19.1.9 Endocrine.

Anyone with thyroid problems?
Anyone with diabetes?
Anyone who is overly heavy or thin?

3.19.1.10 Immune System.

Anyone with frequent infections or hospitalizations, or difficulties healing?

3.19.1.11 Reproduction.

Have any relatives had miscarriages or babies who died, severe pregnancy complications, or infertility?

3.19.1.12 Neurological/Neuromuscular.

Anyone with muscle weakness, or with problems with walking?
Do any family members use a cane or wheelchair? (If there are muscle problems, inquire as to the age at which the problems began and what type of testing was done, such as a muscle biopsy, nerve conduction velocity, or brain imaging.)
Anyone with strokes or seizures? (If so, at what age did they begin, and what medications were given.)
Anyone with uncontrolled movements, tics, difficulties with coordination, or spasticity? (If so, at what age did they begin? Were medications given?)
Anyone with slurred speech?

3.19.1.13   Mental Functioning.

Anyone in the family with mental or intellectual impairment or severe learning disabilities? Did anyone attend special classes or school, or need help to finish school? (Note that the term *mental retardation* is no longer in favor, although this is a term that is still used commonly by medical professionals and even used in the family.) Intellectual disability is the preferred description.

If yes, describe the level of functioning and any dysmorphic features. Was the mother taking any drugs, alcohol, or medications during the pregnancy, or did she have an illness?

Does anyone have a diagnosis of autism or autistic-like features?

Are there any relatives with problems with thinking or judgment, mental illness, or severe depression? (If so, have the patient describe the relative's symptoms, the age symptoms began, and any known medications.)

3.19.2   General Interview Questions

3.19.2.1   Occupation.   Asking about a patient's occupation helps develop rapport. It also may be a clue to a potential environmental exposure that is contributing to a disease.

3.19.2.2   Congenital disabilities.   I also ask near the end of the interview if any relatives have a problem present from birth, particularly of the heart, spine, hands or feet.

3.19.2.3   Drug and Alcohol Abuse.   Knowing about drug and alcohol abuse in the patient and other family members is important for many reasons, If there are abnormal ultrasound findings in a pregnancy or if a child has birth defects with or without intellectual delay, there could be a maternal teratogenic etiology for the problems. Neurological problems can also be related to, or exacerbated by, maternal drug and alcohol use. The known and suspected human teratogens are listed in Table 3.2. For comprehensive information on agents that are potentially teratogenic and their effects, refer to REPRORISK (www.micromedex.com/products/reprorisk) and TERIS (Teratogen Information System at http://depts.washington.edu/terisweb/teris/subscribe.htm). A human teratogen is defined as an agent that can cause abnormalities of form, function, or both, in an exposed embryo or fetus (Friedman and Hanson, 2007). Counseling regarding human teratogens goes beyond memorization of a list of teratogenic agents and requires knowledge of the overall exposure of the agent (dosage and other concurrent exposures, gestational timing, and route of delivery). The biological susceptibility of the mother and the embryo to the agent are other factors which whether a potential teratogen will have a harmful effect (Friedman and Hanson, 2007).

The specific areas to note when inquiring about possible maternal teratogens include

- What is the drug or medicine? (For medications, ask the patient to bring her prescription to the appointment.)

TABLE 3.2   Potential Human Teratogens

Agent

Radiation
  Atomic weapons
  Radioiodine
  Therapeutic radiation
Maternal infections
  Cytomegalovirus (CMV)
  Herpes simplex virus I and II (primary)
  Parvovirus B-19
  Rubella virus
  Syphillis
  Toxoplasmosis
  Varicella virus
  Venezuelan equine encephalitis
Maternal and metabolic factors
  Alcohol
  Autoimmune disorders
  Early amniocentesis (before day 70 post-conception)
  Early chorionic villus sampling (before day 60 post-conception)
  Cretinism, endemic
  Insulin dependent diabetes (poorly controlled)
  Folic acid deficiency
  Hyperthermia
  Phenylketonuria
  Virilizing tumors
Drugs and environmental chemicals
  Alcohol
  ACE inhibitors
  Aminopterin
  Androgenic hormones
  Bisulfan
  Captopril
  Chlorobiphenyls
  Cocaine
  Coumarin anticoagulants
  Cyclophosphamide
  Diethylstilbestrol
  Enalapril
  Etretinate
  Iodides
  Isotretinoin (Accutane)
  Lithium
  Mercury, organic
  Methotrexate (methylaminopterin)
  Methylene blue (via interamniotic injection)
  Misoprostol
  Methimazole
  Pencillamine
  Phenytoin (Hydantoin)
  Polychlorobiphenyls (PCBs) (ingested)
  Tetracyclines

(Continued)

TABLE 3.2   (*Continued*)

Thalidomide
Toulene (abuse)
Trimethadione
Valproic acid
Possible Teratogens
  Binge alcohol use
  Carbamazepine
  Cigarette smoking
  Colchine
  Disulfiram
  Ergotamine
  Fluconazole
  Lead
  Primidone
  Quinine
  Streptomycin
  Vitamin A
  Zinc deficiency
Unlikely Teratogens
  Agent Orange
  Anesthetics
  Aspartame
  Asprin
  Bendectin
  Hydroxyprogesterone
  LSD
  Marijuana
  Medroxyprogesterone
  Metronidazole
  Oral contraceptives
  Progesterone
  Rubella vaccine
  Spermicides
  Video display terminals and electromagnetic waves
  Ultrasound

Source: Adapted from Cohen, 1997; Shepard and Lemire, 2007.

- Why was the medication taken? (This may give additional information regarding a maternal condition, such as diabetes or seizures, which could pose an increased recurrence risk in offspring of an affected individual.)
- When was the medication taken, and for how long? (Ask for specific dates because gestational age may not be correct and/or the patient may be counting the weeks of pregnancy incorrectly.)
- How much did you take?

When inquiring about a patient's drug and alcohol use, remember that people invariably underestimate usage. Do not ask, "Are you a heavy drinker?" Your patient will not want to be judged, and will probably reply "no. Instead ask, "How much alcohol do (did) you use?" or "What drugs do (did) you take?" You can also give an example of an amount used that is more than what you might believe was actually taken. It is rare that a patient would ever admit to an amount used greater than you give as an example.

For patients with a history of substance abuse who are currently pregnant or at risk for pregnancy, you should also assume the patient is continuing to use the substance and counsel accordingly. If they have actually stopped using the substance, great, but if they are continuing to use, then they have the correct information. (I usually buffer this by saying "You said that you were no longer using this, but if you were, this would be the consequences to the baby."

3.19.2.4 Cancer. I usually specifically ask about cancers in the family, because this information may not be volunteered in the medical systems review. Inquire about any family members with cancer, the types of primary cancers, the age of onset, and treatments if known (such as a mastectomy, colectomy, chemotherapy). Also ask about potential environmnental exposures (such as smoking) or occupational exposures. The details of inquiring about specific familial cancer syndromes are outlined in Chapter 5.

3.19.2.5 Ancestors' Origins (ethnicity). Among the last questions to ask is, "Do you know which countries your ancestors are from? What do you consider your ethnic background?" Certain genetic conditions, particularly autosomal recessive disorders, are more common in certain populations (Table 3.3; see also Chapter 2). For some genetic disorders, the sensitivity of DNA testing depends on the person's ethnic heritage because of the ability of the test to identify founder mutations. Ethnicity refers to a group of people who identify with a common racial, national, tribal, religious, linguistic, or cultural origin or background.

Usually this information is placed at the top of the pedigree, for all four grandparents, if known. If the country of origin is unknown, you can draw a question mark or write "unknown" at the top of the lineage.

Patients may wonder why you are inquiring about their ethnic background. They may fear that you have singled out their ethnic group for genetic screening or testing. I usually say, "Information about the origins of your ancestors can help us offer you the most appropriate genetic information and testing. Do you know your country of origin—where your ancestors were from originally? You may get a reply of "South Dakota or Nebraska," to which I reply "Can you be more specific? For instance, were your ancestors African American, Japanese, Chinese, Native American, English, or French?" Knowing the village name from small communities is helpful. If someone is Native American, Alaskan Native or First Nation, it is helpful to ask the tribal background.

Because an increasing number of genetic tests are becoming available to people of Ashkenazi heritage (individuals who are Jewish of eastern European ancestry), I specifically ask, "Is anyone in your family of Russian, German, or Jewish heritage? Because of atrocities against Jews that surrounded World War II and in other periods of history, it is not unusual to find that this ancestry was hidden in the family.

Never assume a person's country of origin by dress, skin color, or language. I learned this the hard way when I requested a Spanish interpreter for a non-English speaking client. When a Japanese gentleman arrived from interpreter services, I said, "You must be in the wrong clinic." He politely informed me that I was the one who was misinformed.

TABLE 3.3   Examples of Genetic Disorders with a High Carrier Frequency in Certain Ancestral Groups[a]

Population Group	Condition	Inheritance Pattern[b]	Approximate Carrier Rate
African (Americans)	Sickle cell anemia	AR	1 in 12
Amish (Old Order of eastern Pennsylvania)	Ellis van Creveld	AR	1 in 7
	Glutaric aciduria I	AR	1 in 10
Ashkenazi Jews	Breast-ovarian cancer syndrome	AD	1 in 40
	Gaucher type 1	AR	1 in 18
	Cystic fibrosis	AR	1 in 30
	Tay-Sachs disease	AR	1 in 31
	Familial dysautonomia	AR	1 in 31
	Canavan disease	AR	1 in 41
	Bloom syndrome	AR	
	Ashkenazi U.S. (New York)		1 in 231
	Ashkenazi Poland		1 in 101
European (northern)	Phenylketonuria	AR	1 in 50
	Cystic fibrosis	AR	1 in 25
Finnish[c]	Congenital nephrotic syndrome	AR	1 in 14
	Aspartylglucosaminuria (AGU)	AR	1 in 30
Hispanic (Americans)	Sickle cell anemia	AR	1 in 18
Hutterite	Carnitine palmityl transferase	AR	1 in 16
French Canadian Saguenay-Lac Saint-Jean	Tyrosinemia 1	AR	1 in 66 / 1 in 20
Inuit Indian	Propionic acidemia	AR	1 in 16
Iranian Jewish	Inclusion body myopathy 2	AR	1 in 15
Mediterranean (Italy, Greece, Cyprus, Portugal, southern Spain)	Sickle cell anemia / β-thalassemia	AR / AR	1 in 40 / 1 in 30
Mennonite (Pennsylvania)	Maple syrup urine disease	AR	1 in 7
Ojibway Indian (Canadian)	Glutaric aciduria 1	AR	1 in 10
South African (white)	Porphyria variegate	AD	1 in 300
Southeast Asian	α-thalassemia (2 gene deletion)	AR	1 in 20
Swedish	Glutaric aciduria I	AR	1 in 85
Turkish	PKU	AR	1 in 19
Yemenite Jewish	PKU	AR	1 in 35
Yupik Eskimo	Congenital adrenal hyperplasia	AR	1 in 10
	Carnitine palmityl transferase 1A	AR	1 in 4
Zuni (New Mexico)	Cystic fibrosis	AR	1 in 15

[a]Some disorders are not of particularly high incidence in a certain ethnic group but because of founder mutations, carrier screening can be reliable and cost effective (e.g., screening for mutations for Niemann-Pick type A or mucolipidosis type IV in the Ashkenazi Jewish population).
[b]AR = autosomal recessive; AD = autosomal dominant.
[c]For a summary of other genetic disorders that are common and/or are associated with founder mutations in the Finnish population See www.findis.org
Sources: Boycott et al., 2008; Clarke, 2006; Kessler et al., 2008; Pletcher et al., 2008; OMIM, 2008; Sinnreich and Karpati, 2006; Watson et al., 2006

I am encountering a growing number of people who have used DNA for genealogy ancestry testing. The basic types are tests of the Y chromosome to trace paternal ancestors and tests of mitochondrial DNA (mtDNA) to trace the maternal lineage. Thomas Shawker provides a nice summary of this type of testing in *Unlocking Your Genetic History* (2004).

3.19.3 It's All Relative: Consanguinity

One of the final family history questions is: "Are you and your partner, or your parents or grandparents related as cousins?" Often you are greeted with a nervous laugh, and an answer of, "Not that we know of." In the United States, people seem to be sensitive to questions about unions between relatives, probably because of misinformation about the risks to offspring of such unions (Bennett et al., 2002, Bittles, 2008). Marriage between first cousins is legal in about half of the states in America. In some parts of the world, particularly in the Middle East, at least half the population is married to a cousin or more distant relative. It is estimated that 1,000 million persons live in countries where 20–50% of marriages are between couples related as second cousins or closer (Bittles, 2008). Double first cousins are common (where two siblings marry another set of siblings, such as two brothers marrying two sisters).

Documenting consanguineous relationships is important for disease risk assessment, particularly for autosomal recessive disorders, because couples who are cousins are more likely to share deleterious genes in common than a non-related couple. Noting consanguinity also has increasing importance in cancer risk assessment (see Chapter 5).

People are often confused by the terms describing kinship. For example, a *second cousin* is often confused with *a first cousin once removed* (Figure 3.10). It is important

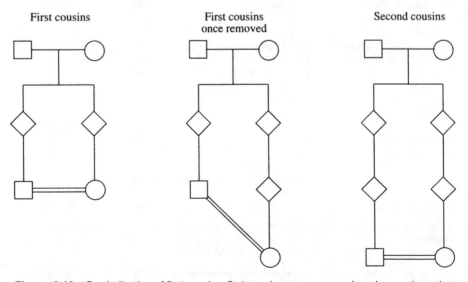

Figure 3.10 *Symbolization of first cousins, first cousins once removed, and second cousins.*

to work backward through the family history to document exactly how the couple is related. For example, the clinician might say, "Let me see if I have this correct, your father and your wife's mother are brother and sister, therefore you are first cousins." If the degree of relationship is not implicit from the pedigree, it should be stated above the relationship line as shown in the pedigree of the prestigious Darwin and Wedgwood families (Figure 3.11).

Individuals from different branches of the family with the same last name may be distantly related. Ancestors from the same small tribes or villages may also be distantly consanguineous.

Documenting that you have inquired about consanguinity should be noted on every pedigree. The information "consanguinity denied" or "consanguinity as shown" can be incorporated in the key or written near the top of the pedigree.

3.20 THE CLOSING QUESTIONS

Before I finish the interview, I always end with these questions:

- Aside from the information that you have given me, are there an conditions that people say run in your family?
- Do you have any other questions about something that you are concerned may be genetic or inherited in your family?
- Is there anything that I have not asked you about that you feel is important for me to know?

Patients always seem to save their burning questions for the last few minutes of their appointment! Perhaps it takes them some time to warm up to the interview. Maybe they are embarrassed about something in their family history. Or possibly nervousness just causes temporary memory loss. Regardless of the reason, always provide the consultand with a final opportunity to think about additional concerns in his or her medical-family history.

3.21 THE FAMILY PHOTO ALBUM

If a person in the family is described as having unusual facial or other physical features, have your patient raid the family photo album. Pictures from a wedding or family reunion are an easy way to see if people resemble each other. Such pictures are also a way to determine if any individual is unusually tall or short for the family. Summer pictures of a beach outing show more flesh, if you are trying to investigate unusual skeletal features or skin findings. Looking at chronological pictures of the same individual over a several year period can be useful; some syndromes may be difficult to identify in childhood, or may be less obvious in an adult than in a child. Obtain pictures presurgery for persons undergoing any corrective craniofacial surgery or for repair of hand or feet anomalies.

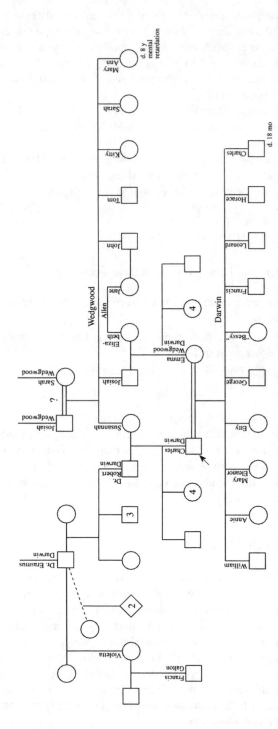

Figure 3.11 *A pedigree of first cousins; Charles Darwin and his wife, Emma Wedgwood Darwin. Their mutual grandparents, Josiah and Sarah Wedgwood were also related as cousins.*

TABLE 3.4   Possible Explanations for a Seemingly Unremarkable Family History

Individual has a new mutation (dominant, mitochondrial)
New X-linked mutation (in a male)
Affected person is not the biological child of parent(s) (e.g., misattributed paternity,
    adoption, donor egg or donor sperm)
Sex-limited inheritance (e.g., ovarian cancer, prostate cancer)
Seemingly unaffected parent actually has subtle expression of disease/syndrome
Delayed age of onset of symptoms
Reduced penetrance
Small family size
Failure of the clinician to take a three-generation pedigree
Person giving history to clinician lacks knowledge about his/her family history
Intentional withholding of information by historian (e.g., person may feel guilty or
    embarrassed or fear discrimination)

3.22   WHAT'S REMARKABLE ABOUT AN UNREMARKABLE FAMILY HISTORY?

Many times when you take a family history there are no obvious genetic diseases or familial aggregation of disease. Table 3.4 reviews some common reasons that a family history of a genetic condition is missed. Clinicians often note in the medical record that the family history is negative or the person has no family history. I prefer stating the family history is unremarkable or noncontributory. The word *negative* may be misconstrued as a value judgment. All humans have a family history, though the medical-family history may not affect the current indication for seeing a health professional.

3.23   CONFIDENTIALITY AND FAMILY HISTORY

A pedigree recorded for clinical purposes should contain key information needed for risk assessment, and documentation of disease status in relatives. It's also important to recognize that pedigrees document sensitive information that should be collected and maintained with the utmost protection for privacy and confidentiality. Initials or first names (in lieu of full names) may be enough to identify persons where medical records are documented and for orientation of discussions with the patient. Use of birth year or age, year of death or age at death, rather than birth date or date of death, would be compliant with HIPAA guidelines where exact dates are viewed as private and protected information (Bennett et al., 2008)

There are no formal guidelines as to whether a family history that is brought to you by the patient, which may contain an abundance of family identifiers, should become part of the patient's permanent medical record. While technically information provided to you by the patient can be included in the patient's medical record, in reality, it is probably wise to be cautious in directly including this chart, as compared to a pedigree you have created.

3.24   WHEN IS A GENETIC FAMILY HISTORY SIGNIFICANT?

This is a tough question to answer. My feeling is that a significant medical family history is one that the patient is concerned about or one that the patient should be concerned about. A 22-year-old woman with an abnormal ultrasound finding at 16 weeks may have a strong family history of breast and ovarian cancer, but a desire for information about the inherited cancer susceptibility testing is probably the farthest thing from her mind at that moment. Instead, delving further into this information at a future visit is warranted and might be communicated to the woman in a follow-up letter.

3.25   THE ULTIMATE PEDIGREE CHALLENGE

The following fictitious family history is provided for you to practice drawing each standardized pedigree symbol. This teaching scenario is republished with permission from the *American Journal of Human Genetics* (Bennett et al., 1995). The answer is in Appendix A.1.

The consultant, Mrs. Feene O'Type, present to your office with a pregnancy at 16 weeks of gestation. She has question about risks to her fetus because of her age. She is 35 years old, and her husband, Gene O'Type, is 36 years old. Mrs. O'Type had one prior pregnancy, an elective termination (TOP) at 18 weeks, of a female fetus with trisomy 21.

Mrs. O'Type's Family History

- Mrs. O'Type had three prior pregnancies with her first husband. The first pregnancy was a TOP, the second, a spontaneous abortion (SAB) of a female fetus at 19 weeks of gestation, and the third, a healthy 10-year-old son who was subsequently adopted by her 33-year-old sister, Stacy.
- Stacy had three pregnancies, two SABs (the second a male fetus at 20 weeks with a neural tube defect, and a karyotype of trisomy 18) and a stillborn female at 32 weeks.
- Mrs. O'Type has a 31-year-old brother, Sam, who is affected with cystic fibrosis (CF) and is infertile.
- Her youngest brother, Donald, age 29 years, is healthy and married. By means of gametes from Donald and his wife, an unrelated surrogate mother has been successfully impregnated.
- Mrs. O'Type's father died at age 72 years, and her mother died at age 70 years, both from "natural causes." Mrs. O'Type's mother had five healthy full sibs who themselves had many healthy children.

Mr. O'Type's Family History

- Mr. O'Type has two siblings, a monozygotic twin brother, Cary, whose wife is 6 weeks pregnant by donor insemination (donor's history unknown), and a 32 year-old sister, Sterrie).

- Sterrie is married to Proto, her first cousin (Sterric's father's sister's son), who has red-green color blindness. She is carrying a pregnancy conceived from Proto's sperm and ovum from an unknown donor. Sterrie and Proto also have an adopted son.
- The family history of Sterrie's mother, who has Huntington disease (HD) is unknown.
- Mr. Gene O'Type's father has a set of twin brothers, zygosity unknown, and another brother and sister (Proto's mother), who also are twins.

3.26 SUMMARY

The guidelines in this chapter are a gold standard of taking a medical-family history. No clinician will have time to ask all of these questions. The use of standard methods and symbols in recording a pedigree will become more important with the incorporation of pedigrees into the electronic medical record. Listening to the client's story; acknowledging significant life events; and respecting cultural belief systems of kinship, health, and wellness are just as important as the medical information recorded.

3.27 REFERENCES

Abboud FE. (1998). *Health Psychology in Global Perspective*. Thousand Oaks: Sage.

Barlow-Stewart K, Yeo SS, Meiser BM, et al., (2006). Toward cultural competence in cancer genetic counseling and genetics education: Lessons leaned from Chinese-Australians. *Genet Med* 8:24–32.

Bennett RL, Motulsky AG, Bittles AH, ct al. (2002). Genetic counseling and screening of consanguineous couples and their offspring: Recommendations of the National Society of Genetic Counselors. *J Genet Couns* 11(2):97–119.

Bennett RL, Steinhaus KA, Uhrich SB, et al. (1995). Recommendations for standardized human pedigree nomenclature. *Am J Hum Genet* 56:745–752.

Bennett RL, Steinhaus French, KA, Resta RG, Doyle DL. (2008). Standardized human pedigree nomenclature: Update and assessment of the recommendations of the National Society of Genetic Counselors. *J Genet Couns* 17(5):424–433.

Bittles AH (2008). A community genetics perspective on consanguineous marriage. *Comm Genet* 11(6):324–330.

Boycott KM, Parboosingh JS, Chodirker BN, et al. (2008). Genetics in the Hutterite population: A review of Mendelian disorders. *Am J Med Genet, Part A* 146A:1088–1098.

Clarke JTR. (2006). *A Clinical Guide to Metabolic Diseases*, 3rd ed. Cambridge: Cambridge University Press.

Cohen LH, Fine BA, Pergament E. (1998). An assessment of ethnocultural beliefs regarding the cause of birth defects and genetic disorders. *J Genet Couns* 7:15–29.

Cohen MM. (1997). *The Child with Multiple Birth Defects*, 2nd ed. New York: Oxford University Press.

Fisher NL, ed. (1996). *Cultural and Ethnic Diversity: A Guide for Genetics Profssionals*. Baltimore: Johns Hopkins University Press.

Fisher N, Lew L. (1996). Culture of the countries of Southeast Asia. In: Fisher NF, ed., *Cultural and Ethnic Diversity, A Guide for Genetics Professionals*. Baltimore: Johns Hopkins University Press, pp. 113–128.

Friedman JM, Hanson JW. (2007). *Clinical Teratology*. In: Rimoin DL, Connor MJ, Pyeritz RE, Korf BR, ed., *Emery & Rimoin's Principles and Practice of Medical Genetics*, 5th ed. Philadelphia: Elsevier, pp. 900–930.

Green JW. (1999). *Cultural Awareness in the Human Services: A Multi-Ethnic Approach*, 3rd ed. Boston: Allyn & Bacon.

Hauck L., Knoki-Wilson Um. (1996). Culture of Native Americans of the Southwest. In: Fisher NF, ed., *Cultural and Ethnic Diversity: A Guide for Genetics Professionals*. Baltimore: Johns Hopkins University Press, pp. 60–85.

Hill CE, O'Brien KM. (1999). *Helping Skills: Facilitating Exploration, Insight, and Action*. Washington, DC: American Psychological Association.

Kalofissudis IA. (2003). Evil eye, creative metaphors and the postmodern nursing. *ICUS NURS WEB J* 13:1–4.

Kessler D, Moehleenkamp C, Kaplan G, et al. (2008). Detection of cystic fibrosis carrier frequency for Zuni Native Americans of New Mexico. *Clin Genet* 49(2):95–97.

Lynch EW, Hanson MJ. (2004). *Developing Cross-Cultural Competence. A Guide for Working with Young Children and Their Families*, 3rd. ed. Baltimore: Brookes.

Marazita ML. (1995). Defining "proband." *Am J Hum Genet* 57:981–982.

McCarthy Veach P, LeRoy BS, Bartels DM. (2003). *Facilitating the Genetic Counseling Process: A Practice Manual*. New York: Springer.

McConkie-Rosell A, Finucane B, Cronister A, et al. (2005). Genetic Counseling for Fragile X Syndrome: Updated Recommendations of the National Society of Genetic Counselors. *J Genet Couns* 14:249–270.

OMIM (Online Mendelian Inheritance in Man). (2009). Available at http://www.ncbi.nlm.nih.gov/omim. Accessed November 28, 2009.

Pletcher BA, Gross SJ, Monaghan KG, et al. (2008). The future is now: carrier screening for all population. *Genet Med* 10(1):33–36.

Resta RG. (1993). The crane's foot: the rise of the pedigree in human genetics. *J Genet Counsel* 2(4) 235–260.

Resta RG. (1995). Whispered hints. *Am J Med Genet* 59:131–133.

Schwartz PJ, Stramba-Badiale M, Crotti L, et al. (2009). Prevalence of congenital Long-QT syndrome. *Circulation* 120(18):1761–1767.

Shawker TH. (2004). *Unlocking Your Genetic History*. Nashville, TN: Rutledge Hill Press.

Shepard TH, Lemire RJ. (2007). *Catalog of Teratogenic Agents*, 12th ed. Baltimore: Johns Hopkins University Press.

Sinnreich M, Karpati G. (2006). Inclusion body myopathy 2. May 24, 2006. Available at genereviews.org. Accessed February 15, 2009.

Stanion P, Papadopoulos L, Bot R. (1997). Genograms in counseling practice: Constructing a genogram (part 2). *Counsel Psychol Q* 10:139–148.

U.S. Department of Health and Human Services. (2009). HHS-U.S. Surgeon General's Family History Initiative. Available at https://familyhistory.hhs.gov. Accessed November 17, 2009.

Watson MS, Lloyd-Puryear MA, Mann MY, et al. (2006). Newborn screening: Toward a uniform panel and system. *Genet Med* 8(5)Suppl:12S–252S.

Wing Sue D, Sue D. (2002). *Counseling the Culturally Diverse: Theory and Practice*. New York: Wiley-Liss.

Chapter 4

Directed Medical-Genetics Family History Questions: Separating the Trees from the Forest

Genetic cases sometimes hide in a chiaroscuro of common disease patterns.... Generalists
will usher the millennium with genetic tests for cancer predisposition and Alzheimer disease.
Genetic risk is a new axis of disease, requiring critical test interpretation, skillful counseling,
and dedicated follow-up of families.... Do today's peculiarities in medical genetics presage
tomorrow's primary care?
—Wendy S. Rubenstein (1997)

4.1 THE APPROACH: LOOK FOR THE RARE BUT REMEMBER THE ORDINARY

Patients and family members often inquire about the heritability of common medical conditions. This chapter provides suggestions for directed family history questions related to many of the everyday medical diseases encountered in the typical family history. By supplementing general family history screening questions (as reviewed in Chapter 3) with a more targeted query, the clinician can probe deeper into the medical-family history and identify individuals who may benefit from a more extensive genetic evaluation and genetic counseling. To borrow from the common proverb, these screening questions are a method of distinguishing the unusual trees from the vast forest. As with any field guide, often it is best to look to the experts for final identification. Resources for making a patient referral for genetic services can be found in Chapter 9. Some of the red flags in a medical-family history that suggest a genetic etiology of disease are reviewed in Table 4.1.

Instead of discussing the potential genetic disorders associated with every common medical condition, this chapter focuses on a selection of medical-family history signposts representative of medical conditions with a potential hereditary etiology. For example, leukemia, although a rare complication of Down syndrome, is not a useful signpost for recognizing this condition because an infant with Down syndrome is more readily diagnosed by other clinical clues. In contrast, leukemia is a cancer that can occur in children and adults in the familial cancer syndrome Li-Fraumeni (see Chapter 5). In this instance, knowing more about the family history can aid the clinician in deciding on genetic testing and health management strategies for relevant family members. The patient's answers to such targeted queries can be transposed into a medical pedigree and used as an investigative map to assist with diagnosis and disease risk appraisal.

In this chapter I provide suggestions for medical-family history queries for the following broad categories of disease: birth anomalies (Section 4.2), hearing loss (Section 4.3), visual impairment (Section 4.4), intellectual delay (formerly referred to as mental retardation) (Section 4.5), autism (Section 4.6), cerebral palsy (Section 4.7), neurological and neuromuscular conditions (Section 4.8), seizures (Section 4.9), stroke, (Section 4.10), dementia (Section 4.11), mental illness (Section 4.12), cardiac disease (Section 4.13), chronic respiratory disease (Section 4.14), renal disorders (Section 4.15), skeletal anomalies and disorders of short stature (Section 4.16), diabetes (Section 4.17), male and female infertility and multiple miscarriages (Section 4.18), and sudden infant death (Section 4.19). Family history markers for identifying individuals with an inherited susceptibility to cancer are discussed in Chapter 5. The decision to include these general groupings of disease in this chapter is based on my experience with some of the questions people have asked me most frequently regarding disorders in their family.

I do not provide information on the diagnostic tests and the clinical signs and symptoms of the many genetic disorders mentioned in this chapter, nor do I discuss the essential genetic counseling and psychosocial issues for each condition. I do mention several situations where obtaining a medical-family history poses special challenges (such as obtaining a history from a person with profound hearing loss or from an individual with severe learning disabilities). In Appendix A.5 I provide general Internet references for learning more about various genetic disorders and genetic testing. Appendix A.7 is a reference for genetic disorders, the genes symbols and names, and the associated pattern of inheritance.

The key to teasing out potential genetic variables in a patient's family history is to look for unusual and infrequent features against a background of common diseases and normal physical variation. Male infertility is common, but a man with infertility, small testes (hypogonadism), and absence of the sense of smell (anosmia) may have a rare inherited condition called Kallmann syndrome. Diabetes mellitus is a common

TABLE 4.1   The Red Flags of Medical-Family History Suggestive of a Genetic Condition or an Inherited Susceptibility to a Common Disease

- Multiple closely related individuals with the same medical or psychiatric condition, particularly if the condition is rare
- Common disorders with earlier age of onset than typical (especially if onset is early in multiple relatives). For example:

  Breast cancer < age 45–50 years (premenopausal)

  Colon cancer < age 45–50 years

  Prostate cancer < age 50–60 years

  Uterine cancer < age 50 years

  Vision loss < age 55 years

  Hearing loss < age 50–60 years

  Dementia < age 60 years

  Stroke < age 60 years

  Heart disease < age 40–50 years
- Bilateral disease in paired organs (e.g., eyes, kidneys, lungs, breasts)
- Sudden cardiac death in a person who seemed healthy
- Three or more pregnancy losses (e.g., miscarriages, stillbirths)
- Medical problems in the offspring of parents who are consanguineous (first cousins or more closely related)

A Person With

- Two or more medical conditions (e.g., hearing loss and renal disease, diabetes and muscle disease, two primary cancers, mental illness and neurological condition)
- Two or more major birth anomalies (Table 4.3)
- Three or more minor birth anomalies (Table 4.3)
- One major birth anomaly with two minor anomalies
- A cleft palate, or cleft lip with or without cleft palate
- Congenital heart defect
- A medical condition and dysmorphic features
- Developmental delay with dysmorphic features and/or physical birth anomalies
- Developmental delay associated with other medical conditions
- Progressive intellectual delay and/or loss of developmental milestones
- Autism or pervasive developmental disorder (particularly with dysmorphic features)
- Progressive behavioral problems
- Unexplained hypotonia
- Unexplained seizures
- Unexplained ataxia
- Progressive neurological condition, movement disorder, and/or muscle weakness
- Unexplained cardiomyopathy
- Hematological condition associated with excessive bleeding or clotting
- Unusual birthmarks (particularly if associated with seizures, learning disabilities, or dysmorphic features)
- Hair anomalies (hirsute, brittle, coarse, kinky, sparse or absent)
- Congenital or juvenile deafness

(Continued)

TABLE 4.1   *(Continued)*

- Congenital or juvenile blindness
- Cataracts at a young age
- Primary adrenocortical insufficiency (male)
- Primary amenorrhea
- Ambiguous genitalia
- Proportionate short stature with dysmorphic features and/or delayed or arrested puberty
- Disproportionate short stature with dysmorphic features and or/delayed or arrested puberty
- Premature ovarian dysfunction
- Proportionate short stature and primary amenorrhea
- Male with hypogonadism and/or significant gynecomastia
- Congenital absence of the vas deferens
- Oligozoospermia/azoospermia

A Fetus With

- A major structural anomaly
- Significant growth retardation
- Minor anomalies

chronic disorder, but a person with diabetes, seizures, hearing loss, and an unsteady gait may have a mitochondrial myopathy.

As clinicians, when we recognize a set of "peculiarities" as a "genetic case" (paraphrasing the Rubinstein quotation that introduced this chapter) it is natural to swell with a peacock's pride at our diagnostic prowess. It is easy for us to lose sight of the person behind the peculiar signs and symptoms. As observed by a parent of a child with a rare condition, a condition is rare only when it happens in someone else's family. Carolyn, a woman with multiple birth anomalies wept after her astute genetic counselor remarked on her beautiful feet (Resta, 1997). She recalls the profound impact of constantly having clinicians point only to her peculiarities:

> Over the years I've seen a lot of doctors. Every one of them has described in excruciating detail what was wrong with me. After a while, I began to feel like no part of me was normal. But deep down inside, I always felt I had beautiful feet. I knew my arm was misshapen, and I knew I didn't have periods like other women, and even my kidneys, which worked fine and people couldn't see, were abnormal. But my feet ... from the knees down, I thought I looked like every woman. As odd as it sounds, having that little bit of security has helped me get through some tough days. Then, 5 years ago, a doctor casually mentioned that my feet look abnormal. His words were not said cruelly, but they cursed me. The last part of me which I had clung to as normal had been destroyed by what that doctor said. When you just told me now that my feet look normal, it brought back the memory of that day when my whole self-image collapsed.

Behind each genetic case is a person and family with normal dreams, thoughts, and feelings.

4.2 PHYSICAL BIRTH ANOMALIES AND VARIANTS

A family history of birth malformations is usually a major concern to a couple making reproductive choices. It is not unusual to encounter a family history of a significant birth anomaly; an estimated 3% of newborns have one or more major physical anomaly. As many as a third of congenital anomalies are characterized as being genetic in origin. Known environmental teratogens (see Table 3.2) are surprisingly few, and they are implicated as causal factors in approximately 1 in 400 birth anomalies (Winter et al., 1988). The etiology of many birth malformations remains unknown. Refer to Section 3.19.2 for the approach to inquiry regarding human teratogenic agents.

Physical anomalies that are recognized at birth or in infancy are categorized as major or minor. Major anomalies (such as an omphalocele, most congenital heart malformations, or a facial cleft) are of medical and or cosmetic significance. Table 4.2 gives examples of major congenital anomalies. Minor malformations (usually involving the face, ears, hands and feet) affect somewhere between 4% and 15% of the population (Cohen, 1997). Minor anomalies do not have substantial medical or cosmetic consequences. A minor anomaly seen without other physical differences may represent the spectrum of normal variation, and it may be inherited. Learning disabilities and congenital intellectual disabilities are often associated with syndromes involving birth anomalies. Before a minor variation is considered significant, the parents (and other family members) should be examined to see if the characteristic is simply a normal familial variant. For example, syndactyly of the second and third toes is often familial.

The identification of minor birth anomalies and differences is an essential component of syndrome recognition (a syndrome is a combination of causally related physical variants). A simian crease (a single line across the palm as compared to the more usual pair of transverse parallel creases) is a normal finding in 3% of the general population but is seen in almost half of all persons with Down syndrome (Jones, 2005). A person who has three minor birth anomalies or a major anomaly with two minor anomalies is likely to have a syndrome. An individual with three or more minor anomalies should also be evaluated for underlying major malformations (such as a heart defect) (Cohen, 1997). Table 4.3 provides examples of minor physical differences detectable at birth or shortly thereafter that may be seen in isolation or as part of a syndrome.

Examining the parents of a child with one or more congenital anomalies is useful for syndrome diagnosis and for determining recurrence risks and prognosis. A child's unusually formed ears may be evident in a parent as a normal familial characteristic. Alternatively, the parent's remarkably shaped ears can be minor manifestations of a variably expressed autosomal dominant syndrome with a more severe presentation evidenced in the child. If both parents of a child with a major birth anomaly have normal physical evaluations, the clinician can be more comfortable quoting chances of recurrence from empirical risk tables than if the child is evaluated in isolation from the parents. Comparing photographs of the child, parents, and other family members is an inexpensive and important method for distinguishing

TABLE 4.2 Examples of Major Congenital Anomalies[a]

Brain malformations
  Holoprosencephaly
  Microcephaly
Cleft lip with or with out cleft palate (CL/P)
Cleft palate (CP)
Esophageal atresia
Microtia, or anotia
Micropthalmos, or anophatlmos
Congenital heart defects
  Atrial septal defect (ASD)
  Coarctation of the aorta
  Double-outlet right ventricle
  Ebstein anomaly
  Ectopia cordis
  Endocardial cushion defect
  Hypoplastic left-heart syndrome (HLHS)
  Tetralogy of Fallot
  Transposition of the great arteries (TGA)
  Ventricular septal defect (VSD)
Neural tube defects (NTD)
  Anencephaly
  Spina bifida
  Encephalocele
  Myelomeningocele
Omphalocele
Gastroschisis
Diaphragmatic hernia
Duodenal atresia
Imperforate anus (anal atresia)
Polydactyly
Absence of thumb or other digits
Arthrogryposis
Limb anomalies
Absence (agenesis) of any organ
  Renal agenesis
  Gonadal agenesis

[a]All terms are defined in the Glossary.

normal variation from subtle syndromic expression of a familial characteristic (see Section 3.21).

Most isolated birth anomalies (major and minor) have a polygenic or multifactorial etiology (see Section 2.7.6). The parents of a child with an isolated congenital malformation usually have a relatively low recurrence risk (in the range of 3–10%). The risk of recurrence rises if there is another affected child in the family. If a parent has more than one child with the same congenital anomaly, or if there is a family history of similar birth anomalies, a single-gene etiology should be investigated. *This includes examining the parents for physical signs of subtle expression of the*

TABLE 4.3 Examples of Minor Physical Differences That Can Be Within Normal Variation or a Feature of a Syndrome (Inherited or Environmental)

Variant Physical Feature	Representative Syndromes
Hair	
Low posterior hairline	Turner syndrome (s.), Noonan s.
Upward sweep of hair ("cowlick")	Several syndromes; may reflect defective brain (frontal lobe development and primary microcephaly)
Widow's peak	May be associated with ocular hypertelorism
White streak (forelock of hair)	Waardenburg s. I and II
Synophrys	Sanfilippos s., deLange s., fetal trimethadione
Hirsuitism	Mucopolysaccharidoses, deLange s.; may be teratogenic effect (e.g., fetal alcohol, hydantoin, or fetal trimethadione)
Sparse fine hair	Hypohidrotic ectodermal dysplasia
Ears	
Simple	Fetal alcohol s., fetal hydantoin s.
Protruberant ears	Fragile X syndrome
Ear tags	Mandibulofacial dysostosis
Ear pits	Branchio-oto-renal s.
Microtia	Mandibulofacial dysostosis
Creases in ear lobe	Beckwith-Wiedemann, familial hyperlipidemia
Eyes	
Iris coloboma	Several chromosome anomalies
Blue or gray sclerae	Normal in newborns, osteogenesis imperfecta
Heterochromia	Waardenburg syndrome I and II
Brushfield spots	Seen in 20% of normal newborns, Down s.
Epicanthal folds	Normal finding in infancy, several chromosome anomalies, other syndromes
Ptosis	Myotonic muscular dystrophy
Hypertelorism	Seen with many craniosynostosis syndromes and chromosomal syndromes
Dystopia canthorum	Waardenburg s.
Hypotelorism	Seen in many syndromes with holoprosencephaly
Downslanting palpebral fissures	Seen in many syndromes
Short palpebral fissures	Seen in many syndromes
Long palpebral fissures	Kabuki s.
Nose	
Prominent, bulbous	22q11.2 deletion s.
Broad nasal bridge	Seen in many syndromes
Philtrum	
Long/flat	Fetal alcohol s.
Oral region	
Micrognathia	Can be seen as deformation from uterine constriction; associated with >100 syndromes
Enamel hypoplasia	Osteogenesis imperfecta I
Wide-spaced teeth	Several syndromes
Peg-shaped teeth	Incontinentia pigmenti
Conical teeth	Hypohydrotic ectodermal dysplasia
Lip pits (in lower lip)	Van der Woude s.
Lip pigmentation	Peutz-Jeghers s.

(Continued)

TABLE 4.3 *(Continued)*

Variant Physical Feature	Representative Syndromes
Neck	
Webbed	Turner s., Noonan s.
Hands and feet	
Polydactyly (postaxial)	Several syndromes; can be inherited as a autosomal dominant syndrome with no other anomalies
Polydactyly (preaxial)	Several syndromes
Brachydactyly	Several syndromes; can be autosomal dominant syndrome with no other anomalies
Metacarpal hypoplasia (short 3rd, 4th, and/or 5th fingers)	Albright osteodystrophy
Digital asymmetry	Oro-facial-digital s. (multiple types)
Clinidactyly	Many syndromes
Tapered fingers	22q11.2 deletion s.
Arachnodactyly	Marfan s.
Single palmar (simian) crease	Several syndromes, including Down s.
Hyperconvex nails	Fetal valproate s.
Nail hypoplasia	Several syndromes
Broad thumbs/toes	Several syndromes
Syndactyly (mild)	Several syndromes
Gap between big toe (hallux) and 2nd toe	Down s.
Chest	
Wide spaced nipples	Turner s.
Supernumerary nipples (accessory or extra)	Multiple syndromes
Skin	
Areas of skin hypopigmentation	Tuberous sclerosis complex
Café au lait spots	Neurofibromatosis 1
Abdominal	
Umbilical hernia	Several syndromes
Genitalia	
Shawl scrotum	Aarskog s.
Hypoplastic labia	Prader-Willi s.
Small penis	Several syndromes
Hypospadias	Several syndromes
Skeletal	
Cubitis valgus	Turner s.
Pectus excavatum	Marfan s.
Pectus carinatum	Marfan s.

condition. Parental consanguinity is another clue suggesting single-gene causation (primarily in relation to autosomal recessive disorders).

Some congenital anomalies are more common in certain ethnic groups. In the United States, cleft lip and palate is more common in people of Asian and Native American descent (1.7–2.1 in 1,000 births and 0.6 in 1,000 births, respectively) than in African Americans (0.3 in 1,000 births) (Cohen, 2007). Postaxial polydactyly occurs in approximately 1 in 500 African Americans and is often inherited in an autosomal dominant pattern within this population. In providing risk assessment, such ethnic variables are important to consider.

Multiple birth defects (major and minor) are often associated with chromosome anomalies (see Section 2.7.8). Thus it is important to inquire about a family history of miscarriages, infertility, mental delay (intellectual disability or mental retardation), and other birth defects. Birth defect(s) associated with other features suggest a single-gene disorder. Exposure to certain prescription drugs or alcohol during critical periods in embryonic development is associated with various birth defects. Remember to explore the mother's history of use of alcohol and street and prescription drug use during the pregnancy. Several infectious agents are teratogenic during pregnancy. Table 3.2 reviews known and potential fetal teratogens. When inquiring about a potential teratogenic agent, remember to document when in the pregnancy the agent was given (or when an infection occurred) as well as the dosage or amounts of drug taken (see Section 3.19.2).

Although environmental factors are rare causes of birth anomalies, it is common for parents to attribute an environmental cause to their child's problems—for example, a difficult birth may be the parents' explanation for the cause of their child's intellectual disability. It is important to listen to these beliefs and not dismiss them with a professional wave of the hand; doing so will only alienate the parents. You can provide an alternative perspective such as, "Yes, we know that complicated labor can cause certain developmental problems, but your child has some physical findings such as a small head size and unusually shaped ears that make me think there may be other causal factors."

Birth defects are divided into three general classifications: *malformations, deformations*, and *disruptions* (Cohen, 1997; Jones, 2005). The distinction among these categories may assist the clinician in determining prognosis, recurrence risk, and appropriate therapeutic interventions.

Malformations are defects in an organ, or part of an organ, resulting from an intrinsically abnormal developmental process. Examples of malformations include syndactyly (webbing of the fingers or toes), polydactyly (extra fingers or toes), congenital heart malformations, cleft lip, and cleft palate. Malformations usually occur early in embryonic development. They often require surgical correction and are associated with perinatal mortality. Malformations are widely heterogenous in their etiology. For example craniosynostosis (an abnormally shaped skull due to premature fusion of the cranial bones) occurs in at least 150 syndromes (Cohen, 2007).

Deformation refers to an abnormal shape or position of a part of the body caused by mechanical forces in utero. Examples of deformations include limb positioning defects (such as clubfoot or congenital hip dislocation) and minor facial deformities (such as a small chin—micrognathia) or facial asymmetry. Deformations usually occur during the third trimester and often represent intrauterine molding from mechanical constraint (e.g., breech presentations, decreased or lack of amniotic fluid, or multigestation pregnancy). Many deformations due to these factors spontaneously correct themselves once the fetus is no longer subjected to intrauterine constraints. However, deformations secondary to an intrinsic cause (such as abnormal formation of the central nervous system, renal or neurological dysfunction) are associated with neonatal morbidity. These intrinsic factors often have a genetic etiology such as hereditary neuropathies and myopathies or renal malformation.

Disruptions are the result of interference with an originally normal developmental process. There is extensive clinical variability in disruptions. Examples of disruptions include digit amputation or facial clefting from amniotic bands. Structural abnormalities due to disruptions often have a vascular etiology such as the rare occurrence of limb reduction anomalies after chorionic villus sampling (Evans and Wapner, 2005; Golden et al., 2003). Maternal factors such as infections and teratogens can be at the root of birth defects from disruptions. The clinician should obtain a detailed pregnancy history regarding the mother of the affected child. For congenital anomalies due to disruptions, the recurrence risk for the parents to have another child is usually small.

Although the separation of birth anomalies into singular categories of malformations, deformations, and disruptions is a valuable clinical tool for determining the etiology of birth defects, the three categories are interrelated. A single extraneous variable can have different physical effects. Decreased amniotic fluid (oligohydramnios) in the third trimester can result in minor deformations (e.g., clubfoot, micrognathia), whereas oligohydramnios in early embryonic development can lead to the disruptive limb-body wall complex (thoracoabdominal wall deficiency with craniofacial anomalies). Micrognathia caused by intrauterine constraint in early fetal development can lead to failure of the tongue to descend, resulting in a developmental malformation—cleft palate. The malformation spina bifida may produce leg paralysis, leading to the deformation of congenital hip dislocation and clubfoot (Cohen, 1997).

Table 4.4 summarizes the general medical-family history questions to pose when there is a family history of one or more birth defects. The medical-family history inquiry is similar for any history of birth anomalies. Brief discussions on three categories of malformations (cleft lip with and without cleft palate, neural tube defects, and congenital heart defects) follow.

4.2.1   Cleft Lip with and without Cleft Palate

Orofacial clefting is the second most common class of congenital anomaly after congenital heart defects (Cohen, 2007); the overall general population frequency is 1 in 700 births. The general types of oral clefting are cleft lip with or without cleft palate (CL/P), cleft palate (CP), median clefts, and alveolar clefts. Cleft palate is a different condition from cleft lip with or without cleft palate. The formation of the palate and lips do not occur at the same time in embryologic development; consequently, CP and CL/P are associated with different genetic risks. Overall the CL/P and CP syndromes are categorized by whether they are syndromic (orofacial clefting associated with other clinical findings) or nonsyndromic (no other obvious clinical findings aside from orofacial clefting). Recently at least three genes have been identified where

TABLE 4.4   Medical-Family History Questions for Congenital Anomalies

Inquiries Related to Child/Adult with a Birth Variant or Anomaly
Does the child/adult have
- Other birth anomalies (particularly of the hands, feet or limbs)? Explain.
- Anything unusual about his or her facial appearance, such as unusual placement or appearance of the eyes, nose, mouth, or ears (inquire about lip pits in relation to CL/P or CP)?[a]
- Are there problems with the hair, teeth, or nails? If yes, describe.
- Any birthmarks? If yes, describe their color, number, shape, size, and locations.
- Any hearing problems? If yes, see Section 4.3.
- Any visual problems? If yes, see Section 4.4.
- Any learning disabilities or problems with schooling? If yes, see Section 4.5.
- Any delays in achieving developmental milestones?
- Any medical problems, particularly neurological or muscle weakness? Explain.
- Does he or she resemble other family members in appearance?
- Is this person of normal stature? Are the limbs in proportion? If not, see Section 4.16.

Pregnancy history for the mother of the affected person
- Were there any problems in the pregnancy (e.g., premature rupture of membranes, placental problems)?
- Was the pregnancy full term? Premature?
- What was the fetal presentation at delivery (e.g., breech, vertex)?
- What was the mode of delivery (e.g., a C-section may have been for breech presentation or fetal distress)?
- Did the mother have any infections or illnesses during the pregnancy? If so, obtain information about timing and length of illness during pregnancy.
- Does the mother have any medical problems such as diabetes, cardiovascular disease, obesity, or a seizure disorder?
- Did she take any medications (particularly for seizures) during the pregnancy? If so, obtain specific information about the medication, dosage and timing.
- Did the mother drink alcohol or use tobacco products? If so, obtain information about usage and timing in pregnancy.
- Did the mother use street drugs (particularly cocaine)? If so, obtain information about usage and timing in pregnancy.
- What are the results of any prenatal testing (such as ultrasound, maternal serum marker testing, amniocentesis, or chorionic villus sampling)?

Family history questions
- Does anyone have a history of pregnancy losses such as miscarriages or stillbirths?
- Have other babies been born with birth anomalies? If so, describe the problems
- Does anyone in the family have
  - Mental delays or learning disabilities? If yes, see Table 4.13.
  - A neurological condition or muscle weakness? If yes, explain and note the age of onset of symptoms (see Table 4.16).
  - Hearing loss? If yes, note the severity and age of onset (see Table 4.7).
  - Vision loss? If yes, note the age and nature of visual problems (see Table 4.9).
- Are the parents of the affected individual blood relatives? If so, what is their exact relationship (i.e., the mother's father and the father's father are brothers, therefore they are first cousins)?

[a]CL/P = cleft lip with or without cleft palate; CP = cleft palate.

families can have mixed clefting in the same family (CP and CL/P; they may have tooth anomalies as well): *MSX1, FGR1, and IRF6.*

Associated birth anomalies occur in a significant number of individuals with clefts (estimates ranges from 44% to 64%) (Cohen, 2007). Anywhere from 13% to 50% of newborns with cleft palate have an associated malformation, and between 7% and 13% of individuals with cleft lip are born with associated birth anomalies, as are 2–11% of individuals with both cleft lip and palate (Firth and Hurst, 2005). More than 350 syndromes are associated with orofacial clefting (Cohen, 2007). Chromosome anomalies, particularly trisomy 13 and trisomy 18, are common causes of CL/P and CP. A medical geneticist should evaluate newborns with a clefting condition to see if a syndrome can be identified. Likewise, individuals with a clefting condition who are interested in genetic risk assessment for reproductive planning should be offered a genetic evaluation, preferably *before* conception.

Cleft lip and palate has been associated with several teratogens in pregnancy, including alcohol abuse (Romitti et al., 2007). The prescription drugs hydantoin, trimethadione, amniopterin, and methotrexate are associated with CL/P. Hyperthermia in the mother (early in pregnancy) is associated with cleft palate. Maternal tobacco use in pregnancy seems to increase the risk of orofacial clefting (Honein, et al., 2007; Little et al., 2004). Some studies suggest that vitamin supplementation with folic acid may help prevent orofacial clefting (Bilek et al., 2008; Wilcox et al., 2007).

Van der Woude syndrome is estimated to account for approximately 2% of all individuals with CL/P. Van der Woude syndrome (with mutation in *IRF6*), is an autosomal dominant syndrome with reduced penetrance and extremely variable expression; the clinical manifestations vary from pits in the lower lips to severe cleft lip. If one of the parents has lip pits, than the couple's chance to have a child with cleft lip is about 26% (not everyone who inherits the gene alteration has clefting). This compares to an 4–6% recurrence risk of CL/P if the parents have a normal examination and there is no other family history of clefting. The popliteal ptergium syndrome is allelic (mutation within the same gene) to van der Woude syndrome and is associated with CL/P, lip pits, syndactyly, syngnathia (a congenital adhesion of the maxilla and mandible by fibrous bands), and popiliteal ptergium (webbing behind the knee), distinct nail anomalies (a skinfold on the nail of the hallux), and genitourinary malformations. It is estimated that variations in the *IRF6* gene explain 10–15% of isolated cleft lip and/or palate (Murray and Schutte, 2004).

Velocardiofacial or DiGeorge syndrome properly refered to as 22q11.2 deletion syndrome is an autosomal dominant syndrome characterized by cleft palate or palatal insufficiencies, cardiac anomalies (conotruncal defects, which include tetraology of Fallot, interrupted aortic arch, ventral septal defect, and truncous arteriosus), frequent infections, thymic hypoplasia, parathyroid dysfunction, typical facies, and learning disabilities. The syndrome may be the most common cleft palate syndrome. Shprintzen and colleagues (1985) reported that 22q11.2 deletion syndrome accounts for about 8.1% of children with palatal clefts. Bipolar disorder and schizophrenia have been described in up to 18% of adults with 22q11.2 deletion syndrome (Firth and Hurst, 2005). It is estimated that less than 2% of persons with schizophrenia have 22q11.2 deletion syndrome (Firth and Hurst 2005).

Most first instances of CL/P or CP in a family follow a multifactorial threshold model of causation. Risk of recurrence for the healthy parents of an affected child to have another affected child are gleaned from empirical risk tables, and range from 5–6% for CL/P (with the risk being slightly higher for bilateral CL/P) to 2–3% for CP. A parent with apparently isolated CL/P has an approximately 4% chance to have a child with CL/P, with a similar risk for a parent with CP to have a child with CP (Firth and Hurst, 2005).

There are at least 15 different genes that are believed to contribute to nonsyndromic cleft lip and/or palate (Cohen, 2007). Mutations in *MSX1* account for about 2% of persons with nonsyndromic CL/P (Jezewski et al., 2003). Mutations in this gene are inherited in an autosomal dominant pattern and thus this testing should be considered in a family with more than one generation of CL/P; tooth anomalies may occur as well.

4.2.2 Congenital Heart Defects

Congenital heart defects (CHD) are the most common form of birth anomaly, affecting more than 7 in 1,000 newborns worldwide (Burn and Goodship, 2007). Between 20% and 45% of infants with CHD have other noncardiac abnormalities. A specific genetic cause is identified in about 1 in 5 children with a cardiac malformation. Usually CHDs occur sporadically, with about 10% occurring as part of a syndrome. Congenital heart malformations are associated with close to 400 syndromes. Burn and Goodship (2007) provide a comprehensive list of syndromes associated with cardiac malformation as well as a listing by major features (e.g., dysmorphic features and intellectual disability, limb reduction defects, polydactyly, skeletal defects, ear and eye anomalies, genitourinary defects).

A chromosome anomaly should be considered in any newborn (or fetus) with a CHD especially if the child has other congenital anomalies or dysmorphic features. The autosomal dominant 22q11.2 deletion syndrome is associated with a wide spectrum of CHD and accounts for at least 2% of all heart defects (Burn and Goodship, 2007).

There are several known teratogenic influences on the developing heart (Table 4.5). Maternal alcohol use is the most significant environmental cause of CHD (mainly tetralogy of Fallot, VSD and/or ASD). Maternal use of anticonvulsants and retinoic acid are linked to an increased risk of CHD, and there may be a link with maternal use of lithium and a slight increase risk of Ebstein anomaly. Maternal illnesses associated with an increased risk for CHD include uncontrolled maternal diabetes, rubella infection, and maternal systemic lupus erythematosus. Maternal obesity in pregnancy has been associated with CHD and other malformations (Prentice and Goldberg, 1996; Watkins et al., 2003). Folic acid supplementation is likely to play a significant role in the reduction of conotruncal defects (Burn and Goodship, 2007).

4.2.3 Neural Tube Defects

Neural tube defects (NTDs) (e.g., anencephaly, exencephaly, iniencepphaly, encephalocele, meningocele and myelomeningocele, and spina bifida occulta) are

TABLE 4.5   Common Cardiac Teratogens

Teratogenic Agent	Heart Defect[a]
Maternal Factors	
Maternal alcohol abuse	VSD, ASD, PDA, double-outlet right ventricle, tetralogy of Fallot
Maternal diabetes (particularly if poorly controlled)	TGA, VSD, coarctation of aorta, HLHS
Maternal epilepsy	TGA
Maternal PKU (poorly controlled)	VSD, PDA, tetraology of Fallot, HLHS
Maternal rubella	VSD, ASD, PDA, peripheral pulmonary stenosis
Maternal systemic lupus erythematosus	Fetal heart block
Drug Exposure	
Androgenic hormones	Tetraology of Fallot, TGA
Cocaine	Heteterotaxic heart malformations
Hydantoin	VSD
Lithium	ASD, Ebstein anomaly, tricuspid atresia
Retinoic acid/isotretinoin (Accutane, excessive vitamin A)	VSD, coarctation of aorta, HLHS, tetraology of Fallot, TGA
Thalidomide	ASD, VSD, tetralogy of Fallot, truncus arteriosus
Trimethadione	TGA, HLHS, tetraology of Fallot
Valproic acid	TGA, HLHS, tetraology of Fallot, VSD

[a]Abbreviations: ASD = atrial septal defect; HLHS = hypoplastic left heart syndrome; PDA = persistent ductous arteriosis; PKU = phenylketonuria; TGA = transposition of the great arteries; VSD = ventricular septal defect
Sources: Burn and Goodship, 2007; Robinson and Linden, 1993; Sanders et al., 2002.

central nervous system birth defects involving problems with closure of the neural tube. Most neural tube defects occur as isolated defects (nonsyndromic) and are sporadic; they are thought to occur through the cumulative effects of multiple genetic and environmental risk factors. If a child with a NTD has dysmorphic features with or without other major or minor anomalies, a chromosomal or single-gene syndrome should be considered. The secondary medical consequences of a primary neural tube defect (e.g., hydrocephalus, scoliosis, dilated urinary tract, and clubfoot) are not considered primary malformations (Finnell and Mitchell, 2007). For the majority of individuals with a neural tube defect, the cause for the anomaly is unknown. The empiric recurrence risk for parents to have another child with a neural tube defect range from 3% to 5%; the chance is likely lower with folic acid supplementation, but this does not prevent 100% of neural tube defects (Finnell and Mitchell, 2007).

It is estimated that 50–70% of all neural tube defects would be eliminated if pregnant women were to consume 0.4 mg folic acid daily (Czeizel et al., 1996). The problem is that the neural tube closes before 28 days after conception, usually earlier than a woman knows she is pregnant. Because in the United States as many as 40–50% of pregnancies are unplanned, the Food and Drug Administration (FDA) mandates supplementation of grains with folic acid. (World Health Organization, 2004; U.S. Food and Drug Administration, 1996), and fortification of food with folic acid has been implemented in many other countries. Women who have a previous child with an isolated NTD should consume 4.0 mg folic acid daily, preferably 3 months before conception and during pregnancy. The total daily intake of folic acid should not exceed 1.0 mg unless prescribed by a physician.

The major teratogenic influences on neural tube defects are valproic acid, poorly controlled insulin-dependent diabetes mellitus, and maternal hyperthermia (from febrile illness in the first trimester); the antiseizure medication carbamazepine also is likely to be a risk factor for neural tube defects (Finnell and Mitchell, 2007). These exposures must occur before the closure of the neural tube at 28 days of pregnancy. There is growing evidence that women who are obese (with a body mass index, BMI, greater than 29 kg/m^2) are more likely than average-weight women to have an infant with anencephaly or spina bifida (Watkins et al., 2003).

4.2.4 The Detection of Fetal Anomalies on Routine Ultrasound Examination

Fetal malformations are usually identified serendipitously during a routine ultrasound. Clinicians challenged with making a precise fetal diagnosis are limited by a snapshot glimpse of the fetus, instead of the luxury of the full-system review that can be done after birth. Certainly a family history can assist with attempts at diagnosing a fetal condition; although the pedigree may not influence immediate management decisions. The songraphic finding of a malformation necessitates an *immediate* discussion with the patient about further testing to determine the fetal chromosome pattern or even array CGH (i.e., by obtaining amniotic fluid or fetal cord blood). This is true regardless of the parental family history or any potential maternal exposures to fetal teratogens. When a fetal anomaly is detected, it is reasonable to obtain an abbreviated family history from the parents, as is outlined in Table 4.6. A more thorough family history can be initiated once the chromosome results are available. Reviews by Benacerraf (2007), Paladini and Volpe (2007), and Sanders et al. (2002) provide practical approaches to the many differential diagnoses to consider with specific ultrasound findings.

There is a distinction between true fetal anomalies (e.g., cystic hygroma, clefting, and heart defects) and variants of normal anatomy that, in the absence of a chromosome anomaly, are clinically insignificant (e.g., echogenic intracardiac foci, and mild pylectasis). There are other variants that in a chromosomally normal fetus still need further evaluation because the ultrasound variant may be a response to fetal stress (such as hyperechogenic bowel and cystic fibrosis).

The identification of a potential fetal abnormality in what was thought to be a normal pregnancy is a crisis for the unsuspecting parents. The parents usually experience shock, worry, grief, guilt, even emotional detachment from the pregnancy when confronted by this news. They may have little tolerance for the probing questions required to take an exhaustive three-generation pedigree. Through their fog of grief and worry, the parents may even feel the health professional is asking questions to assign blame (especially with questions about teratogens and consanguinity). Family members may not know about the pregnancy; inquiring about the extended family may be viewed as a threat to privacy, further compounding the difficulties in obtaining an extensive pedigree.

TABLE 4.6   Minimal Medical-Family History Information to Obtain from the Parents after an Abnormal Fetal Ultrasound

Current Obstetrical History

- What have you been told about the ultrasound findings?
- What is the date of your last menstrual period?
- Have there been any complications during the pregnancy (e.g., bleeding)?
- Have you had other testing during the pregnancy (e.g., maternal serum screening, prior ultrasounds)?
- Is the father of the baby involved with the pregnancy? (Ask this question if he is not present at the visit.)
- Was this a planned pregnancy? (If not, the mother may not have had early prenatal care, or the fetus may have been exposed to teratogens before the mother knew she was pregnant.)

Past Obstetrical History

- How many pregnancies have you had altogether? (Include miscarriages, terminations of pregnancy, live births and delivery mode.)
- For any pregnancy terminations, was the termination due to a fetal anomaly or medical indication?
- Were any of the pregnancies with a different partner?
- What are your children's ages?

Mother's Health

- Do you have any health problems? (Specifically inquire about diabetes and high blood pressure, colds, fever, and illnesses in the pregnancy especially if the fetal problems could have a viral etiology. Document timing during pregnancy.)
- What medications do you take on a regular basis?
- Have you taken any prescription or over-the-counter drugs or herbal medicines during the pregnancy?
- Are you taking prenatal vitamins?
- Do you use any recreational drugs? (Note amount and timing.)
- Do you smoke or chew tobacco?
- How much alcohol have you had during the pregnancy? (Note quantity, type of beverage, and how often.)

Father's Health

- Does the father of the baby have any medical problems?
- Has the father of the baby had children or pregnancies (including miscarriages) with any previous partners? Do his children have any medical problems?

Maternal and Paternal Family History
If the patient answers yes to any of these questions, a more extensive family history is warranted, asking directed questions as appropriate.

- Is there anyone in your family, or the family of the baby's father who has had a baby with a birth defect, mental delay (retardation), or learning problems?
- Does anyone in the family have any major medical problems?
- Are the two of you related as blood relatives? For example, are you cousins?
- Has anyone in either family had a miscarriage, a stillborn baby, or a baby who died?

Is there anything I have not asked you or anything else in your family history that you think is important for me to know about?

4.3 DEAFNESS/HEARING LOSS

4.3.1 Genetic Causes of Deafness and Hearing Loss

Given that nearly 50% of individuals have significant hearing impairment by age 80, uncovering a family history of hearing loss is not surprising. The prevalence of severe hearing loss in children under the age of 3 years is approximately 2 in 1,000 births (Khoury et al., 1997). About 4 in 1,000 children under age 19 years are hearing impaired (Falk et al., 2007). Hearing loss can be conductive, sensorineural, or a combination of both (mixed). It is further categorized by being syndromic or nonsyndromic, and prelingual (before language development) or postlingual (after language development). Genetic factors account for about half of all prelingual hearing loss, with the majority being autosomal recessive and nonsyndromic. Several hundred different genes causing nonsyndromic and syndromic hearing loss and deafness have been discovered (Van Camp and Smith, 2009). Acquired causes and unknown reasons equally subdivide the remaining etiological factors in hearing loss, at 35% and 30%, respectively (Falk et al., 2007).

Because 90% of persons who are deaf have children with a partner who is also deaf, careful genetic counseling for these couples is important (Reardon et al., 2004). With more than 400 inherited syndromes associated with hearing loss, determining the etiology of hearing loss for an individual or family often proves quite a conundrum, particularly because about 90% of individuals with congenital hearing loss have hearing parents (Reardon et al., 2004). Nonsyndromic deafness has no other signs or symptoms and accounts for the majority (about 70%) of inherited hearing loss (Falk et al., 2007).

Of nonsyndromic hearing loss, autosomal recessive mutations account for the majority (75–80%), particularly in profound prelingual (before speech) hearing loss (Ballana et al., 2009). Mutations in the gene connexin 26 or nonsyndromic neurosensory deafness (DFNB1 with mutations in *GJB2*) and/or connexin 30 (DFNA3 with mutations in *GJB6* or *GJB2*) probably account for 20% of all childhood hereditary hearing loss and 50% of autosomal recessive nonsyndromic hearing loss (Falk et al., 2007). Autosomal dominant inheritance is more often seen with postlingual hearing loss and with moderate or progressive hearing loss. An autosomal dominant pattern of inheritance is the etiology of 15–25% of nonsyndromic hearing loss. Only 1–2% of nonsyndromic inheritance is attributed to X-linked inheritance (Ballana et al., 2009). Given the rarity of X-linked deafness syndromes, two brothers with nonsyndromic hearing loss or deafness are more likely to have autosomal recessive gene mutations than an X-linked mutation (Falk et al., 2007). Less than 1% of nonsyndromic hearing loss is due to mitochondrial mutations (Ballana et al., 2009).

Although mitochondrial inheritance is a small contributor to the overall prevalence of hearing loss, sensorineural hearing loss is an extremely common finding in several mitochondrial myopathies (Table 2.6).

With more than 100 different genes causing nonsyndromal hearing loss, it is easy to confuse the syndrome nomenclature (Falk et al., 2007). The gene locus for nonsyndromic deafness is abbreviated DFN (for DeaFNess) followed by the inheritance pattern—*A* for autosomal dominant (DFNA), *B* for autosomal recessive (DFNB), and no suffix notation for X-linked (DFN)—and a number indicating the order the gene was discovered—(DFNA11, DFNB1, and DFN4). DFNM is used for mitochondrial and modifying loci. Syndromic hearing loss is named after the researchers who described the syndrome (e.g., Waardenburg syndrome) or by descriptive terms (e.g., branchio-oto-renal syndrome).

Individuals with chromosome anomalies often have hearing impairment (Falk et al., 2007). Hearing loss is rarely a presenting clinical feature in recognizing children with chromosome anomalies, nor is hearing loss prominent in their family histories.

4.3.2   Classification of Hearing Loss and Deafness Syndromes

The questions to ask in obtaining a medical-family history for deafness are extensive (Table 4.7) because almost any organ system can be involved in syndromic deafness. There are six major parameters that help classify hearing loss (Reardon et al., 2004; Falk et al., 2007):

1. Severity of hearing loss (Table 4.7)
2. Type of deafness
   a. *Sensorineural deafness* (neural or nerve deafness, perceptive deafness); the abnormality lies between the hair cells of the cochlea and the auditory regions of the brain. The problem is usually with the hair cells themselves. Rarely the problem is with the auditory nerve (*auditory neuropathy*).
   b. *Conductive deafness*; the problems lies in the external or middle ear.
3. Deafness associated with other features (syndromic deafness) as compared to isolated (undifferentiated) nonsyndromic deafness
4. Age of onset (congenital/prelingual, and postlingual childhood or adult onset)
5. Progressive or nonprogressive hearing impairment
6. Acquired (either prenatal or postnatal) or genetic

These classification systems often shift as the molecular etiology of the various forms of deafness is defined.

Medical record documentation of hearing studies and medical problems is essential for accurate genetic assessment. The diagnostic evaluation of hearing loss is extensive and includes otologic, audiologic, and physical examinations as well as CT or MRI examination of the temporal bone and molecular genetic analysis. Numerous syndromes involve hearing loss and eye disorders, so it is important to obtain records of ophthalmologic evaluations. Renal anomalies are also frequently associated with hearing loss. The branchio-oto-renal syndrome (BOR) with gene mutations in *EYA1* (or less commonly *SIX5*) is seen in 2% of deaf children, and Alport syndrome (perceptive deafness and chronic nephritis with mutations in *COL4A5*, *COL4A3*, or *COL4A4*) accounts for about 1% of all genetic hearing loss; BOR is seen in about 2% of persons undergoing renal transplants (Falk et al., 2007). Pendred syndrome

TABLE 4.7 Medial-Family History Questions for Deafness/Hearing Loss

For the person and/or relative with hearing loss or deafness document:

- What is the type of hearing loss?
  - *Conductive* (external ear defects involving pinna and/or outer ear canal, and/or middle ear defects involving tympanic membrane, ossicles or eustachian tube): Speech is often good because person hears his or her own voice well; person hears sounds well but sounds are quieter.
  - *Sensorineural* (perceptive or neuronal type involving inner ear/cochlear defects): Sounds are distorted (particularly consonants) and quieter; person has problems hearing his or her own voice, so speech is impaired.
  - *Mixed*
- How severe is the hearing loss?
  - Mild (20–49 dB)
  - Moderate (40–60 dB)
  - Severe (60–80 dB)
  - Profound (> 80 dB)
- At what age was the hearing loss detected?
  - Prelingual (onset before speech development)
  - Postlingual (onset after speech development)
- What is the hearing impaired individual's method of communication?
  - Sign language
  - Lip reading
  - Tactile (for deaf-blind)
  - Speech (note that nasal speech suggests velopharyngeal insufficiency)
- Is the hearing loss progressive or stable?
- Has the individual had chronic exposure to noise? (occupational or environmental)
- Has the individual had any chronic diseases or trauma to the ear?
  - Chronic ear infections
    - Was the person treated with an aminoglycoside? (tends to be steep, high-frequency hearing loss)
  - Meningitis
  - Mastoiditis
  - Kernicterus (bilirubin encephalopathy, often associated neurological and learning problems)
  - Myxedema (hypothyroidism)
- Did the individual's mother have any Illnesses or problems during her pregnancy? If yes, what is the timing in pregnancy and length of the exposure?
  - Rubella
  - Alcohol (amount)
  - Cytomegalovirus
  - Toxoplasmosis
  - Retinoic acid
  - Quinine
  - Maternal diabetes
  - Oligohydramnios (possible fetal kidney problem)

(Continued)

TABLE 4.7 *(Continued)*

- Has the individual had any problems with learning? (Inquire about special education, see Section 4.5.)
  - Intellectual disability

    Progressive (regression in skills)

    Nonprogressive
  - Learning disabilities
- What medical evaluations have been done and what specialists has the person with hearing loss seen? (Obtain reports of audiograms, BAER, ophthlamological evaluations, electroretinograms, EEG, ECG, brain scans, etc.)
- Does the person have any unusual physical features?
  - *Eyes (physical)*
    - Placement

      Hypertelorism (wide spaced)

      Hypotelorism (close together)

      Dystopia canthorum (short palpebral fissures with displacement of inner canthi giving the impression of hypertelorism, seen in Waardenburg syndrome type 1)
    - Shape (small, absent, down slanting)
    - Eyelid coloboma (notched; common in mandibulofacial dysostosis)
    - Ptosis
    - Coloring

      Heterochromia (different colored; seen in Waardenburg syndrome)

      Blue sclerae (white of eyes has blue tint; common in osteogenesis imperfectas and Ehlers-Danlos syndrome VI/kyphoscoliosis type)
  - *Visual problems* (include age at onset and note any treatments, see Section 4.4)
    - Progressive
    - Stable
    - Glaucoma
    - Cataracts (see Tables 4.9 and 4.10)
    - Retinitis pigmentosa (frequently associated with syndromic hearing loss, particularly with the Usher syndromes, Refsum syndrome)
    - Optic atrophy
  - *Ears* (external anomalies are extremely common in syndromic hearing loss)
    - Physical shape and size (describe: cupped, crumpled, etc.)
    - Absent
    - Placement (e.g., low set, rotated)
    - Ear tags (common in oculo-auriculo-vertebral dysplasia)
    - Ear pits (common in branchio-oto-renal syndrome)
  - *Nose*
    - Unusual shape
    - Pear or bulbous (common in tricho-rhino-phalangeal syndrome)
    - Depressed nasal bridge
    - Wide nasal bridge
    - Inability to smell (anosmia) (Kallmann syndrome, Refsum syndrome)
  - *Mouth*
    - Cleft lip
    - Cleft palate
    - High arched palate
    - Lip pits (seen in van der Woude syndrome and popliteal ptergium syndrome)

TABLE 4.7   *(Continued)*

- *Chin*
  - Micrognathia (small; seen in mandibulofacial dysostosis)
  - Prognathic (large)
- *Face*
  - Asymmetric
  - Unusual shape (e.g., long, seen in tricho-rhino-phalangeal syndrome; triangular, in the osteogenesis imperfectas)
  - Coarsening of facial features (common in lysosomal storage disorders)
- *Head*
  - Microcephaly (small)
  - Macrocephaly (large)
- *Hair*
  - White streaks (seen in Waardenburg syndrome; don't mistake artificial hair coloring)
  - Sparse or patchy (several syndromes, including ectodermal dysplasias)
  - Coarse (common in storage disorders)
- *Teeth*
  - Conical
  - Malocculusion
  - Discoloration
  - "Brittle" (common in osteogenesis imperfecta)
- *Hands and feet*
  - Short fingers/toes (brachydactyly)
  - Long fingers/toes (arachnodatyly)
  - Syndactyly (webbed or fused; describe if both hands and feet and which digits)
  - Polydactyly (extra fingers/toes; describe if extra digit is on side of thumb or 5th finger)
  - Other digit anomalies
  - Abnormal nails (ectodermal dysplasias)
- Does the person have other health problems, or is there a family history of health problems such as the following?
  - *Cardiovascular*
    - Conduction defects (common in Jervell and Lange-Nielsen syndrome, Refsum syndrome)
    - Congenital heart defect (describe anomaly)
  - *Gastrointestinal*
    - Enlarged liver or spleen (common in lysosomal storage diseases)
  - *Renal anomalies* (common in Alport syndrome and branchio-oto-renal syndrome)
  - *Skeletal*
    - Tall stature
    - Short stature (common in many skeletal dysplasias)
    - Limbs proportionate
    - Limbs disproportionate
    - Scoliosis
    - Congenital hip dislocation
    - Multiple fractures (common in the osteogenesis imperfectas)
    - Loose joints

(Continued)

TABLE 4.7 *(Continued)*

* *Skin*
  * Unusual birthmarks (describe)
  * Albinism
  * Scaling/ichthyosis (several syndromes)
  * Ectodermal dysplasia
  * Branchial cysts/fistulas (present on lower neck) (seen in branchio-oto-renal syndrome)
* Neurological (note age at onset)
  * Gait problems (common in hereditary motor-sensory neuropathies, Friedreich ataxia, mitochondrial diseases, and several rare ataxia syndromes)
  * Brain "tumors" (describe) (common in neurofibromatosis type 2)
  * Muscle weakness
  * Spasticity
  * Seizures (see Section 4.9)
  * Stroke-like episodes
  * Episodic vomiting/headaches (common in metabolic and mitochondrial disorders)
  * Dementia (note age at onset; see Section 4.11)
  * Movement disorder
* Endocrine
  * Diabetes (see Section 4.17)
  * Thyroid disease (seen in Pendred syndrome)
* Fertility problems
  * Hypogonadism (seen in Kallmann syndrome, Norrie disease)
* Is there a history of sudden death or fainting? (seen in Long QT syndrome)
* Are the parents of the child blood relatives? (e.g., first cousins or more closely related)

Sources: Smith and Camp, 2007; Tewfik et al., 1997; Toriello et al., 2004.

or DFNB4 (bilateral prelingual sensorineural hearing loss with goiter, and Mondini dysplasia—presence of a dilated vestibular aqueduct associated with dilation of the apical turn of the cochlea, resulting in an abnormal 1.5 turns replacing the normal 2.5 turns, and mutations in *SLC26A4* or *FOXI1*) is thought to account for about 5% of severe/profound congenital deafness (Chang et al., 2009). Excellent reviews of the syndromes and conditions associated with hereditary deafness can be found in Falk et al. (2007), Kochar et al. (2007), and Toriello et al. (2004) and at Hereditary Hearing Loss Homepage (webh01.ua.ac.be/hhh). The Deafness Research Group provides current information on the connexin-deafness genes (http://davinci.crg.es/deafness). Some of the more common syndromic causes of hearing loss are listed in Table 4.8.

4.3.3 Acquired Forms of Hearing Loss and Deafness

Acquired hearing loss in children can be due to congenital TORCH infections (**t**oxoplasmosis, **r**ubella, **c**ytomegalovirus, and **h**erpes), perinatal asphyxia, prolonged hyperbilirubinemia, and postnatal infection (bacterial meningitis). Sensorineural hearing loss also occurs as a complication of congenital syphilis. Pinna

TABLE 4.8 Common Inherited Hearing Loss Syndromes: Their Features and Patterns of Mendelian Inheritance

Syndrome	Features[a]	Pattern of Inheritance	Gene (s)
Alport syndrome	*Males:* Progressive SNL (beginning in adolescence), progressive glomulonephritis (end-stage renal failure often by 20s), anterior cataract (lenticonus; onset teens/adult); *Females:* 1–2% similarly affected as males	XL	*COL4A5*, 85% XL, 15% due to new mutations
Alport syndrome with leiomyomatosis	*Males:* Progressive SNL (beginning in adolescence), renal failure, esophageal dysfunction, genital leiomyomas, sometimes posterior cataract, intellectual disability	XL (contiguous gene deletion)	Deletion of *COL4A5* to 2nd exon of *COL4A6*
Alport syndrome with intellectual disability (AMME complex)	Progressive SNL, intellectual disability, midface hypoplasia, elliptocytosis	XL (contiguous gene deletion)	Deletion of *COL4A5* and *FACL4*
Alport syndrome, recessive type	Progressive SNL, renal failure in males and females before age 30	AR	Homozygotes or compound heterozygotes for *COL4A3* or *COL4A4*
Alport syndrome, dominant type	SNL progressive, renal failure of varying severity	AD	Dominant-negative mutations in *COL4A3* or *COL4A4*
Biotinidase deficiency	Identified by newborn screening in many parts of world; treated with dietary biotin, screening in United States; if untreated SNL, seizures, ataxia, optic atrophy	AR	*BTD*
Branchiootorenal syndrome (BOR)	SNL, mixed, CHL; branchial cleft cysts or fistulae, external ear malformation, preauricular pits, renal anomalies	AD	*EYA1, SIX1* Other
Jervell and Lange-Nielsen syndrome	Congenital deafness and prolonged QT interval	AR	*KCNE1, KCNQ1*
Mandibulofacial dysostosis (Treacher-Collins syndrome)	CH, external oar anomalies, abnormalities of the jaw and facial bones (hypoplasia of the mandible and zygomatic bones), lower eyelid coloboma, dental anomalies, sometimes cleft palate or cleft lip and palate	AD	*TCOF1*

(Continued)

TABLE 4.8   *(Continued)*

Syndrome	Features[a]	Pattern of Inheritance	Gene (s)
Neurofibromatosis 2 (NF2)	Hearing loss in 3rd decade due to vestibular schwannoma (other rare tumors: meningioma, astrocytoma, ependymomas)	AD	*NF2*
Pendred syndrome	Severe to profound SNL (associated with abnormalities of bony labyrinth—Mondini dysplasia or dilated vestibular aqueduct), euthyroid goiter (develops in puberty or adulthood)	AR	*SLC26A4*, Other
Refsum (adult) syndrome	Severe progressive SHL, RP, ataxia, ichthyosis (onset childhood/adolescence); treatable with dietary modification and plasmapharesis	AR	*PHYH, PEX7*
Stickler syndrome (hereditary anthro-ophthalmopathy)	Progressive SNL, cleft palate, spondyloepiphyseal dysplasia, osteoarthritis (severe myopia and retinal detachment in STL1 and STL2), marfanoid habitus, characteristic facies; STL is considered the non-ocular type	AD	STL1 (*COL2A1*) STL2 (*COL11A1*) STL3 (*COL11A2*)
Usher syndrome	SNL, development of retinitis pigmentosa (type I: congenital severe to profound SNL and abnormal vestibular function, RP onset childhood; type II: congenital mild-severe SNL and normal vestibular function, RP onset adolescence or later; type III: progressive hearing loss and progressive loss of vestibular function, later onset RP)	AR	Multiple loci for each type
Waardenburg syndrome (WS1, WS2, WS3, WS4)	SNL, pigmentary changes, white forelock, heterochromia (dystropia canthorum in WS1; WS2 same as WS1 but no dystropia canthorum; limb anomalies in WS3; Hirschprung disease in WS4)	AD	WS1 (*PAX3*) WS2 (*MITF*) WS3 (*PAX3*) WS4 (*EDNRB, EDN3, SOX10*)

[a]Abbreviations: CHL = conductive hearing loss; SNL = sensorineural hearing loss; RP = retinitis pigmentosa.
Sources: Falk et al., 2007; Firth and Hurst, 2005.

anomalies and serous otis media occur frequently with fetal alcohol syndrome and with consequent conductive hearing loss. Noise exposure in adults is a major cause of acquired hearing loss. Hearing loss can also be due to aminoglycoside ototoxicity. This is more likely in individuals with A-to-G transition at position 1555 (A1555G) in the mitochondrial genome (Falk et al., 2007).

4.3.4 Genetic Assessment and Counseling for Persons with Hearing Loss and Deafness

Providing genetic assessment to a person who is deaf or a couple in which one or both are deaf can be challenging at many levels (Israel et al., 1996). Because of communication barriers, a health provider with average hearing may have trouble obtaining medical-family history from a client who is deaf. Individuals who are deaf may use any combination of skills to communicate, such as a sign language like American or British Sign Language (ASL and BSL, respectively), lip reading, a tactile communicator (for persons who are deaf-blind), writing on paper, or using a laptop computer. Phone conversation between an individual with hearing loss and the hearing health provider can be accessed through a TTY message-relay system. The service operator relays word-for-word the communication between the message typed by the deaf person to the hearing person and vice versa. A certified ASL interpreter (preferably one with medical knowledge) should interpret during clinical visits.

An individual with a hearing impairment may have difficulty communicating with his or her relatives with average hearing. Thus the consultand may have more limited knowledge about the health of family members. The clinician may be able to obtain additional family history information by contacting a hearing family relative (with permission of the consultand) and, of course, respecting the privacy of the client who is nonhearing and his or her relatives.

From the perspective of the health professional with average hearing, the translated speech or rapidly scrawled words of the patient who is non-hearing may seem terse and choppy. American Sign Language is not merely a codification of English; ASL does not directly translate into English. Difficulties with translation are compounded by the fact that many individuals with deafness have had barriers to quality education. For these reasons, unfortunately, a professional who is hearing may falsely perceive that the individual with deafness is intellectually disabled.

Often individuals with hearing impairment identify themselves as "deaf"—a descriptive name for a unifying culture, not a medical label describing a handicapping condition that needs to be treated or cured (Israel et al., 1996; Middleton et al., 1998). Health professionals need to determine the client's preferred terminology for his or her hearing difficulties (e.g., hearing impairment, deafness, hard-of-hearing) and use this terminology in discussion with the client. Couples in which one or both individuals are deaf may have few concerns about having a child who also is deaf. In fact, they may worry about parenting a child who is hearing (Middleton et al., 1998). They may take offense to medical lingo that describes "risks" of having a "hearing impaired," "abnormal" or "affected" child as compared to a "normal" hearing child. The clinician should choose words reflecting *chances* over risks, and describe children as *hearing* and *nonhearing*. (Israel et al., 1996).

4.4 VISION IMPAIRMENT

With better control of nutrition and of maternal and childhood infections (such as smallpox and maternal rubella), inherited disorders account for a large fraction of congenital and childhood visual impairment. Estimates are that half of all visual impairment before the age of 45 years has a genetic etiology; all inheritance patterns are represented, including single-gene, mitochondrial, and chromosomal. Obtaining medical documentation of the type and degree of visual disturbance is absolutely essential to provide genetic counseling. Retinal dystrophies are the most common form of genetic blindness (accounting for more than 50%) (Heckenlively and Daiger, 2007). More than 200 inherited disorders involve retinal degeneration (usually presenting as night blindness and eventual loss of central vision) (Heckenlively and Daiger, 2007). Conversely, 10% of all inherited disorders involve the retina directly or indirectly (Heckenlively and Daiger, 2007). The important medical-family history features to document when an individual has congenital blindness or later-onset visual loss are presented in Table 4.9.

TABLE 4.9   The Medical-Family History Approach to Visual Loss

- What was the person's age at the onset of blindness or visual loss?
- Document with ophthalmologic records the area of visual pathology (some conditions will overlap in more than one area):
  - Retina (e.g., retinitis pigmentosa, macular degeneration, retinoblastoma)
  - Choroid (e.g., choroidermia)
  - Optic nerve or disc (e.g., atrophy hypoplasia)
  - Lens (e.g., cataract, ectopia lentis)
  - Eyeball or globe (e.g., high myopia, glaucoma, structural defect such as microphathlamos or anopthalmos)
  - Iris (uvea) and uveal tract (e.g., aniridia or iris hypoplasia, coloboma, chorioretinitis)
  - Nystagmus (common in disorders of hypopigmentation such as albinism)
- Is the visual disturbance bilateral or unilateral? (bilateral disease is more likely to have a genetic etiology)
- Did the mother of the person with visual impairment have any infections during the pregnancy?
- Are the parents of the person with visual impairment related as cousins, or more closely? (suggests autosomal recessive inheritance)
- Does the person (or other family members) have other diseases or medical conditions? Focus on:
  - Dysmorphic features with or without other birth anomalies (see Section 4.2)
  - Hearing loss (see Section 4.3). The various forms of the autosomal recessive Usher syndrome (retinitis pigmentosa with sensorineural hearing loss) account for 8% of profound deafness in children. Among the deaf-blind population, RP has a prevalence estimated at 50% (Toriello et al., 2004)
  - Intellectual (mental) disability or learning disabilities (see Section 4.5)
  - Neurological disease (see Section 4.8)
  - Dementia (see Section 4.11)
  - Pigmentary and skin abnormalities
  - Short stature (see Section 4.16)
  - Diabetes (see Section 4.17)
  - Reproductive anomalies including hypogonadism (see Section 4.18)

Sources: Arnould-Devuyst et al., 2007; Toriello et al., 2004.

4.4.1   Early-Onset Cataracts

Approximately 1 in 250 infants is born with a cataract (though not all cataracts are clinically significant), and an estimated 23% of congenital cataracts are familial (Bashour 2008; Rabinowitz, et al., 2007). Worldwide, 10% of all blindness is attributed to congenital cataracts (Rabinowitz et al., 2007). Cataracts seem to be involved in the aging process, for all humans will develop cataracts (referred to as senile cataracts) that can impair vision if they live to an advanced age. The upper age limit that is considered "early" for the onset of cataracts is debatable (Rabinowitz, et al., 2007).

Determining the significance of a family history of cataracts can be sorted by the age of presentation of the cataracts—congenital, infancy: younger than 12 months; childhood: 1–15 years; adult: >15 years). Approximately 70–75% of congenital cataracts are nongenetic in etiology. Worldwide, maternal infections (e.g., rubella, varicella, toxoplasmosis) are an important cause of congenital cataracts. Diabetes mellitus is a frequent fundamental metabolic factor in the development of childhood cataracts. Presenile cataracts can be secondary to an underlying lens anomaly, which may have a hereditary etiology (Rabinowitz et al., 2007) such as:

- *Ectopia lentis* (dislocated lens). Can occur as a result of a traumatic blow to the head, as an isolated hereditary condition (autosomal dominant or recessive), or as a feature of an inherited syndrome (such as Marfan syndrome or homocystinuria).
- *Iris colobomas* (notching). Are associated with several chromosomal anomalies and CHARGE association. Colobomas may occur after an injury or surgery.
- *Multiple lenticonus* is a bulge in the front or back of the lens.
- *Retinal degeneration* is associated with retinitis pigmentosa and usually develops after the age of 30 years.

There are several familial forms of isolated congenital/infantile cataracts. These are classified by their morphology as zonular, polar, total (mature), and membranous (Rabinowitz et al., 2007). The zonular cataracts are further subdivided into nuclear, lamellar, sutural, spear-like, coralliform, floriform, and capsular; the lamellar subtype is the most common type of congenital cataracts (Rabinowitz et al., 2007). Dominant, autosomal recessive, and X-linked patterns have been observed for isolated familial cataracts.

Several chromosomal syndromes are associated with the development of cataracts at a young age (Rabinowitz et al., 2007). Early age at onset of cataracts is seen in several inborn errors of metabolism (see Table 4.12) in which the underlying defect is in cholesterol synthesis or metabolism (e.g., galactosemia, mannosidosis, neuraminidase deficiency, Lowe syndrome, Wilson disease, untreated PKU, Smith-Lemli-Opitz syndrome, Zellweger spectrum syndrome, cerebrotendinous xanthomatosis, melavolonic aciduria) (Rabinowitz et al., 2007).

There are multiple rare syndromes with early-onset cataracts (Table 4.10); referral to a medical geneticist is recommended. The family-medical history questions for cataracts are reviewed in Table 4.11.

TABLE 4.10   Examples of Hereditary and Environmental Syndromes Associated with Early-Onset Cataracts

Age at Presentation	Syndrome	Inheritance Pattern[a]	Other Cardinal Features[a]
Birth	Cockayne syndrome B	AR	LD/ID (progressive), dysmorphic features, hearing loss, retinal degeneration, premature aging, short stature
	Lowe (oculocerebrorenal) syndrome	XL	Short stature, sebaceous cysts, ID, hypotonia, dysmorphic features, renal aminoaciduria (females may have only the characteristic "punctuate spoke-like cataracts")
	Marshall syndrome	AD	Hearing loss, dysmorphic features, skeletal anomalies, ectodermal dysplasia
	Oculomandibulofacial syndrome (Hallerman-Streiff)	?AD or AR	Dysmorphic features including characteristic thin/beaked nose and small chin, variable LD/ID, dental anomalies/congenital teeth, dermatologic findings, hypotrichosis
	Rhizomelic chondrodyplasia punctata	AR	ID, limb shortening (humeri and femora), coronal vertebral clefts, ichthyosis
	Zellweger syndrome spectrum (cerebrohepatorenal syndrome, perioxisome biogenesis disorders)	AR	Perioxisome malfunction, seizures, dysmorphic features, joint contractures, hepatomegaly, hypotonia (heterozygote carriers have curvilinear lens opacities)
Newborn (1–4 wk.)	Fetal rubella	Maternal infection	ID, deafness, chorioretinitis, glaucoma, patent ductus arteriosis, peripheral pulmonic stenosis, myocardial disease
	Fetal varicella	Maternal infection	ID, seizures, chorioretinitis, limb/digit anomalies, growth deficiency
	Galactosemia	AR	Successful dietary intervention with lactose-free diet, but may still have LD, growth delays, ovarian failure; identified by newborn screening in many countries
	Galactokinase deficiency	AR	Cataracts may be only manifestation

TABLE 4.10 *(Continued)*

Age at Presentation	Syndrome	Inheritance Pattern[a]	Other Cardinal Features[a]
Infancy (1–12 mo.)	Chondrodysplasia punctata (Conradi-Hunermann)	XL (often lethal in males)	asymmetric limb shortness, early punctuate mineralization, growth deficiency, distinctive face, sparse coarse hair, thick scales on infant skin, red skin with large pores, some with ID/LD
	Lysosomal storage disorders	AR, XL	Coarsening facies, ID/LD, hepatosplenomegaly, bony changes (dystosis multiplex)
	Smith-Lemli-Opitz syndrome	AR	ID, short stature, dysmorphic features, genitourinary and limb anomalies
Childhood (1–15 y)	Fabry disease	XL	cornea verticillata, lenticular "Fabry cataract" (neither interfere with vision), tortuous conjuctival and retinal vessels, left ventricular hypertrophy, problems with sweating, skin findings (angiokeratoma), pain (acroparesthesias), anhidrosis, cerebrovasular manifestations, renal involvement, gastrointestinal problems
	Incontinentia pigmenti	XL (lethal in males)	ID/LD, neurological deficits, skin lesions that are replaced by hyperpig-mented/hypopigmented areas, dental anomalies
	Nance-Horan syndrome (cataract-dental syndrome)	XL	microcornea, dental anomalies (cone-shaped incisors, supernumerary teeth), some with DD. Females may have posterior Y-sutural cataracts with small corneas and teeth anomalies.
	Neurofibromatosis 2	AD	Hearing loss, bilateral vestibular schwannomas, brain tumors (meningiomas, gliomas)
	Pseudohypoparathyroidism	XL	LD, short stature, brachydactyly, hypocalcemia

(Continued)

TABLE 4.10 *(Continued)*

Age at Presentation	Syndrome	Inheritance Pattern[a]	Other Cardinal Features[a]
	Rothmund-Thomson	AR	Pokiloderma, sparse hair/eyelashes/eyebrows, small stature, skeletal and dental anomalies, osteosarcoma
	Stickler syndrome	AD	LD, dysmorphic features, retinal detachment, myopia, hypotonia, hyperextensible joints, skeletal anomalies, cleft palate, hearing loss
	Wilson disease	AR	Liver disease from copper accumulation, psychiatric disease, neurological deterioration
Adulthood (>15 y)	Alport syndrome	AD, XL	Anterior lenticonus, sensorineural hearing loss, renal disease
	Cerebrotendinous xanthomatosis	AR	Xanthomas, thickening tendons, spasticity, dysarthria, dementia and neurological deterioration, cardiovascular disease
	MYH9RD[b]	AD	Congenital thryombocytopenia and large platelets, high-frequency sensorineural hearing loss (presentation 1st–6th decade), glomerulonephritis (onset 20–40 y)
	Myotonic muscular dystrophy	AD	Myotonia, muscle weakness, ptosis
	Nail-patella syndrome (hereditary oncho-osteodysplasia)	AD	Congenital glaucoma, underdeveloped kneecaps and thumbnails, dental anomalies, renal disease, constipation
	Werner syndrome	AR	Characteristic facies and dermatologic pathology, short stature, hypogonadism, premature aging

[a]Abbreviations: LD = learning disabled; DD = developmental delay; ID = intellectual disability (formerly mental retardation); AD = autosomal dominant; AR = autosomal recessive; XL= X-linked: ? = unknown.
[b]Formerly called Epstein, Fechter, May-Hegglin, or Sebastian syndrome.
Sources: Clarke, 2006; Jones, 2005; Rabinowitz, et al., 2007; Saudubray and Charpentier, 1995; Savoia and Balduini, 2008; Sybert, 2010.

TABLE 4.11 Medical-Family History Queries for Cataracts

- At what age were the cataracts diagnosed?
- Are the cataracts in both eyes? (unilateral cataracts more likely from maternal infection)
- Did the mother of the person with cataracts have any infections in pregnancy?
- What evaluations have been done? (e.g., CBC, BUN, TORCH titers, VDRL, urine for reducing substances, red cell galactokinase, urine for amino acids, calcium phosphorous, chromosome studies, DNA studies, brain scans, hearing tests)
- How are the cataracts described? (e.g., location, color, density, shape) Obtain ophthalmologic records.
- Does the person with cataracts have any unusual facial or physical features?
- What is the height of the person?
  - Is the person unusually tall or short compared to other family members?
  - Record historian's estimate of parental and sibling heights.
- Does the person with cataracts, or his or her relatives have:
  - Other medical problems? Explain.
  - Learning disabilities or developmental delays?
  - Unusual skin findings or hair texture, or patchy hair? Describe.
  - Unusual sun sensitivity?
  - Hearing loss? (note severity and age at onset; see Section 4.3)
  - Heart disease (see Section 4.13)
  - Muscle weakness? Describe and note age at onset.
  - Skeletal anomalies?
  - Any neurological problems? (e.g., slurred speech, unsteady gait, seizures) Describe problems, age at onset, any evaluations. (see Section 4.8)
  - Psychiatric disease, dementia, or significant behavioral problems? (see Section 4.11 and 4.12)
  - Any kidney disease? (see Section 4.15)
  - Do other relatives have cataracts or other eye diseases?
- Are the parents of the person with cataracts related as first cousins or more closely related?

Sources: Bashour, 2008; Firth and Hurst, 2005; Rabinowitz et al., 2007.

4.5 INTELLECTUAL DISABILITY

Mental retardation is not something you have, like blue eyes or a bad heart, nor is it something you are, like short or thin. It is not a medical disorder or a mental disorder.... Mental retardation reflects the "fit" between the capabilities of individuals and the structure and expectations of their environment.

—American Association on Mental Retardation (1992), now the American Association on Intellectual Development and Disabilities

Concern about a family member with intellectual disability is frequently the impetus for a person or couple to seek genetic counseling. The term *intellectual disability* is synonymous with the term *mental retardation* and is the preferred terminology

(Schalock et al., 2007). The prevalence of severe intellectual disability (an IQ less than 50) is in the range of 3.8 in 1,000, but much higher (29.8 in 1,000) if mild intellectual disability is included (Raymond, 2007; Roveland et al., 1997). Severe intellectual disability is more likely to have a genetic etiology (30–40% as the result of single-gene or chromosomal disorders) than are milder forms of intellectual disability (Raymond, 2007). Chromosomal syndromes are responsible for the majority of the identifiable causes of severe intellectual disability. (See Table 2.1 for family history features suggesting a chromosomal syndrome.) Down syndrome is believed to be the etiology for 1 in 3 of all individuals with moderate intellectual disability. In persons with developmental delay who were not considered to have a syndrome, an estimated 11% will have a microdeletion.

Between 25% and 50% of all intellectual disability is attributed to mutations in X-linked genes, with fragile X syndrome accounting for 40% of all individuals with X-linked intellectual disability (Raymond, 2007). Molecular testing for fragile X should be considered in any male or female with unexplained intellectual disability in the absence of minor or major malformations. Stevenson, Scwartz and Schroer (2000) provide an excellent review of more than 100 X-linked syndromes associated with intellectual disability, and the Greenwood Genetic Center provides an online source of new X-linked intellectual disability syndromes and nonsyndromic X-linked intellectual disabilities (www.ggc.org/xlmr.htm). Close to 100 nonsyndromic X-linked intellectual disability mutations (MRX) mutations have been described. Autosomal recessive or X-linked inborn errors of metabolism are responsible for about 5% of all severe postnatal intellectual disability (Jones, 2005). See Table 4.12 for clinical and family features suggestive of an inherited inborn error of metabolism.

Be wary of the language you use when inquiring about a family member with intellectual disabilities. Families and disability advocates often feel *mental retardation* is a derogatory term. Instead, they may prefer descriptions such as *learning disabled, mentally or educationally challenged, slow learner, special needs*, and even *differently abled* (Finucane, 1998). It is appropriate to say the "child with intellectual disabilities" but not the "mentally retarded child." The use of suitable descriptors of intellectual functioning is extremely important when discussing reproductive risks and choices with a man, woman, or couple with mental delays. Journalist Michael Bérube (1996), the parent of a child with Down syndrome, captures the thoughts of many disability activists regarding sensitivity toward the "language of mental retardation" when he writes:

> I'm told that intelligence has obvious survival value, since organisms with a talent for information processing "naturally" beat out their competitors for food, water, and condos, but human history doesn't convince me that *our* brand of intelligence is just what the world was waiting for.

Mild intellectual disability may run in the family, and have both an environmental and genetic etiology. Asking about the parents' mental abilities is important. Although it is often difficult to determine the cause of mild intellectual disability, a family history of "normal intelligence" can be very reassuring to the inquiring family member.

TABLE 4.12   Features Suggesting a Metabolic Genetic Disorder

- Failure to thrive
- Hypotonia
- Loss of developmental milestones
- Cognitive delay (mental retardation)/global developmental delay
- Head circumference that is normal at birth then fails to follow the growth curve
- Neurological deficits in more than one part of the nervous system (e.g., central nervous system disease and peripheral neuropathy)
- Episodic symptoms, such as:
  - Vomiting
  - Ataxia
  - Coma
- Progressive worsening of symptoms (particularly if acute onset), such as:
  - Movement disorder
  - Cognitive decline
  - Psychiatric illness
  - Muscle weakness or neurodegeneration
  - Visual loss
  - Dysarthria
- Metabolic acidosis
- Chronic diarrhea
- Recurrent infections
- Symptoms brought on by infectious illness or fasting
- Symptoms began with weaning
- Abnormal behavior (irritable, impulsive, aggressive, hyperactive, self-mutilation)
- Seizures
- Stroke (in infancy or childhood)
- Cataracts in infancy or childhood
- Hair anomalies
  - Excessive body hair (hirsute)
  - Brittle, fragile hair
  - Stiff, kinky, or coarse hair
  - Sparse or absent hair (alopecia)
- Coarsening of facial features
- Dysostosis multiplex
- Enlarged liver and/or spleen
- Unusual odor (particularly when ill), such as:
  - Sweaty feet, cheese (isovaleric academia, glutaric academia type 2)
  - Rancid, fishy, rotten cabbage (tyrosinemia)
  - Musty, mousy (untreated PKU)
  - Sweet (maple syrup urine disease)
  - Fishy (trimethylaminuria)
  - Hops, beer, dried celery (methionine malabsorption)
  - Poor feeding
- Unusual dietary pattern (e.g., avoids protein)
- Parental consanguinity (suggests autosomal recessive inheritance)
- Autosomal recessive or X-linked inheritance patterns are typical

Sources: Berry and Bennett, 1998; Clarke, 2006; Raymond, 2007; Saudubray and Charpentier, 1995.

It is not unusual for a person with mild intellectual disability to consider child-bearing. Myriad environmental, social, and family history variables complicate the assessment of reproductive risks for these individuals (Finucane, 1998). Individuals with mild intellectual disability may live under impoverished conditions due to the limited ability to earn income, adding potential environmental deprivation to the at-risk child's developmental milieu. There is a good likelihood that the partner of the affected individual is also learning disabled. This leads to the added complication of needing to make a genetic risk assessment based on two parents affected with learning disabilities that most likely have different etiologies (Finucane, 1998). The incidence of sexual abuse perpetrated against women with developmental disabilities is high. Because a significant proportion of this abuse is committed by blood relatives, there can be the added component of risk for autosomal recessive conditions because of parental incest (Finucane, 1998).

There are many unique issues in providing genetic counseling to individuals with mild intellectual disability. The potential parent with learning disabilities may be less concerned about having a child "like me," who also has learning delays, than having a child with physicial birth anomalies (Finucane, 1998). These individuals may be unreliable family historians as well as concrete thinkers who may have difficulty conceptualizing the multitude of facts and figures that are traditionally reviewed in a typical genetic counseling visit. Finucane (1998) suggests that the content of such counseling should shift from "facts to feelings."

When a family history of intellectual disability is identified, there are several key historical questions that can help with identification of syndromes and assist with determining recurrence risks. These family history features are summarized in Table 4.13.

A simple question to begin with is, *What diagnostic testing has been done.* Any child or person with unexplained intellectual disability and dysmorphic features should have a chromosome study, particularly if there is a family history of intellectual disability and miscarriages (suggesting a chromosome translocation). Individuals born before the 1970s may not have had a banded chromosome study. If an adult with features characteristic of a chromosomal syndrome had a normal chromosome study before the early 1990s, it is worth redoing the cytogenetic study using more sophisticated techniques. A normal chromosome study does not eliminate a genetic diagnosis. Comparative genomic hybridization (CGH) is a technology that may replace chromosomal analysis, but it is currently usually done in conjunction with chromosomal analysis (Sagoo et al., 2009).

Were any metabolic studies done? (Such as plasma amino acids, urine organic acids, lactate, or pyruvate). *Has any neurological testing been done?* (including brain imaging). Major brain malformations are more likely to have a genetic etiology than are minor structural abnormalities (Raymond, 2007).

How severe is the learning disability? Do you have the results of any formal developmental testing? About 30–40% of individuals with severe intellectual disability have a single-gene or chromosomal disorder, in contrast to only 10% of those with mild intellectual disability (Raymond, 2007). Severely aberrant mental development is usually clearly identified by 3–6 months of age. Documentation of actual IQ scores

TABLE 4.13   Features to Document in the Medical-Family History When a Family Member Has Intellectual Disability[a]

- Severity of cognitive delay (DSM IV classification)
  - Mild (IQ 50–55 to ~70)
  - Moderate (IQ 35–40 to 50–55)
  - Severe (IQ 20–25 to 35–40)
  - Profound (IQ < 20–25)
- The age that the delays were noted
- Static or progressive mental impairment
- Intellectual abilities of parents of affected child
  - Ask about learning disabilities, secondary education, any special assistance in classes
- Pregnancy and health history of affected child's mother:
  - Full gestation or premature
  - Traumatic delivery or asphyxiation (e.g., cord accident)
  - Teratogenic exposure (specifically ask about alcohol and recreational drugs)
  - Seizure medications
  - Maternal infections (syphilis, rubella, toxoplasmosis cytomegalovirus, HIV, herpes simplex)
  - Maternal disease (PKU, myotonic dystrophy)
- History suggesting early postnatal trauma (abuse, neglect, severe malnutrition)
- Any episodes of severe childhood illness, including:
  - Recurrent infections
  - Episodic vomiting
  - Intermittent coma
  - Episodes of hypoglycemia
  - Chronic diarrhea
- Anything unusual about the person's dietary pattern
- Unusual body odor, particularly when ill
- Abnormal behavior
- Hearing deficits (type and severity)
- Vision deficits (type and severity)
- Height of the individual, and height of parents and siblings
- Birth anomalies
- Physical and dysmorphic features:
  - *Head size* (microcephalic or macrocephalic)
  - *Eyes*
    - Unusual placement
    - Abnormal movements
  - *Ears*
    - Large or unusually shaped
  - *Face*
    - Dysmorphic features
    - Coarsening of facial features
  - *Hair*
    - Patchy, sparse, balding
    - Unusual texture (brittle, kinky)
    - Excessive body hair

(Continued)

TABLE 4.13   *(Continued)*

- Unusual skin pigmentation
- Skeletal anomalies
- Joint laxity
- Enlarged liver or spleen
- Large testes
- Neurological/neuromuscular findings, including:
  - Seizures
  - Weakness
  - Hypotonia or hypertonia
  - Gait disturbances
  - Involuntary movements
- Family history of:
  - Intellectual/learning disabilities
  - Miscarriages
  - Multiple birth defects
- Parental consanguinity

[a]Formerly referred to as mental retardation.
Sources: Raymond, 2007; Sutherland et al., 2007.

from affected family members is important. In the absence of medical records, descriptive information about the individual is useful. For example, *What life skills does the person have?* (e.g., feeding and dressing self, the ability to make change, living on own, driving a car or taking a bus, reading). *Were the problems present from birth?* Developmental delays noted from birth or shortly thereafter suggest a teratogenic exposure in pregnancy, or a chromosomal problem. *Are the delays remaining static or progressing? If progressive, at what age did the changes begin?* Normal development, followed by a loss of developmental milestones or progressive decline in school performance suggests an inherited biochemical disorder (usually autosomal recessive or X-linked recessive; refer to Table 4.12) or a mitochondrial disorder. Persons with chromosomal problems usually do not regress in their development. Other causes of developmental delay and failure to thrive that should not be overlooked include severe malnutrition, abuse, and neglect. Apparent regression may be attributed to environmental factors such as poorly controlled seizure activity, overmedication with anticonvulsants, intercurrent illness, emotional problems, or depression (Clarke, 2006).

Were there problems in pregnancy or with birth? Was the birth premature or delivered full term? Did the mother take any medications during pregnancy? Does the mother have any medical problems? Answers to these questions can help determine whether the child's delays are due to genetic or environmental causes (Robinson and Linden, 1993) such as the following:

- Maternal factors (e.g., maternal PKU, maternal muscular dystrophy)
- Teratogens (e.g., alcohol and/or recreational drugs, fetal hydantoin syndrome)

- Prematurity
- Prenatal or perinatal infections or illness
- Birth trauma (e.g., intracerebral hemorrhage)
- Asphyxia (e.g., abruption placentae, cord prolapse, meconium aspiration)
- Kernicterus (neonatal jaundice/hyperbilirubinemia)

Children with intellectual disability secondary to a prenatal infection (such as rubella, cytomegalic virus, and toxoplasmosis) usually have one or more of the following features: microcephaly, chorioretinitis, prenatal onset growth deficiency, hepatosplenomegaly, neonatal petechiae, jaundice, and deafness (Jones, 2005).

Family lore often focuses on birth trauma or drug use in pregnancy as the cause of intellectual disability in a family member; obtaining prenatal and birth records can help elucidate whether or not this is a factor in the etiology of an individual's cognitive delays.

Did the parents of the individual with learning disabilities have any problems in school? Were they ever in special classes to provide extra help in learning? What types of employment has either parent had? Have other people in the family required extra assistance with learning? The answers to these questions will give you an idea of the intellectual abilities of the parents of the affected individual or if there is a family history of learning disabilities.

Has the person had episodes of severe illness requiring hospitalization? Has the individual had episodes of excessive vomiting, coma, or low blood sugar (hypoglycemia)? Has the individual been hospitalized for frequent infections or chronic diarrhea? Any of these symptoms can be seen in inborn errors of metabolism (Table 4.12).

Does the person have poor feeding or an unusual dietary pattern? Avoidance of certain foods (particularly protein) can be a symptom of some of the inborn errors of metabolism (Table 4.12). Excessive eating can be seen in Prader-Willi syndrome (imprinting/microdeletion). *Does the person have an unusual body odor, particularly when he or she is ill?* A few of the inborn errors of metabolism are associated with a specific body odor (Table 4.12).

Are there extreme or unusual behavior problems? Destructive behavior may indicate a biochemical genetics problem such as Sanfilippo syndrome or Lesch-Nyan syndrome (both autosomal recessive), or Hunter syndrome (X-linked). Mental illness is seen in some of the other autosomal recessive enzyme deficiency disorders, including homocystinuria, methylene tetrahydrofolate reductase deficiency, and Krabbe disease. Outbursts of inappropriate laughter may be seen in Angelman syndrome (imprinting/microdeletion). Boys with X-linked adrenoleukodystrophy may present with gait disturbances associated with irritability, withdrawal, obsessive behaviors, and school failure (Clarke, 2006). Schizophrenic-like symptoms can be seen in individuals with 22q11.2 and other chromosomal syndromes.

Does the person look the same as or different from other family members? Would you be able to tell from a photograph that there is something different about him or her? Many syndromes with intellectual disability have associated dysmorphic features. By inquiring if the person in question has facial features similar to others in the family, it may help you discern whether or not the characteristics are simply familial variation or a unique syndromic feature. Pictures from a family gathering are invaluable.

How tall is this individual? What are the heights of his or her parents and brothers and sisters? Unusual stature (particularly short stature) is a feature of many syndromes associated with intellectual disability/learning disabilities.

Does the person with intellectual disability/learning disabilities have any birth anomalies or are there birth malformations in other family members? Does the person or other family members have other medical problems (including hearing, speech or visual deficits)?

Is there anything unusual about the person's hair; for example, is it unusually coarse, curly, or brittle? Is the hair absent, patchy, or sparse? Many syndromes are associated with intellectual disability and hair anomalies (Sybert, 2010). Several of the inborn errors of metabolism are associated with differences in the texture and/or fullness of scalp hair.

Are there any unusual birthmarks or skin problems? Cutaneous manifestations and varying degrees of intellectual disability are often seen in association (which is not surprising given the common embryonic ectodermal origins of the skin and nervous system). There are at least a hundred syndromes associated with cutaneous findings and intellectual disability (Jones, 2005; Sybert, 2010). Two of the most common causes of intellectual disability and unusual birthmarks are neurofibromatosis 1—associated with café au lait spots, learning disabilities, and sometimes a large head—and tuberous sclerosis complex—associated with hypopigmented macules ("ashleaf" spots), and angiofibromas clustering on the face, cheeks nose, and mouth, and shagreen patches (pink, yellow or whitish plaques). Both are autosomal dominant conditions. Telangiectasias are a major feature of the autosomal recessive condition ataxia telangiectasia.

Are there neurological or muscular symptoms associated with the intellectual disability? For example, does this individual have seizures, problems with coordination and/or walking, poor muscle tone (hypotonia), or muscle weakness? Congenital myotonic dystrophy is associated with hypotonia, and intellectual disability with a family history of muscle weakness. Individuals with tuberous sclerosis complex may have a seizure disorder, intellectual disability, hypopigmented spots, and periungual fibromas of the nails. Epilepsy with progressive muscle weakness is a common feature of the mitochondrial encephalopathies.

4.6 PERVASIVE DEVELOPMENTAL DISORDERS (PDD)/AUTISM SPECTRUM DISORDER (AUTISM)

The pervasive developmental disorders (PDDs) make up of a group of disorders that are classified based on impairments in social interaction and communication, in the presence of repetitive or stereotypical behaviors. These disorders include autistic disorder (or classic autism), childhood disintegrative disorder (early normal development, including speech followed by severe regression between ages 2 and 10 years affecting language, social skills, cognition, and daily life skills), Asperger syndrome, Rett syndrome, and PDD not otherwise specified (children are less severely affected and do not meet classifications of classic autism or Asperger syndrome). Autism disorder is among the most common developmental disorders. Estimates of the prevalence of all autism spectrum disorders has been estimated as high as 10–60 in 10,000, with males being more commonly affected than females (Rutter and Simonoff, 2007; Sikich et al., 2006). The diagnosis is usually made in the first 3 years of life, though development in the 1st year may appear normal (Rutter and Simonoff, 2007). Characteristic features include impairments in processing social and environmental information, language abnormalities (30% have no speech), and repetitive or stereotyped behaviors. Severe intellectual disability (IQ below 70) is seen in about 75% of autistic individuals. Persons with Asperger syndrome may have normal intelligence or be considered gifted. Strengths are usually in visuospatial skills, with larger deficits in verbal, abstraction, and conceptualization skills (Rutter and Simonoff, 2007). Other features associated with PDD/autism include a head circumference above that of the 98th percentile (macrocephaly, which may occur postnatally), epilepsy (affecting about 25%), a history of minor obstetric complications (unexplained by environmental risk factors), and minor congenital anomalies particularly involving the external ear. Environmental agents such as rubella are also a cause. (Schaefer and Mendelsohn, 2008).

Autism has a heterogeneous etiology. A genetic etiology has been identified in 6–15% of persons with autistic-like features, suggesting that all patients with autistic-like features would benefit from a genetic evaluation (Abdul-Rahman and Hudgins, 2006, Shaefer and Mendelsohn 2008). Autistic features seem to be a marker for abnormal brain development, and the current classification of the pervasive developmental disorders seems most useful for treatment and less important in determining etiology. In determining a genetic etiology of autism, it is important to first confirm the diagnosis of autism. Hearing loss can be mistakenly diagnosed for autism (Shaefer and Mendelsohn, 2008).

Chromosomal analysis with high-resolution prometaphase karyotype (band level greater than 550) produces the greatest yield, particularly if the individual has any minor physical anomalies. FISH analysis is recommended for 22q11.2 deletion (velocardiofacial/DiGeorge syndrome) and 15q duplication (the Prader-Willi/Angelman syndrome critical region) or deletion. In fact, 15q aberrations may be among the most common cause of autism. Use of subtelomeric FISH analysis or aCGH (microarray-based comparative genome hybridization) for people with autism is still being evaluated for efficacy of detecting anomalies, but given the relatively low cost and the ability to test for a variety of putative loci for autism, aCGH is likely to become a standard part of an autism evaluation (Schaefer and Mendelsohn, 2008).

To date, the most common single-gene disorders associated with autistic-like features include:

- Rett syndrome, an X-linked condition with lethality in males, is associated with mutations in *MECP2*. This diagnosis should be considered in females with developmental delay who are identified before age 4 years, particularly if there is normal early development followed by global regression, developing microcephaly, and loss of purposive hand movements with characteristic "midline hand washing." Limited studies suggest that 3–13% of female children with autistic features and developmental delay will have an *MECP2* sequence mutation. (Schaefer and Mendelsohn, 2008). Mutation in *MECP2* is not universally lethal in males and is a cause of autism and developmental delay in males.

- Fragile X syndrome, an X-linked disorder, affects less than 3% of persons with autism.
- Tuberous sclerosis complex, an autosomal dominant condition, affects an estimated 3–4% of individuals with autism (Rutter and Simonoff, 2007). Approximately 25% of persons with tuberous sclerosis complex have autism.
- Persons with macrocephaly (a head circumference greater than 2.5 standard deviations above the mean) and autism spectrum disorder should have *PTEN* genetic analysis even without additional clinical or family history features suggesting Cowden syndrome (Buxbaum et al., 2007; Herman et al., 2007; Orrico et al., 2008).
- Virtually 100% of persons with Smith-Lemli-Opitz syndrome have autism. Studies testing for 7-dehydro-cholesterol levels in persons with idiopathic autism have not been done, but this may become part of the screening protocol for autism (Sikora et al., 2006).
- For people with an X-linked pattern of neurobehavioral and nerurodevelopmental disorders and cognitive defects, genetic testing for neuroligin3 (*NGN3*) and neuroligin 4 (*NGN4*) are a consideration (Schaefer and Mendelsohn, 2008).

Autistic disorder is considered to have a polygenic/multifactorial etiology. The chance that parents of a child with autism will have another affected child is 3–6% (unless a genetic syndrome is identified) (Sikich et al., 2006), with the risks to second- and third-degree relatives being in the range of 0.13% and 0.05%, respectively (Jorde et al., 1991). The recurrence risk increases to up 50% with a second affected child (Schaefer and Mendelsohn, 2008). The siblings of an individual with autism are also at slightly increased risk to have behavioral problems as well as subtle deficits in speech, language, and social functioning (Rutter and Simonoff, 2007). The medical-family history questions related to autism are reviewed in Table 4.14.

4.7 CEREBRAL PALSY

Cerebral palsy is a heterogenous collection of clinical conditions that describe a nonprogressive physical disorder that affects movement and posture (Raymond,

TABLE 4.14   Medical-Family History Questions for Autism

- Were there any complications with the pregnancy or birth of the child?
- Did the mother take any medications, alcohol, or street drugs in the pregnancy? (specifically alcohol exposure, valproic acid)
- Did the mother have any illness in the pregnancy? (rubella, cytomegalovirus)
- At what age were the problems with language/socialization/behavior noted?
- Do you know the individual's IQ? (obtain records)
- Has normal hearing been confirmed?
- Are there any food intolerances?
- Has there been regression/loss of skills? (Consider *MECP2* in females; metabolic screening such as urine mucopolysaccharides and organic acids, serum lactate, amino acids, ammonia, and acyl-carnitine profile, depending on what has already been tested for in the newborn screening panel.)
- What type of diagnostic testing has been done? (obtain any reports)
  - Has the individual had a routine karyotype and/or fragile X (*FMR1*) DNA studies? (confirm band-level of karyotype)
  - Have comparative genomic hybridization (aCGH) studies been done?
  - What conditions were screened for in the newborn screening test?
  - Have neuroimaging studies been done? (particularly in instances of macrocephaly, microcephaly, and seizure disorder)
- Does the individual or any relatives have:
  - A large head (2.5 standard deviations greater than the mean)? (consider *FMR1, PTEN*)
  - Small head? (fetal rubella, Smith-Lemli-Opitz, many chromosomal syndromes; deceleration in head growth seen in Rett syndrome)
  - Any unusual facial characteristics?
  - Any minor physical anomalies?
  - A history of seizures? (obtain EEG)
  - Any unusual birthmarks or skin problems? (ashleaf-hypopigmented spots, Shagreen patch, adenoma seabaceum, angiofibromas, and periungual fibromas in tuberous sclerosis complex; trichelemmomas, acral keratoses, lipomas, and papillomatous papules in Cowden syndrome; large areas of hypopigmented streaks or whorls along the lines of Blaschko in hypomelanosis of Ito)
  - Any other medical problems?
- Is there a family history of:
  - Miscarriages?
  - Cognitive delay (mental retardation), learning disabilities, or autism?
  - Behavioral problems?
  - Seizures?
  - Cancer? (particularly thyroid, breast, uterine, or kidney cancer as seen in Cowden syndrome)
- Are the parents related as blood relatives?

Sources: Abudul-Rahman and Hudgins, 2006; Rutter and Simonoff, 2007; Schaefer and Mendelsohn, 2008.

2007). There is no on-going pathological process, though the clinical features can change with age and brain maturity (Firth and Hurst, 2005). The main classifications of cerebral palsy (Firth and Hurst, 2005; Wilson and Cooley, 2006) include:

- *Spastic cerebral palsy* (decreased muscle strength with increased muscle tone and brisk reflexes)
  - *Spastic hemiplegia* (nonsymmetrical)
  - *Spastic diplegia* (symmetrical with the legs affected more than the arms; there is a higher incidence of intellectual disability)
  - *Spastic quadriplegia* or *tetraplegia* (all four limbs are affected)
- *Athetoid cerebral palsy* (characterized by involuntary movements and loss of control of posture; includes dyskinetic, dystonic, extrapyramidal, choreathetoid)
- *Ataxic cerebral palsy* (generally reflects cerebellar involvement with poor coordination of movements and wide-based gait, tremor may be observed)
- *Atonic* or *hypotonic cerebral palsy* (hypotonia, decreased muscle tone beyond the 1st year of life)

Cerebral palsy is a common disorder with a prevalence of approximately 1.5 to 2.5 in 1,000 births (depending on how cerebral palsy is defined) (Raymond, 2007). The spastic forms are the most common. Cerebral palsy is rarely inherited (Firth and Hurst, 2005; Raymond, 2007). Despite popular beliefs, birth trauma is not a frequent cause of cerebral palsy (<5%) (Raymond, 2007). The etiology of cerebral palsy cannot be determined for many persons with cerebral palsy; the most common associations include (Firth and Hurst, 2005; Raymond, 2007; Wilson and Cooley, 2006):

- Prematurity
- Low birth weight (<1,500 g) (confers a 25–30 times increased risk of cerebral palsy)
- Infections (prenatal and postnatal)
- Bleeding in the first trimester (e.g., vascular event, loss of a twin)
- Twin gestation
- Cerebral dysgenesis (alterations in the formation of the central nervous system such as abnormal migration or proliferation leading to congenital malformation in the size, structure, and function of the brain—for example, lissencephaly, agenesis of the corpus callosum)
- Anoxia

There are several genetic conditions that may be misdiagnosed as cerebral palsy, or in which features of cerebral palsy are seen; most of these conditions are neurodegenerative and have other clinical symptoms that aid in diagnosis. Rare inherited conditions to consider (Firth and Hurst, 2005; Raymond, 2007; Wilson and Cooley, 2006) include:

- Mitochondrial disorders
- Inborn errors of metabolism:
  - Arginase deficiency (AR)
  - Abetalipoproteinemia (AR)
  - Fatty aldehyde dehydrogenase deficiency (Sjögren-Larsson syndrome)
  - Ornithine translocase deficiency or hyperornithemia-hyperammnomeia-homocitullinuria
  - Pyruvate dehydrogenase deficiency
- Perioxisomal disorders
  - Zellweger spectrum
- Dopa-responsive dystonia (most are autosomal dominant with mutations in *DYT5*)
- Rett syndrome due to *MECP2* mutations (X-linked)
- Angelman syndrome (imprinting defect)
- X-linked intellectual disability due to *ARX* mutations
- Biallelic factor V mutations (perinatal stroke)
- Leukodystrophies:
  - Metachromatic leukodystrophy (AR)
  - Krabbe disease (AR)
  - Adrenoluekodystrophy (X-linked)
- Movement disorders:
  - Wilson disease (AR)
  - Ataxia telangiectasia, (AR)
  - Lesch-Nyhan syndrome (X-linked)

Suggested medical-family history questions for cerebral palsy are given in Table 4.15. Even if an etiology for cerebral palsy is not determined, it is often comforting to parents to point out that they did not cause their child's problems because this is a common belief. This is another condition where it is particularly important to hear the parents' and family's beliefs about causality of the problem (such as birth trauma), and then respectfully provide some more likely explanations.

4.8   NEUROLOGICAL AND NEUROMUSCULAR DISORDERS

Molecular diagnosis is creating an upheaval in the classification systems of genetic neurological diseases. The spinocerebellar ataxias (SCA) are now classified into more than 30 subtypes, depending on the molecular etiology; some types have been described in only one family. The nomenclature flip-flops back and forth between the hereditary motor sensory neuropathies (HMSN) and the subtypes of Charcot-Marie-Tooth (CMT) as molecular diagnosis refines the phenotypes. Many of the forms of muscular dystrophy can now be distinguished by molecular testing. Not

TABLE 4.15   Medical-Family History Questions for Cerebral Palsy

Pregnancy history for the mother of the child/person with cerebral palsy:
- Was there anything unusual about the pregnancy? (e.g., infections, bleeding loss of a twin, lack of fetal movement)
- Did the mother have any illnesses in pregnancy? Describe nature of illness, diagnostic evaluation, treatment, timing in pregnancy.

Birth history of the person with cerebral palsy:
- Was the child born prematurely?
- What was the birth weight?
- Do you know the Apgar scores?
- Was the child admitted to the neonatal intensive care unit? Obtain details

For the person with cerebral palsy:
- Is the head circumference normal? (Ideally obtain growth charts and charts of growth of head circumference.)
- What evaluations have been done?
  - Brain imaging? (MRI can identify any lesions compatible with asphyxia, prematurity, congenital stroke, structural brain anomalies, basal ganglia lesions, agenesis of the corpus callosum, and lissencephaly.)
  - Karyotype and/or array CGH?
- Any abnormalities on newborn screening? (particularly for amnio acid and organic acid disorders)
- Is there progression (worsening) of symptoms?
- Does the person with cerebral palsy look like other relatives? Is there anything unusual about the way the person looks? (If so, consider syndromic conditions, karyotype and/or array CGH.)

Does the person with cerebral palsy and/or his or her relatives have a history of:
- Intellectual impairment?
- Seizures?
- A movement disorder?
- Ataxia?
- Unusual birth marks or skin disorder?
- Congenital anomalies?

Are the parents of the child/person with cerebral palsy related as cousins or more closely related? (suggests autosomal recessive inheritance)

Sources: Firth and Hurst, 2005; Raymond, 2007; Wilson and Cooley, 2006.

only is this flurry of molecular advances recasting the stage of how we think about neurological disorders but molecular genetic blood tests may also save a person from invasive procedures such as muscle or nerve biopsies. The family-medical history is often the first step in decision making for a diagnostic evaluation. Coupled with the findings from the patient's neurological exam, the medical-family history guides the clinician in choosing from the myriad diagnostic tools available for neurological diagnosis. One third of single-gene defects are associated with diseases that affect the nervous system (Gallagher, 2005). For references surveying the ever-changing field of neurogenetics see Lynch (2006), Rosenberg et al. (2007), the Winter–Baraitser Neurogenetics Database (http://imdatabases.com), and the disease specific reviews in GeneReviews (www.genereviews.org) (See also Appendix A.5).

Many hereditary neurological disorders are clinically complex because the nervous system is intimately intertwined with other organ systems; therefore, the family history approach to helping identify inherited neurological conditions must be broad. Table 4.16 outlines the medical-family history questions for a neurological condition.

This section is followed by more specific inquiries for directed medical-family histories for seizures, stroke dementia, and mental illness. Several hereditary conditions with neurological impairment also include hearing loss (see Section 4.3) and/or visual impairment (see Section 4.4). Cardiomyopathies are common in the muscular dystrophies (see Section 4.13). Inherited metabolic disorders are a frequent inherited cause of progressive neurological conditions, particularly in children. Table 4.12 reviews some of the medical-family history indicators of an inborn error of metabolism.

4.9 SEIZURES

Epilepsy is a group of disorders with many causes. Approximately 1% of the world population has recurrent seizures (Prasad and Prasad, 2007). Epilepsy is a disorder of the brain, characterized by recurrent, unprovoked, transient episodes of cortical neuronal activity, manifesting as a motor, sensory, autonomic, cognitive, or psychic disturbance (Prasad and Prasad, 2007). Myoclonic epilepsy is a common feature of inborn errors of metabolism and mitochondrial disorders (characteristics of mitochondrial disorders are summarized in Table 2.5). Acquired epilepsy accounts for one third of seizure disorders (Prasad and Prasad, 2007) and can result from any brain injury such as head trauma, meningitis or encephalitis, asphyxia (prenatal or postnatal), and hypoxia-ischemia from cerebrovascular disease. Seizures can also be related to tumors and drug use.

Epilepsy may occur in isolation or as part of a syndrome (single gene, chromosomal, or mitochondrial). More than 200 inherited syndromes are associated with seizure disorders, but they account for less than 1% of all cases of epilepsy (Prasad and Prasad, 2007). A general epilepsy syndrome may be associated with several different varieties of seizures. For example, generalized tonic-clinic, myoclonic, and absence seizures may occur in juvenile myoclonic epilepsy.

The classification of seizure types is complex, and the nomenclature is changing and is beyond the scope of this discussion. The International League against Epilepsy has the most current updates on classifications and genetic syndromes (www.ilae-epilepsy.org). The classification is based primarily on age of onset, seizures types,

TABLE 4.16 Medical-Family History Questions for Neurological Disorders[a]

- Describe the problems. Are they with strength? With sensation? With weakness? With coordination? With intellect? With walking? With speech?
- At what age did these problems begin?
- What parts of the body are affected? For example, are there problems with weakness in the following:
  - *Hands*: Does the person drop things or have trouble holding a pen/pencil?
  - *Feet*: Does the person trip frequently or have trouble lifting his or her feet such that they make a "slapping" sound when walking? Are the feet unusually shaped? For example, does anyone have high arches, claw or hammer toes? (common in CMT/HMSN)
  - *Face*: Are there problems with smiling, whistling, using a straw (common in FSHMD and MMD)?
  - *Arms*: Does the person have trouble lifting things? Does the person have problems combing his or her hair?
  - *Legs*: Do you notice anything unusual about the shape of the legs? (e.g., unusually large calves are seen in Duchenne-Becker muscular dystrophy; thin calves are seen in the hereditary neuropathies)
- At what age did the individual begin walking? (normal is between 10 and 15 months)
- Was the individual ever able to run?
- Did (does) he or she participate in sports? Explain.
- Are the problems getting worse over time or are the stable? If worse, over what period time? (e.g., 5 years ago, past 5 months)
- Is the person able to walk on his or her own or does he or she require assistance? (e.g., cane, wheelchair)
- Is there anything unusual about the way this person looks compared to other family members? If yes, explain.
- Are there other neurological disorders in this individual or in other family members such as
  - Seizures? (see Section 4.9)
  - Dysarthria (slurred speech)? (common in many of these disorders but particularly in the hereditary ataxias)
  - Intellectual disability or learning disabilities? (see Section 4.5)
  - Problems with thinking or judgment? (note age at onset)
  - Problems with memory? (note age at onset)
  - Uncontrolled movements? (common in Huntington disease)
  - Gait disturbances?
  - Spastic movements?
  - Stiff movements?
  - Depression or mental illness (see Section 4.12)
- Does this person or do other family members have a problem with alcohol abuse of chemical dependency?

TABLE 4.16   *(Continued)*

* Does the person, or other family members have other diseases or medical conditions? Focus on

  * Hearing loss? At what age? (common in NF2, several of the cerebellar ataxias, mitochondrial myopathies, associated with some forms of HMSN/CMT; see Section 4.3)

  * Visual impairment? At what age? (visual disturbances are frequently associated with neurological disorders, particularly retinopathies with or without mental retardation; early onset cataracts are common in MMD; see Section 4.4)

  * Skeletal anomalies, including problems with posture?

  * Short stature (see Section 4.16)

  * Heart disease? (particularly myopathies and cardiac conduction detects; see Section 4.13)

  * Diabetes (see Section 4.17)

  * Thyroid disease

  * Any unusual birthmarks or pigmentary changes? (common in tuberous sclerosis complex, NF, cerebrotendinous xanthomastosis, and some of the rarer cerebellar ataxias)

  * Cancer? (occult carcinoma may cause symptoms of an acquired ataxia)

* What studies have been done? (e.g., nerve biopsy, muscle biopsy, nerve conduction studies, spinal taps; imaging of the brain and/or spinal cord by MRI/ PET, or CT scans; metabolic testing such as organic and/or amino acids, molecular testing)

* What is the family's ethnic background/country of origin? (For some neurological conditions there is a founder effect such that certain gene alterations are easier to identify in certain groups or the disorder may occur more frequently in individuals of certain ancestries)

* Are the parents of the individual related as cousins or more closely related?

---

[a]Abbreviations: CMT = Charcot-Marie-Tooth disease; FSHMD = fascioscapulohmeral muscular dystrophy; HMSN = hereditary motor-sensory neuropathies; MMD − myotonic muscular dystrophy; NF = neurofibromatosis.

EEG signatures, common anatomy, and pathophysiology. The seizure types are broadly divided into self-limited and continuous seizures and into focal (partial) and generalized seizures.

Questions to ask for a family history of seizures are listed in Table 4.17. Seizures are a presenting sign or an evolving feature of many of the inborn errors of metabolism (particularly the storage disorders). Some of the common symptoms of inborn errors of metabolism are listed in Table 4.12. It is important to obtain documentation of any medical evaluations such as EEGs, brain imaging studies (CT, MRI, PET scans), ophthalmologic testing, metabolic testing (plasma amino acids, urine organic acids), and pathology reports from biopsies of skin lesions. Several anticonvulsant agents are toxic to the fetus during pregnancy (see Table 3.2). Seizure control and the potential teratogenic effects of medication on a developing fetus are important considerations in

TABLE 4.17   Medical-Family History Questions for a Seizure Disorder[a]

- Do you know the type of seizures? (e.g., focal—formerly called partial, local, focal neocortical without local spread, clonic, myoclonic, inhibitory motor, sensory, aphasic, focal neocortical with local spread, hippocampal and parahippocampal, generalized absence, generalized absence myoclonic, generalized with tonic and/or clonic manifestations, atonic.) Obtain EEG data.
- Were the seizures single or repeated?
- Did the seizure occur with an illness or fever?
- At what age did the seizures begin? (neonatal, infancy, childhood, adolescence, as an adult)
- Did the individual with seizures have any type of brain trauma or infection?
- What medications does the individual with seizures take?
- Did the mother of the person with seizures have any infections in pregnancy? (can be seen in fetal toxoplasmosis, rubella, herpes, and CMV)
- Does any other family member have seizures? Who?
- What studies have been done? (brain imaging, biochemical screening, chromosome analysis)

Does the person with seizures or any relatives have:

- Unusual facial features? (coarsening of facial features, with ID, can be seen in storage diseases—AR or XL; dysmorphic facial features, with ID, seen in several chromosome anomalies and single-gene disorders)
- Large head, protruding jaw and ears (with ID)? (characteristic of fragile X syndrome—XL-trinucleotide repeat)
- Microcephaly? (can be seen with chromosome disorders, multiple single-gene disorders)
- Unusual facial acne? (angiofibromas are characteristic of tuberous sclerosis complex—TSC—AD with variable expressivity)
- Impaired hearing? (see Section 4.3)
- Problems with vision? (see Section 4.4)
- Unusual skin findings?
  - White (ashleaf) spots, common in TSC
  - Brown (café au lait) spots, common in neurofibromatosis 1 (NF1—AD with variable expressivity)
  - Swirls of patchy hypopigmentation (with ID) characteristic of hypomelanosis of Ito (chromosomal mosaicism/unknown)
  - Marbled, swirly patches of skin, characteristic of incontinentia pigmenti (XL dominant)
  - Red/purple (port wine) stains (nevus flammeus) seen in Sturge-Weber syndrome (sporadic)
  - Yellow/orange tan nevi seen in sebaceous nevus sequence (sporadic)
  - Fatty benign tumors (lipomas)
- Unusual lumps or growths? (neurofibromas in NF1; angiofibromas in TSC)
- Growths under nails? (periungual fibromas are pathognomonic for TSC)
- Cognitive delay (ID) or learning disabilities? (can be seen with NF1, TSC, fragile X syndrome, maternal teratogens, chromosome anomalies and inborn errors of metabolism including storage disorders; see Section 4.5)

TABLE 4.17 *(Continued)*

- Developmental regression? (can be seen with metabolic disorders particularly storage disease, mitochondrial disease)
- Problems with walking (gait disturbance)? At what age? (can be seen with several of the hereditary ataxias, mitochondrial myopathies, and inborn errors of metabolism; see Section 4.8)
- Difficulty with coordination?
- Muscle weakness?
- Problems with behavior, thinking, or judgment? (see Sections 4.11 and 4.12)
- Are the parents of the individual with seizures blood relatives—for example, are they cousins?

[a]Abbreviations: ID = intellectual disability; NF1 = neurofibromatosis 1; TSC = tuberous sclerosis complex; AD = autosomal dominant; AR = autosomal recessive; XL = X-linked.
Sources: Fernandez and Bird, 2002; Sybert, 2010.

managing the pregnancy of a woman with a seizure disorder and should be discussed in genetic counseling.

4.10 STROKE

Strokes are the third most common cause of death in the United States. *Stroke* is an umbrella term describing several different disease processes, including large vessel atherosclerosis, small vessel or lacunar disease, and cardioembolism, all of which result in focal or sometimes global cerebral damage due to disruption of blood flow to the brain (Francis et al., 2007). An estimated 85% are due to cerebral ischemia and 15% are due to primary intracerebral hemorrhage (Francis et al., 2007).

There are several risk factors for stroke, some of which are modifiable, which including tobacco use, oxidized LDL, hyperglycemia/diabetes, hypertension, and periodontal disease. Substance abuse (cocaine and heroin) is another cause. Obesity is a risk factor for stroke and several of the other risk factors associated with stroke (such as diabetes and hypertension). The genetic etiology of stroke is likely multigenic with influence by other risk factors such as tobacco use. Polymorphisms in the phosphodiesterase 4D gene (*PDE4D*) seem to increase stroke risk particularly in association with tobacco use (Munshi and Kaul, 2008).

There are several single-gene disorders of which stroke is part of the multisystem disorder. Although these are rare, they are important to consider in the evaluation of person with stroke, particularly if the stroke is below age 55. Fabry disease may account for 1% of all unexplained (acute cryptogenic) stroke. Although this is an X-linked disorder, women are affected as well. Single-gene disorders associated with early stroke are reviewed in Table 4.18. The family history questions in relation to stroke are reviewed in Table 4.19. Stroke can also be seen with congenital heart disease; rheumatic valve disease; endocarditis; arrhythmias; and after cardiac surgery, vasculitis, and hypercoagulable states (such as antiphospholipid syndrome, antithrombin III/protein C deficiencies) (Francis et al., 2007).

TABLE 4.18   Inherited Disorders Associated with Early-Onset Stroke

Disorder/Gene	Features	Inheritance Pattern
CADASIL (cerebral autosomal dominant arteriopathy with subcortical infarcts and leukoencephalopathy)/ NOTCH3	Migraine-like headaches, depression, psychosis, TIA, recurrent lacunar strokes (which may lead to pseudobulbar palsy and subcortical dementia); characteristic white matter lesions in the external capsule and temporal poles; age of onset 30–60 years	AD
CARASIL (cerebral autosomal recessive arteriopathy with subcortical infarcts and leukoencephalopa-thy)/HTRA1	Strokes affecting small cerebral vessels, alopecia, pseudobulbar signs, rigidity, spasticity, dysarthria, ataxia; progressive motor and mental deterioration; diffuse white matter abnormalities; to date observed in only persons of Japanese ancestry; onset range 20–44 years	AR
Cerebral amyloid angiopathy/hereditary cerebral hemorrhage with amyloidosis/APP	Intracranial hemorrhage, infarcts due to amyloid deposits in cortical and leptomeningeal vessels; mean age of onset 55 years; rare; first described in Dutch families	AD
CRV and HERNS (cerebro-retinal vasculopathy and hereditary endotheliopathy with retinopathy, nephropathy, and stroke)/TREX1	Microangiopathy of the brain in combination with vascular retinopathy, dysarthria, seizures, punctuate vasculitis skin lesions	AD
Ehlers-Danlos syndrome (vascular type) IV/COL3A1	Thin and translucent skin, easy bruising, fragile arteries and intestines (prone to rupture); 10% show neurovascular complications (intracerebral aneurysms, carotid and vertebral arterial dissection)	AD
Fabry disease/GLA	Lysosomal storage disorders, with large and small vessel disease; neuropathic pain, renal failure, cadiomyopathy; multiple strokes occur in ~25% of patients; strokes from small vessel occlusion by lipid deposition, large vessel disease, or embolism from cardiac disease; age of onset <40 years.	XL
Familial amyloid angiopathy/cystatin (amyloidosis VI)/CST3	Small lobar cerebral hemorrhage, cerebral ischemia, and infarctation due to amyloid deposition in the walls of small and medium blood vessels of cerebral cortex and meninges; spasticity, incoordination, dementia; onset before to age 40; rare; first described in Icelandic families	AD

TABLE 4.18 *(Continued)*

Disorder/Gene	Features	Inheritance Pattern
HHT (hereditary hemorrhagic telangiectasia)/*ENG, ACVRL1*	Embolic stroke, vascular dysplasia with variable expressivity, leading to venous malformations (arteriovenous malformations)	AD
Homocystinuria (cystathionine β-synthase)/*CBS*	Accumulation of homocysteine and premature atherosclerosis, ectopia lentis, high arched palate, developmental delay, skeletal anomalies, psychiatric disorder, thromboembolism; estimated 50% have thromboembolic event by age 30, with about one third being strokes	AR
Marfan syndrome/*FBN1*	Dislocated lens, skeletal involvement with bony overgrowth (tall stature, arachnodactyly, pectus deformity), joint laxity, aortic dilation, aortic aneurysm; 4% show neurovascular (large vessel) disease	AD
MELAS (mitochondrial encephalopathy lactic acidosis and stroke)/mitochondrial	Mitochondrial encephalopathy, lactic acidosis and stroke-like episodes (typically in the occipitoparietal region), migraines, short stature, developmental delay, diabetes mellitus; onset variable	MT
MoyaMoya disease/*MYMY1, MYMY2, MYMY3*	Bilateral intracranial carotid artery occlusion with telangiectatic vessels in the region of the basal ganglia; predominant in East Asian populations; juvenile onset (<5 years) and 30–50 years for the adult type	AD with incomplete penetrance, possibly AR
Pseudoxanthoma elasticum (PXE)/*ABCC6 (MRP6)*	Connective tissue disorder with high prevalence of cardiovascular complications (large vessel disease, calcification), angioid streaks in the retina, visual impairment, skin changes (lax, redundant, and inelastic skin with yellowish papules at neck and axilla), gastrointestinal hemorrhage	AR
Sickle cell disease/*HBB*	Hemolysis and intermittent episodes of vascular occlusion resulting in tissue ischemia and acute and chronic organ dysfunction, chronic anemia, aplastic crisis, stroke (large and small vessel disease), TIA; up to 25% of affected persons have strokes by age 45; onset in childhood	AR

Sources: Bevans and Markus, 2004; Francis et al., 2007.

TABLE 4.19   Family History Questions in Relation to Stroke

At what age did the strokes begin?
What diagnostic evaluations have been done? (obtain records, including brain imaging,
    cardiovascular evaluation: lipoprotein levels, echocardiogram, angiography, Doppler studies)
Does the person have any of the following risk factors:
    Obesity?
    Diabetes?
    Tobacco use? How many cigarettes daily and for how many years?
    Drug use?
    Hypertension?
    Infections?
Does the person or any relatives have a history of:
    Heart disease? (e.g. atherosclerosis, congenital heart defects, valve disease, arrhythmia)
    Visual disturbances? (retinal changes in PXE[a] and CRV/HERNS; dislocated lenses in Marfan
        syndrome)
    Unusual skin findings? (yellowish papules, and lax, redundant skin in PXE, fragile,
        translucent screen in Ehlers Danlos IV, angiokeratomas in Fabry disease)
    Developmental delays? Note if this was present from birth or there is regression in skills.
    Psychiatric disease?
What is the country of origin of each set of grandparents?
Are the parents related as blood relatives (such as cousins or more closely) (suggestion of
    autosomal recessive condition)

Abbreviation: [a]PXE = pseudoxanthoma elasticum.

4.11   DEMENTIA

From past generations we receive a few strands of DNA, sometimes a heritage, a memory
of one sort or another.

—Daniel A. Pollen (1993)

Dementia is a loss of brain function involving problems with memory, behavior,
learning, and communication. It is not one illness and is due to a primary or secondary disease process affecting the brain. The most common causes of dementia are
Alzheimer disease, vascular dementia, or a combination of the two. Alzheimer disease
is the leading cause of dementia over the age of 40. The prevalence of Alzheimer disease is age dependent and varies from 0.3–0.5% in individuals age 69–69 to 11–15%
in the age group over 80 (Pericak-Vance and Haines, 2002).

A neuropathological diagnosis is required to determine the type of dementia. If
your patient has a living first-degree relative with dementia, encourage your patient
to discuss the delicate subject of brain autopsy with his or her family members. For
deceased relatives, it is essential to obtain neuropathology records to provide accurate genetic assessment for other family members. On several occasions I have been
involved with a patient evaluation in which we actually obtained ancient neuropathology slides. These slides were reinterpreted by a neuropathologist, which resulted in
a new diagnosis and an alteration in the genetic counseling.

Most dementia is not inherited. Noninherited causes of dementia include acquired immunodeficiency syndrome, syphilis, central nervous system infections, vascular disease (e.g., strokes), metabolic or nutritional deficiencies (e.g., thyroid and B_{12} deficiency), brain tumors, drug toxicity, and Creutzfeldt-Jakob disease (Pericak-Vance et al., 2007). Inherited disorders associated with adult-onset dementia are included in Table 4.20.

Huntington disease should be considered in any adult with a movement disorder, incoordination, and problems with thinking and judgment. It is inherited as an autosomal dominant trait, so usually there is a family history of the condition. Because this is a trinucleotide repeat disorder (see Chapter 3), an individual who has an apparent new mutation most likely has a parent with a CAG repeat expansion in the intermediate range (30–35 CAG repeats) (Wheeler et al., 2007).

Familial Alzheimer disease (FAD), a rare cause of dementia, has been mapped to several different loci. The major early-onset genes for FAD are *APP*, *PS1* and *PS2* (all autosomal dominant); *APOE* is considered a late-onset dementia susceptibility gene. These four genes explain less than 50% of all causes of Alzheimer disease (Pericak-Vance et al., 2007). The primary history feature that suggests FAD is early-onset dementia and memory loss (before age 60 years) that is inherited in an autosomal dominant pattern.

Other rare causes of Alzheimer-like dementia are included in Table 4.20 These conditions can be distinguished from FAD mainly by neuropathological distinctions and/or DNA testing. Frontotemporal dementia (formerly called Pick disease) is rare but is second to Alzheimer disease as a cause of familial dementia. Of frontotemporal dementias, 20–30% are hereditary, with mutations in the tau gene (*MAPT*) being the most common cause of familial frontotemporal dementia.

There are several uncommon metabolic disorders (all inherited in an autosomal recessive pattern) associated with the development of dementia in childhood (before age 15 years) (Saudubray and Charpentier, 2001):

- Ceroid lipofucinosis
- Gaucher disease III (juvenile or Norrbottnian type)
- Lafora disease
- Niemann-Pick type C
- Proprionic acidemia
- Sandhoff disease
- Sialidosis
- Late-onset Tay-Sachs disease (GM2 gangliosidosis)

Adrenoleukodystrophy is an X-linked disorder of very long chain fatty acids. Affected males can have attention deficit disorder/hyperactivity, dementia, progressive behavioral disturbance, and vision loss (onset between 4 and 8 years). The disease can be milder in males with onset in the late 20s with progressive paraparesis, adrenocortical dysfunction, sphincter disturbances and sexual dysfunction, and there can be an Addison disease-only phenotype with adrenocortical insufficiency usually by age 8

TABLE 4.20   Inherited Disorders Associated with Adult-Onset Dementia[a]

Disorder/Gene	Inheritance Pattern	Other Clinical Features
Aceruloplasminemia/*CP*	AR	Diabetes mellitus, anemia, movement disorder, ataxia, dysarthria, retinal degeneration; dementia about 25% with onset around age 50; general symptom onset between 25 and 60 years
Amyotrophic lateral sclerosis—Parkinsonian features/dementia (possibly *TRPM7*)	? two-allele additive major locus, ? environment	ALS, parkinsonian features, progressive motor function loss, lower motor neuron manifestations, muscle cramps and weakness; unusually high incidence among Chamaroo people of Guam
CADASIL/*NOTCH3*	AD	Relapsing strokes, seizures, migraines, motor disabilities, mood swings/depression, cognitive decline; onset usually between 35 and 50 years
Choreoacanthocytosis/ *VPS13A*	AR	Chorea (progressive), acanthocytes (red cell anomaly), dystonia, seizures, myopathy; mean age of onset 35 years
Creutzfeldt-Jacob diseases/*PRNP*	Sporadic, AD	Ataxia, jerky trembling movements (usually transmitted as a sporadic prion disease; onset between 45 and 75 years
Deafness-dystonia-neuronopathy (Mohr-Tranebjaerb syndrome)/*TIMM8A*	XL, or contiguous gene disruption at Xq22	Males with SNL (prelingual or postlingual); onset in teens of ataxia/dystonia; decreased visual acuity from optic atrophy (onset in 20s); dementia onset in 40s *Females* may have mild SNL and focal dystonia
DRPLA/*ATN1* (trinucleotide CAG repeat expansion)	AD	Seizures, choreoathetosis, ataxia, psychiatric disturbance, intellectual deterioration; mean age of onset 30 years
Fatal familial insomnia (FFI)/*PRNP* (point mutation)	AD	Insomnia, dysarthria, visual disturbances, cognitive capacity relatively good but may have slowed processing and memory impairment, characteristic neuropathology; onset typically in 40s to 50s.
Fragile X-associated tremor/ataxia syndrome (FXTAS)/*FMR1* (CTG trinucleotide repeat premutation)	XL (males primarily affected, but females can be as well)	Cerebellar ataxia, intention tremor, short-term memory loss, executive function deficits, parkinsonism, peripheral neuropathy, lower limb muscle weakness; onset typically age 50 and older

TABLE 4.20 *(Continued)*

Disorder/Gene	Inheritance Pattern	Other Clinical Features
Frontotemporal dementia with parkinsonism-17 (FTDP-17, hereditary Pick disease)/*MAPT* (tau)	AD	Extrapyramidal signs (rigidity, bradykinesia, supranuclear palsy, saccadic eye movements), language disturbances, distinct neuropathology, onset between 40 and 60 years; most common form of frontotemporal dementia
Frontotemporal dementia-CHMP2B-related (FTD-3)/*CHMP2B*	AD	Described in a single family in Denmark; specific neuropathology; onset between 40 and 55 years
Frontotemporal dementia-GRN-related (FTDU-17)/*GRN*	AD	Parkinsonian features, distinct neuropathology; mean age of onset 52–63 years
Gerstmann-Sträussler-Scheinker disease (*PRNP*; several different point mutations)	AD	Cerebellar ataxia, dysarthria, nystagmus, spasticity, increased muscle tone, visual disturbances, deafness, sometimes parkinsonian features; onset between 35 and 55 years
Gliosis, familial subcortical (Neumann type)	? AR, ? AD	Neuropathological distinctions from familial Alzheimer disease
Hallervorden-Spatz disease/*PANK2*	AR, sporadic	Retinitis pigmentosa, gait abnormalities, dystonia, rigidity, chorea, seizures; onset 7–15 years
Huntington disease/*HTT* (CAG repeat expansion 36 and larger)	AD	Chorea (progressive), incoordination, psychiatric (compulsive behavior), anxiety, depression; early age of onset associated with larger CAG expansions, but symptoms typically in 30s and 40s
IBMPFD /*VCP*	AD	Proximal and distal muscle weakness, Paget disease of bone; mean age of onset is 42 years, with frontemporal dementia occurring at mean age of 55
Kearns-Sayres syndrome (varying mitochondrial deletions with hotspot between positions 8469 and 13147)	MT	Cerebellar ataxia, ophthalmoplegia, retinal degeneration, seizures, sensorineural deafness, short stature, headaches, diabetes, cardiac conduction defects; onset younger than 20 years
Lewy body dementia (heterogeneous)	Sporadic, AD	Dysphasia, visual hallucinations, parkinsonian features
MELAS (various mitochondrial point mutations)	MT	Seizures, sensorineural deafness, cortical blindness, renal anomalies, myopathy, short stature, headaches, diabetes (type II), stroke-like episodes, hypertrophic cardiomyopathy, cardiac conduction defects, lactic acidosis; onset before age 40

(Continued)

TABLE 4.20   *(Continued)*

Disorder/Gene	Inheritance Pattern	Other Clinical Features
MERRF (most commonly, mitochondrial point mutation at position 8344)	MT	Cerebellar ataxia, myoclonus, seizures, sensorineural deafness, weakness, short stature, lipomas, hearing loss, cardiomyopathy (onset childhood)
Pick disease	Sporadic, AD	Neuropathological distinctions from familial Alzheimer disease
Spinocerebellar ataxia type 2/*ATXN2* (trinucleotide CAG repeat expansion)	AD	Cerebellar ataxia, dysarthria, peripheral neuropathy, ophthalmoplegia, rarely retinitis pigmentosa, dystonia, chorea; typically onset in 30–40 years
Wilson disease/*ATP7B*	AR	Parkinsonian features, tremor, ataxia, dysarthria, dystonia, Kayser-Fleischer ring (eyes), liver disease, lower serum ceruloplasmin, disturbance in copper metabolism; onset 6–20 years

[a]Abbreviations: CADASIL = cerebral autosomal dominant arteriopathy with subcortical infarcts and luekoendephalopathy; DRPLA = dentatorubro-pallidolusian atrophy; IBMPFD = inclusion body myopathy associated with Paget disease of bone (PDB) and/or frontotemporal dementia; MELAS = mitochondrial encephalomyopathy, lactic acidosis, and stroke-like episodes; MERRF = myoclonic epilepsy and ragged-red fibers.
Sources: Clarke, 2006; Holm et al., 2007; OMIM, 2009; Pericak-Vance et al., 2007.

years. Females can display a milder neurological disability (adrenomyeloneuropathy) with later onset (usually age 35 or later) (Moser et al., (2006).

Refer to Table 4.12 for the medical-family history features suggesting inborn errors of metabolism. Signs to suggest an inborn error of metabolism associated with dementia include onset before age 40 years, presence of neurological signs (particularly extrapyramidal abnormalities, presence of white matter disease, and evidence of executive dysfunction (Clarke, 2006).

Many of the conditions that are associated with childhood or adult-onset dementia are also seen in individuals that have behavioral disorders or mental illness as a frequent presenting manifestation of the disease (see Section 4.12 and Table 4.23). Several of the mitochondrial myopathies (Kearns-Sayres syndrome, MERRF, and MELAS) may also present with dementia in childhood or as an adult (Clarke, 2006).

The medical-family history questions for sorting through a possible hereditary etiology for dementia are reviewed in Table 4.21.

4.12   MENTAL ILLNESS

Individuals with mental illness in the family are often profoundly concerned about their own chances of developing a mental disorder or having affected children. These fears are partly because of the significant aura of stigmatization and shame that

TABLE 4.21 Medical-Family History Questions for Dementia

- At what age did your relative develop dementia? (onset of dementia before age 60 is more likely to have a hereditary component)
- Describe the problems (behavioral, word finding, memory loss, hallucinations)
- If deceased, was a brain autopsy performed? (obtain pathology reports)
- Have any brain imaging studies been done, such as an MRI or CT scan? (obtain reports)
- Does/do the person(s) with dementia drink alcohol or use street drugs? (note type of substance, how much, and for how long)

Does the affected individual or anyone in the family have:
- Problems with speech, for example word finding and/or slurred speech? Describe and note age at onset.
- Difficulty with hearing? Note age at onset and progression. (see Section 4.3)
- Problems with vision? Note age at onset and specific problems. (e.g., retinal degeneration, problems with eye movements, etc.; see Section 4.4)
- Muscle weakness? Describe onset and progression. If so, was a muscle biopsy performed?
- A history of strokes or stroke-like episodes? Note age at onset.
- Uncontrolled movements (chorea) or tremor? Note age at onset.
- Parkinson's disease? Note age at onset and any treatment.
- A seizure disorder? Note age at onset, and type if known (see Section 4.9)
- Were the parents related as close relatives (such as first cousins)? (suggests autosomal recessive disorder)

is traditionally associated with the diagnosis of a mental illness (Kinney, 2007). Providing genetic risk assessment for these individuals is frustrating, mainly because the definitions of mental illness rest on shifting territory. The studies from which empirical risk figures are drawn depend on the criteria chosen for diagnosis of the mental illness, and the classifications of mental illness have changed over time. For example, some investigators use a broad definition of manic depressive illness that is characterized by episodes of persistent elevated and persistent depressed mode. Others use more specific diagnoses such as bipolar disorder type I, in which the elevated mood states are frank mania, and bipolar disorder type II, with less pronounced hypomanic episodes (McInnis et al, 2007). To confuse nosology further, schizophrenia is distinct from manic-depressive disorders, yet mood disorders can have psychotic features. Additional classification dilemmas arise when confronted with the milder clinical spectrum of mood disorders, such as hypomania without major depression, cyclothymia, dysthymia, and seasonal affective depression disorder (Potash, 2006).

Genetic disorders that may present with psychiatric or severe behavioral abnormalities are included in Table 4.22. The genetic etiology of mental illness is likely a combination of single genes, polygenic inheritance involving a few major genes, or a polygenic mixture of major and minor genes (Kinney, 2007). For affective disorders, the empiric risk for a first-degree relative to be affected is in the range of 20–25%, with most of the risk due to unipolar depression (Detera-Wadleigh and Goldin, 2002). The median age of onset of bipolar disease is in the mid-20s, and for unipolar disease about age 30 (Detera-Wadleigh and Goldin, 2002).

TABLE 4.22   Genetic Disorders That May Present with Psychiatric or Severe Behavioral Abnormalities[a]

Condition[b]	Age of Onset of Mental Illness	Behaviors	Inheritance
Adrenoleukodystrophy/ adrenal myeloneuropathy	Childhood–young adults	Social withdrawl, irritability, obsessional behavior, inflexibility, mania, depression	XL
CADASIL	Young adults	Deficits in executive function, narrowing of field of interest, cognitive decline	AD
Cerebrotendinous xanthomatosis[c]	Teens–adulthood	Delusions, hallucinations, catatonia, dependency, irritability, agitation, and aggression	AR
Cobalamin metabolism defects (CblC)[c]	Variable	Chronic or subacute psychiatric symptoms, confusion, behavior problems, visual hallucinations, depression	AR
DRPLA	Adulthood	Psychosis	AD
Fragile X syndrome (*FMR1* CTG repeat expansion)[c]	Childhood	Hyperactivity, hand flapping, hand biting, temper tantrums	
Fragile X tremor ataxia syndrome (FXTAS) (*FMR1* CTG repeat premutation)	50s and older	Executive function deficits, cognitive decline, short-term memory loss	XL
Frontotemporal dementias (includes FTDP-17 or Pick disease)	Adulthood	Disinhibition, loss of initiative, obsessive-compulsive behavior, delusions, hallucinations, verbal aggressiveness, hyperorality	AD
GM2 gangliosidosis (late-onset Tay-Sachs)	Teens–adulthood	Acute psychosis, agitation, obsessional paranoia, mania, depression, hallucinations, stereotypic motor movements	AR
Hartnup disorder[c]	Variable	Emotional instability, psychosis	AR
Homocystinuria (MTHF reductase deficiency)[c]	Variable	Acute "schizophrenia," confusion, behavior problems, catatonia, visual hallucinations, depression	AR
Homocystinuria (cystathionine B-synthase deficiency)[c]	Teens–adulthood	Hallucinations (auditory and visual), paranoia, personality disorder, anxiety, depression, obsessive-compulsive behavior	AR

TABLE 4.22 *(Continued)*

Condition[b]	Age of Onset of Mental Illness	Behaviors	Inheritance
Huntington disease	Adult	Depression, personality changes, agitation, irritability, apathy, anxiety, disinhibition, euphoria, hallucinations	AD
Juvenile Huntington disease	5–15 years	Similar to adult with rapid decline	AD
Kufs disease (adult-onset neuronal ceroid lipofuscinosis, ANCL)	15–50 years	Thought disorder, flat affect, paranoia, hallucinations	AR
Lafora type, progressive myoclonus epilepsy	6–17 years	Visual hallucinations, depressed mood, agitation, dementia	AR
Leigh disease or NARP[c] (neurogenic muscle weakness, ataxia, retinitis pigmentosa)	Early childhood	Mild anxiety disorder	MT, AR
Lesch-Nyhan syndrome[c]	Childhood	Severe self-injurious behavior, aggressiveness, coprolalia	XL
Metachromatic leukodystrophy, late-onset (arylsulfatase A deficiency)	20 + years	Anxiety, depression, emotional lability, social withdrawl, disorganized thinking, poor memory, mimics schizophrenia	AR
Neuronal ceroid lipofuscinosis (Kufs disease)	Variable	Thought disorder, flat affect, paranoia with hallucinations, delusions, inappropriate behavior	AR, ?AD
Niemann-Pick type C	Teens–adulthood	Depression, schizophrenia	AR
Nonketotic hyperglycinemia[c]	Variable	Behavior problems, episodes of confusion; may be triggered by febrile illness	AR
Ornithine transcarbamylase deficiency (late onset)	Variable	Periodic acute agitation, anxiety, confusion, hallucinations, paranoia; may be triggered by high protein intake or situation of high protein catabolism (e.g., illness, injury, surgery)	XL
Phenylketonuria (poor dietary control)	Adults	Depression, anxiety, phobias	AR
Porphyrias (acuto intermittent porphyria, coproporphyria, porphyria variegata)	Teens–adult	Chronic anxiety, depression, restlessness, insomnia, depression, paranoia, hallucinations (during acute crisis); may be triggered by porphryogenic drugs, alcohol, or infection	AD

(Continued)

TABLE 4.22 *(Continued)*

Condition[b]	Age of Onset of Mental Illness	Behaviors	Inheritance
Sanfilippo syndrome[c]	Childhood	Hyperactivity, impulsivity, aggression, insomnia	AR
22q11.2 deletion syndrome (velocardiofacial syndrome)[c]	Teens–adult	Disinhibition, impulsivity, attention deficit, perseveration, schizophrenia, bipolar disorder, depression, anxiety	AD
Wilson disease	Variable	Anxiety, depression, schizophrenia, manic-depressive psychosis, antisocial, catatonia	AR
Wolfram syndrome (DIDMOAD)[c]	Teens–adult	Depression, paranoia, hallucinations (auditory and visual), violent behavior, sometimes dementia	MT, AR

[a]Abbreviations: AD = autosomal dominant; AR = autosomal recessive; XL = X-linked; MT = mitochondrial; CADASIL = cerebral autosomal dominant arteriopathy with subcortical infarcts and leukoencephalopathy; DID-MOAD = diabetes insipidus-diabetes mellitus-optic atrophy-deafness; DRPLA = dentatorubro-pallidoluysian atrophy; FTDP-17 = frontotemporal dementia with parkinsonism-chromosome 17 linked.
[b]See Appendix A.7 for gene symbols and names.
[c]Associated with learning disabilities.
Sources: Clarke, 2006; GeneReviews, 2009; OMIM, 2009; Sedel et al., 2007.

The prevalence of schizophrenia differs around the world and may reflect variations in culture, gene pools, and diagnostic practice (Kinney, 2007). The overall lifetime prevalence is usually quoted as between 0.1% and 1% (Kinney, 2007). There are several known genetic disorders to consider when there is a family history of schizophrenic-like symptoms (see Table 4.22). The 22q11.2 deletion syndrome is estimated to affect just under 2% of persons with schizophrenia (Firth and Hurst, 2005). Two rare but treatable metabolic disorders are autosomal recessive Wilson disease and autosomal dominant acute intermittent porphyria. Hartnup disorder is an autosomal recessive inborn error of metabolism (characterized by light-sensitive skin changes similar to the rash of pellagra) and associated with cerebellar ataxia and episodic psychotic features. Expression seems to be associated with dietary factors and is treatable with oral nicotinamide (Sybert, 2010). Nonhereditary causes of schizophrenic-like disorders include brain injury or malformation (e.g., physical trauma, brain tumor, embolism, or ischemia), viral encephalitis, syphilis, chronic alcoholism, drug abuse (particularly cocaine, crack, LSD, PCP, or amphetamines), and metabolic/systemic disease (e.g., hypoglycemia, vitamin B_{12} deficiency, systemic lupus erythematous, uremic syndrome, hepatic encephalopathy, pellagra (Kinney, 2007).

Empiric risks for schizophrenia are more complicated because they apply to relatives with chronic schizophrenia and, as noted, affective disorders can be mistaken for schizophrenia, and organic brain disorders can have schizophrenic-like symptoms. The lifetime risk of developing schizophrenia is reduced by half at age 30, and the risk of developing schizophrenia after age 50 is remote. The general empiric risk for relatives of a person with schizophrenia are 2% in a first cousin, 6% in half siblings, 9% in full siblings, 17% in dizygotic twins, and 48% in monozygotic twins (Kinney, 2007).

Obtaining medical-family history information for a psychiatric illness can be challenging. The report of which family members are affected with a psychiatric disorder may differ, depending on which relative is interviewed and the diagnosis. There is a greater problem with underreporting psychiatric illness than overreporting of disease, although the classification of mental illness is often accurate (specificity) (Miline et al., 2008). Miline and colleagues (2008) found that women are more likely to report major depressive episodes, conduct disorders, and alcohol dependency than males and that persons also affected with a mental health disorder are more likely to report accurately major depression, anxiety, schizophrenia, and drug dependence in another affected relative. A major study of twins, one of whom had a history of depression and the other did not, suggested that the twin with the major depression was more likely to report depression in their mother than the twin without major depression (Kendler et al., 1991). Family members may be protective of this private information because of fears of ostracism or feelings of shame. The parents of a person with mental illness may fear their parenting styles caused their child's problems; probing questions may exacerbate their feelings of guilt. A parent with profound mental illness may be a poor historian.

Though it is optimal to review medical records on affected family members, psychiatric records are often difficult to obtain on both living and deceased individuals, despite written permission from the affected person or next-of-kin.

Table 4.23 reviews the family-medical history questions for mental illness.

4.13 DISORDERS INVOLVING THE CARDIAC SYSTEM

4.13.1 Classification of Cardiac Anomalies

Molecular genetic techniques continue to redefine the classifications and methods of evaluating cardiac dysfunction. Heart disease can be broadly classified into structural or nonstructural along the following categories:

I. **Structural Cardiac Disease**
   - *Cardiomyopathies (Diseases of the Heart Muscle)*
     - *Hypertropic (HCM).* Hypertrophic cardiomyopathies are common, affecting approximately 1 in 500 individuals. Most are familial (affecting two or more closely related relatives). There are at least 24 known causative genes that predominantly encode sarcomeric proteins (Cowan et al., 2008). Mutations in *MYH7* and *MYPBC3* occur with the greatest frequency (Cowan et al., 2008).
     - *Dilated (DCM).* Dilated cardiomyopathy is characterized by left ventricular dilatation and impaired systolic function (reduction in the myocardial force of contraction with a left ventricular ejection fraction of less than 50%).

TABLE 4.23   Family Medical-History Queries for Mental Illness

- What is the formal psychiatric diagnosis? (try to obtain medical records)
- At what age did the mental illness and/or behavioral problems begin?
- Any medications?
- Does the person have a history of drug or alcohol abuse?
- Is there anything that may have triggered the problems, such as an illness or surgery, or use of medications, drugs or alcohol? Explain.
- Does the person have other medical problems? In particular, is there a history of:
  - Learning disabilities or intellectual disability? If yes, see Section 4.5.
  - Birth anomalies? (cleft palate and/or congenital heart disease with velocardiofacial or 22q11.2 deletion syndrome)
  - Visual disturbances? (retinitis pigmentosa with Hallervorden-Spatz)
  - Any unusual movements? (e.g., Huntington disease, Wilson disease, Hallervorden-Spatz, FXTAS)
  - Problems with coordination or walking? (several of the ataxias, mitochondrial disorders, inborn errors of metabolism)
  - Seizures? If yes, see Section 4.9.
  - Sun sensitivity (photosensitivity)? (e.g., porphyria, Hartnup disorder)
  - Any unusual lumps? (could be xanthomas)
  - Chronic diarrhea? (Hartnup disorder, Sanfilippo syndrome)
  - Acute abdominal pain? (e.g., porphyria)
- Do any family members have mental illness or other medical problems (as above)?
- Have any family members attempted or committed suicide?
- Are the parents of the individual blood relatives?

- Symptoms can include heart failure, cardiac rhythm and conduction disease, and thromboembolic disease (including stroke).
- The most common environmental or acquired cause is injury from myocardial infarction and related coronary artery disease (referred to as ischemic dilated cardiomyopathy), some of which is due to hereditary factors (Hunt, c04+bib+0052). Other environmental causes include congenital heart disease, valve disease, drug toxicity (anthracyclines are the most common), thyroid disease, inflammatory conditions, myocarditis, chronic hypertension, and effects from radiation treatment (Hershberger et al., 2008).
- The nonacquired forms are called idiopathic cardiomyopathy (IDC); an estimated 20–50% have a genetic basis (Hershberger et al., 2008). At least 25–50% are suspected to be inherited, and most of these are autosomal dominant (90%) or X-linked, but autosomal recessive and mitochondrial forms exist. Mutations in over 20 different genes are associated with familial dilated cardiomyopathy (Nauman et al., 2008). Mutation in myosin-7 (*MYH7*) seems to be the most common autosomal dominant form of familial hypertrophic cardiomyopathy (accounting for an estimated 4% of familial dilated cardiomyooathy.

- Dilated cardiomyopathy can be associated with myopathy including the X-linked diseases Duchenne-Becker muscular dystrophy (with mutation in DMD), Emery-Dreifuss muscular dystrophy with mutations in *LMNA* and defect in the LMNA protein (autosomal dominant) or *EMD* with defect in the emerin protein (X-linked). Mutations in LMN account for an estimated 6% of familial dilated cardiomyopathy and should be considered in individuals with dilated cardiomyopathy and prominent conduction system disease (Cowan et al., 2008). Mutations in *TNNT2* are thought to account for 3% of idiopathic dilated cardiomyopathy (Cowan et al., 2008).
- *Arrhythmogenic right ventricular dysplasia/cardiomopathy (ARVD/C).* About 30–50% of persons with ARVD/C have a family history of the condition. At least 7 different genes have been identified; these are usually autosomal dominant, autosomal recessive (homozygote or double heterozygote), or compound heterozygotes. The most common mutations seem to be in *DSP*, *PKP2*, *DSG2* and *TGFB3* (Cowan et al., 2008)
- *Restrictive (RCM).* It is debatable whether this truly represents a distinct category of cardiomyopathy, and how RCM is distinguished from endocardial fibroelastosis is unclear. Heterozygous mutations in Desmin, Lamin A/C, and troponin can cause familial RCM. Late-onset amyloid cardiomyopathy in African Americans is often due to mutations in the gene encoding transthyretin (*TTR*).
- **Congenital Heart Defects (e.g., 22q11.2 Deletion Syndrome, Holt Oram Syndrome, Down Syndrome)**
- **Aneurysms.** An estimated 10–20% of aneurysms have a genetic predisposition. Marfan syndrome, polycystic kidney disease, vascular type (IV) Ehlers-Danlos syndrome, Loeys-Dietz syndrome (TGF-β receptor) (all autosomal dominant), and α-1-antitrypsin deficiency (autosomal recessive), should be considered if there is a history of familial aneurysms.
- **Valve defects.** For example, mitral valve prolapse, bicuspid aortic valve.

II. **Nonstructural Cardiac Disease**
- **Cardiac Conduction Defects/Channelopathies.** Diseases of heart rhythm, such as primary long QT syndrome (multiple autosomal dominant and recessive forms with reduced penetrance) and autosomal recessive Jervell-Lange-Nielsen syndrome associated with long QT and sensorineural deafness (mutations in *KCNQ1* and *KCNE1*); Brugada syndrome (autosomal dominant with reduced penetrance with onset usually in the 3rd decade and typical electrocardiogram of P-R prolongation and ST elevation, 15–20% have *SCN5A* mutations); short QT, which is characterized by sudden death, syncope, and atrial arrhythmia (particularly atrial fibrillation), mutations in *KCNH2*, *KCNQ1*, *KCNJ2*; and catecholaminergic ventricular tachycardia (CPVT; cardiac electrical instability induced by physical exercise or intense emotion that may present as syncope in childhood). Most are autosomal dominant, with over half having mutations in the ryanodine receptor (*RYR2*). Mutations in the *CASQ2* gene account for a rare autosomal recessive form.

• **Dyslipoproteinemias.** Associated with abnormalities in the metabolism of plasma lipoproteins and their associated apoproteins, which in turn significantly increase the risk of atherosclerosis and coronary artery disease. They are among the most common genetic disorders in Westernized countries, and they are inherited in an autosomal dominant pattern.

4.13.2   The Approach to Family History of Cardiac Disease

The person giving you his or her family history is unlikely to separate a relative's heart disease into distinct categories as outlined above. Obtaining medical records—such as echocardiograms (an ultrasound of the heart), electrocardiogram reports (cardiac rhythm studies), studies of vascular function, surgical reports, and pathological reports from surgical specimens, cardiac and muscle biopsies, plasma lipoprotein and apopotein studies, creatine kinase levels, molecular analysis, and autopsy reports—is essential for genetic diagnosis and risk assessment.

The important aspects to document in the medical family history with regard to heart disease are outlined in Table 4.24. When there is a family history of a congenital heart defect, the family history queries are similar to as for other congenital anomalies (as outlined in Section 4.2 and Table 4.4). Cardiomyopathies that present before the age of 4 years are often due to mitochondrial disorders or inborn errors of metabolism (particularly storage disorders), which are inherited in an autosomal recessive or X-linked pattern (Clarke, 2006). Family history features suggesting a mitochondrial disorder or inborn error of metabolism are reviewed in Table 2.5, 2.6, and 4.12, respectively. Clarke (2006) provides a concise discussion of several of the inherited metabolic disorders in which cardiomyopathies are a prominent feature.

4.14   CHRONIC RESPIRATORY DISEASE

Hereditary influences on common respiratory conditions (such as asthma) are just beginning to be elucidated. It is likely that several genes are involved with gene expression influenced by environmental exposures to allergens, air pollutants, and smoking. The major single-gene contributors to respiratory disease are cystic fibrosis and α-1-antitrypsin deficiency (both autosomal recessive disorders). Chronic sinopulonary infections can be seen in individuals with primary ciliary dyskinesia (immotile cilia syndrome or Kartagener syndrome), Young syndrome, and cystic fibrosis (all are autosomal recessive). The carrier frequency of cystic fibrosis is high enough in some ethnic populations that it is not unusual to see cystic fibrosis occur in more distantly related relatives (for example, a cousin, niece or nephew to a person with cystic fibrosis).

Idiopathic pulmonary fibrosis (IPF) is a relatively rare condition. About 10% of persons with familial IPF have mutations in *SFTPC*, *TERT,* or *TERC* (all autosomal dominant with reduced penetrance) (Wise and Scwartz, 2007).

Pulmonary arterial hypertension (PAH) can present with shortness of breath, chest pain, and fatigue. Mutations in *BMPR2* have been identified as a cause of PAH.

TABLE 4.24 Medical-Family History Questions for Cardiac Disease[a]

Note that the noncardiac findings in the person and his or her relatives can be some of the most informative diagnostic clues.

Information on person with cardiac disease:
- What is the nature of the heart disease?
  - Enlarged heart
    - Hypertropic cardiomyopathy (HCM)
    - Dilated cardiomyopathy (DCM)
  - Heart rhythm problems
    - Long QT syndrome (LQTS; heterogenous, AD)
    - Short QT syndrome, Brugada syndrome (AD)
    - Anderson Tawil syndrome (ATS; AD)
    - Catechoalminergic polymorphic ventricular tachycardia (CPVT; AD)
    - Arrthymogenic right ventrical cardiomyopathy (ARVC; heterogeneous, AD)
    - Jervell and Lange Nielsen syndrome (AR)
  - Aortic rupture
    - Marfan syndrome (AD)
    - Loeys-Dietz syndrome (AD)
    - Ehlers-Danlos syndrome, vascular type (AD)
- At what age was the heart disease diagnosed?
  - Cardiomyopathies in an infant are more likely to have a mitochondrial, autosomal recessive (AR), or X-linked (XL) etiology.
  - Autosomal dominant inheritance (AD) inheritance is more common with cardiomyopathies with later age of onset.
  - Cardiac arrhythmias in infants may be a sign of a severe fatty oxidation defect.
- Is the person living or deceased?
- If deceased, was an autopsy done? (obtain report)
- Was the heart disease of sudden onset or had the heart disease been diagnosed for a long time?
- Was there anything that might have triggered the cardiac event (athletic activity, swimming, medications)?
- Has the person ever fainted or passed out during or after exercise, when startled, or during an emotional or stressful situation?
- Did the problems occur during or after a pregnancy?
- Did (does) the person have a history of high blood pressure?
- Did (does) the person use alcohol? Tobacco? How heavily?
- Is/was the person overweight?
- Do you know what medications the person takes/took?
- Do you know what medical/diagnostic studies have been done? Obtain reports of studies such as echocardiograms, exercise tolerance tests, lipid panels, creatine kinase (CK), angiography, cardioversion, and heart and/or muscle biopsies.
- What surgeries (cardiovascular or otherwise) have been performed? (obtain surgical and pathology reports)
- Does the person have other medical problems? (explain)
- Did (does) the person have a history of any chronic infections or autoimmune disease? (seen in Barth syndrome)
- Were there any complications after the birth of this individual, such as floppiness? (hypotonia)

(Continued)

TABLE 4.24   *(Continued)*

Information on person with cardiovascular disease and relatives

- Any history of stroke? If yes, what was the age at onset? (see Section 4.10)
- Any history of sudden death? If yes, what was the age at death? Obtain pathology reports.
- Is there a history of neuromuscular disease? Cardiomyopathy is a component of several neuromuscular disorders such as myotonic muscular dystrophy (AD), Friedreich ataxia (AR), Duchenne-Becker and Emery-Dreifuss muscular dystrophy (both XL), the limb girdle muscular dystrophies (AD, AR), and mitochondrial disorders (such as Kearns-Sayre syndrome, MELAS and MERRF).
- Is there a history of periodic muscle weakness? Periodic paralysis with long QT syndrome seen in Andersen-Tawil syndrome.
- Any history of seizures? (see Section 4.9)
- Any history of hearing loss? Jervell-Lange-Nielsen syndrome, multiple lentigines syndrome (AD), and some of the mitochondrial disorders are associated with hearing loss (see Section 4.3).
- Any history of blood disorders? Neutropenia is seen in Barth syndrome (XL).
- Any unusual skin findings?
  - Xanthomas in many of the dislipoproteinemias
  - Angiokeratomas and restrictive cardiomyopathy in Fabry disease (XL)
  - "Bronze skin" and restrictive cardiomopathy in untreated hemochromatosis (AR)
  - Palmoplantar keratoderma, wooly hair, and ARVC with biventricular cardiomyopathy in Naxos disease (AR)
  - Fragile, translucent, hyperelastic skin in vascular Ehlers-Danlos syndrome (type IV)
  - Velvety, translucent skin, wide and atrophic scars in Loeys-Dietz syndrome
  - Peau d'orange skin in pseudoxanthoma elasticum (AR)
- Any history of unusual bruising? Can be seen in vascular Ehlers-Danlos (type IV-vascular) and Loeys-Dietz syndrome
- Anyone with problems with healing? Can be seen in vascular Ehlers-Danlos (type IV) and Loeys-Dietz syndrome
- Any history of loose or hyperextensible joints? Can be seen in connective tissue disorders such as vascular Ehlers-Danlos syndrome (type IV) and Marfan syndrome
- Anyone unusually tall or short compared to their family?
  - Routinely inquire about parental and sibling heights.
    - Marfan syndrome and homocystinuria (AR) are associated with tall stature.
    - Turner syndrome (CH), Noonan syndrome (AD), Barth syndrome, and Andersen-Tawil syndrome are associated with short stature.
- Is there a history of scoliosis (curvature of the spine)? Can be seen in connective tissue disorders and neuromuscular diseases
- Does anyone have an unusually shaped chest? Pectus excavatum and pectus carinatum can be seen in Marfan syndrome and Loeys-Dietz syndrome
- Anyone with unusually long fingers or toes (arachnodactyly)? Can be seen in Marfan syndrome and Loeys-Dietz syndrome
- Is there anything unusual about the way the person looks? Dilated cardiomyopathy is associated with Noonan syndrome; Timothy syndrome is a rare AR associated with long-QT syndrome, syndactyly, mild facial dysmorphism, congenital heart disease, hypoglycemia, cognitive abnormalities, and autism; Andersen-Tawil is a rare condition associated with long QT syndrome, mild dysmorphic features, and periodic paralysis; craniosynostosis and hypertelorism can be seen in Loeys-Dietz syndrome

TABLE 4.24   *(Continued)*

- Is there a history of cleft palate? Can be seen in Loeys-Dietz syndrome. If bifid uvula consider Loeys-Dietz
- Are there any unusual dental findings? Multiple missing teeth (oligodontia) and persistent primary dentition seen in Andersen-Tawil syndrome; crowded teeth and high palate seen in Marfan syndrome and Loeys-Dietz syndrome
- Is there a family history of learning disabilities or intellectual disability? Myotonic dystrophy, Noonan syndrome, Danon disease, Timothy syndrome, Andersen-Tawil syndrome, lysosomal storage disorders, and homocystinuria are associated with learning disabilities.
- Is there a history of spontaneous pneumothorax? Can be seen in Marfan syndrome
- Is there a history of chronic disease in the person or other family members? Note in particular a history of diabetes, kidney disease, liver disease, and thyroid disease. Renal disease is associated with Fabry disease
- Is there a family history of pregnancy loss, stillborns, sudden infant death syndrome (SIDS), or early childhood deaths? (see Section 4.19)
- Are the parents related as blood relatives?

[a]Abbreviations: AD = autosomal dominant, AR = autosomal recessive, XL = X-linked. See Appendix A.7 for gene symbols and names.
Sources: Clarke, 2006; Firth and Hurst, 2005; Nauman et al., 2008.

Surfactant dysfunction has been recognized as a cause of severe neonatal respiratory distress. Several genes seem to play a role, including *SFTPB*, *SFTPC*, and *ABCA3* (Deterding and Fan, 2005).

An approach to directed medical-family history queries for chronic respiratory disease is shown in Table 4.25.

4.15   RENAL DISEASE

A primary genetic or developmental kidney disorders is identified in at least 10% of adults with renal disease and a higher proportion of pediatric patients (Lifton et al., 2009). Hereditary renal disorders can be divided into six general categories (Lifton et al., 2009).

1. **Malformations of the kidney and urinary tract.** There are several hundred syndromes and single-gene disorders involved in congenital structural disorders of the kidney, urinary tract, and valves (Casas et al., 2007). Approximately 35% of individuals with chromosomal disorders have renal anomalies (Casas et al., 2007). Teratogens known to affect the development of the kidney and ureter include alcohol, alkylating agents, angiotensin-converting enzyme inhibitors, cocaine, maternal diabetes, rubella, thalidomide, trimethadione, and vitamin A derivatives (Casas et al., 2007).
2. **Cystic disease of the kidney**. Kidney cysts (often congenital) are a component of several hereditary syndromes. Multiple renal cysts are associated with single-gene disorders, chromosome anomalies, maternal alcohol use, uncontrolled

TABLE 4.25 Medical-Family History Questions for Chronic Respiratory Disease[a]

- Has the individual had respiratory problems from birth? If not, at what age did the respiratory problems begin?
- Does this person smoke cigarettes, or has he or she smoked cigarettes in the past? How many packs per day and for how long?
- If the person is a nonsmoker, has he or she been exposed to secondhand smoke?
- What is this person's occupation? Could the lung disease be related to occupational exposure? (e.g., silica, asbestos, heavy metals, wood and metal dust, moldy foliage, etc.)
- What studies have been done? Obtain medical records, including:
  - Chest X-rays/lung imaging studies
  - Pulmonary function studies
  - Sinus radiographs (X-rays and/or CT scans)
  - Sweat chloride studies for (CF diagnosis)
  - Bronchoscopy
    - Biopsy and electron microscopy of respiratory epithelium
  - Hearing evaluation (if chronic otitis media)
  - Measurement of serum concentrations of α-1-antitrypsin
- DNA testing (obtain the actual lab results, especially for CF because laboratories use different mutation panels)
- Does the person have a history of fatty, foul-smelling stools? (seen in CF)
- What types of medical interventions have been done? Has the individual had any hospitalizations? Any surgeries?
- Does the individual or any relatives have a history of[b]:
  - Neonatal respiratory distress? (CF, PCD, surfactant dysfunction)
  - Chronic sinusitis? (CF, PCD, Young syndrome)
  - Chronic nasal congestion? (CF, PCD, Young syndrome)
  - Chronic cough? (common in most respiratory syndromes)
  - Emphysema? (AATD)
  - Pulmonary fibrosis? (IPF)
  - Chronic infections (respiratory and/or otitis media)?
  - Nasal polyps? (can be seen in CF, Young syndrome, and PCD)
  - Problems with the ability to smell? (anosmia in PCD)
  - Liver disease? (CF; cirrhosis and fibrosis of the liver can be seen in AATD)
  - Pancreatic disease? (CF)
  - Gastrointestinal disease? (CF)
  - Are there abnormalities in the placement of organs or missing organs?
    - Situs inversus totalis in PCD (mirror image reversal of all visceral organs)
    - Heterotaxy in PCD (situs ambiguous)
    - Asplenia in PCD
  - Congenital heart malformations?
    - Associated with heterotaxy in PCD (e.g., atrial isomerism, transposition of great vessels, double outlet right ventricle, anomalous venous return, interrupted inferior vena cava, bilateral superior vena cava)

TABLE 4.25   *(Continued)*

- Has this person had problems conceiving a pregnancy or have relatives (particularly siblings) had infertility?
  - Obtain reports of semen analysis
    - Azoospermia can be seen in CF (congenital absence of the vas deferens) and Young syndrome (epididymal obstruction)
    - Immotile sperm and cilia with absent or abnormal dynein arms of sperm in PCD
- What is the person's ethnic origin?
  - AATD is rare in persons of Asian or African American ancestry
  - The frequency of (*CFTR*) mutations varies widely based on ethnicity. Knowing the family ancestry can help the clinician interpret DNA testing
- Are the persons related as cousins or more closely related? (suggests autosomal recessive inheritance)

---

[a]Abbreviations: AATD = α-1-antitrypsin deficiency; CF = cystic fibrosis; IPF = idiopathic pulmonary fibrosis; PCD = primary ciliary dyskinesia (Kartagener syndrome). See Appendix A.7 for gene symbols and names.
[b]Note age that symptoms began or age at diagnosis.
Sources: Zariwala et al., 2008; Zhu et al., 2006.

maternal diabetes, and fetal rubella. In adults, autosomal dominant polycystic kidney disease, tuberous sclerosis complex, von Hippel-Lindau disease, and Birt-Hogg-Dubé should be considered (all autosomal dominant conditions with variable expressivity).

3. **Glomerular disorders**

   Congenital nephrosis (nephritic syndrome) (AR)

   Renal amyloidosis (AD)

   Hereditary nephritis. The most common cause of inherited nephritis is *Alport syndrome* (a heterogenous group of disorders, characterized by sensorineural hearing loss with renal diseases that are inherited in AD, AR, and XL patterns).

   Nail-patella syndrome (onchyo-osteodysplasia) (AD)

   Uremic syndromes

4. **Tubular disorders**

   Nephrogenic diabetes insipidus (NDI) (usually X-linked with females often being symptomatic, rarely autosomal recessive)

   Renal tubular acidosis (RTA) (with the exception of Wilson disease, RTA is rarely the presenting feature in persons with an inherited cause of RTA); examples of inborn errors of metabolism with RTA include (Clarke, 2006):

   Carnitine palmitoyl transferase 1 (AR)

   Cystinosis (AR)

   Cytochrome-c-oxidase deficiency (congenital lactic acidosis) (AR)

   Galactosemia (AR)

   Hereditary fructose intolerance (AR)

   Hypophosphatemic rickets (XL with expression in females)

   Lowe syndrome (XL)

   Pyruvate carboxylase deficiency (AR)

    Tyrosinemia (hepatorenal) (AR)
    Wilson disease (AR)
5. **Inborn errors of metabolism**
    Fabry disease (XL condition resulting in renal failure from glycosphingolipid deposition)
    Glutaric academia type II (multiple acyl-CoA-dehydrogenase deficiency)
    Certain *hereditary amyloidoses* (heterogeneous group of disorders all inherited as autosomal dominant disorders)
    Sickle cell disease (AR)
    Peroxisomal disorders (AR or XL) (e.g., Zellweger syndrome spectrum)
6. **Phakomatoses and kidney cancers**
    Tuberous sclerosis complex (AD; with shagreen patches, angiomas, ashleaf spots, cortical tubers, renal cell cancer)
    Von Hippel-Lindau syndrome (AD; with hemangioblastomas and kidney cancer)
    Birt-Hogg-Dubé (AD; with achrocordons, trichodiscomas, spontaneous pneumothorax and kidney cancer)

A general approach to medical-family history queries for renal disorders is shown in Table 4.26.

4.16 SKELETAL ANOMALIES AND DISORDERS OF SHORT STATURE

Good things come in small packages.

                              —My mother

The determinism of what is normal or aberrant when it comes to measuring stature depends on ethnic, familial, and nutritional variables. If, in evaluating a family history, there is concern about a relative with seemingly unusual stature, obtaining growth curves (if available) on the relative is important. Is this person growing along his or her own curve or does growth seem to have reached a plateau? Documenting parental, grandparental, and sibling heights is also useful. Obtaining the radiographic reports and films, including the bone age, is imperative; the radiographic findings are usually essential for making a diagnosis. An excellent review of the radiographic findings in skeletal dysplasias can be found in *Taybi and Lachman's Radiology of Syndromes, Metabolic Disorders and Skeletal Dysplasias* (Lachman, 2006).

For individual with short stature, the first step is determining whether it is proportionate or disproportionate short stature. Person with disproportionate short stature usually have an inherited skeletal dysplasia or metabolic bone disease. As shown in Table 4.27, individuals with proportionate short stature may have a more generalized disorder attributed to factors such as malnutrition, chronic disease (particularly renal disease), a malabsorption disorder, endocrine/metabolic disorders, a genetic or chromosomal syndrome, or a teratogenic exposure (Graham and Rimoin, 2007). If possible, obtain actual measurements of upper to lower body segment ratio, arm

TABLE 4.26   Medical-Family History Queries for Renal Disorders[a]

Prenatal history
- Was there anything unusual about the prenatal history of the individual? (for example oligohydramnios)
- Did this person's mother
  - Use alcohol during the pregnancy? If so, when during the pregnancy, how often and how much?
  - Use cocaine during the pregnancy? If so, when and how often?
  - Have diabetes during the pregnancy?
  - Take any medications during the pregnancy? (especially vitamin A congeners, trimethadione)
  - Have any infections during the pregnancy?
  - Have any testing done in the pregnancy? (such as maternal-fetal marker screening or fetal chromosome studies)

Individual's medical history
- What was the age of onset of the renal disorder?
- What studies have been done? (obtain documentation of renal function studies, abdominal imaging studies, biopsies)
- Does (did) the individual drink alcohol? How much?
- Were there any anomalies noted at birth or shortly thereafter? (e.g., microcephaly, cleft lip/palate, heart defects, neural tube defects, hand and feet anomalies, limb anomalies, skeletal anomalies)
- What is the person's occupation? Could this be a toxic exposure such as lead poisoning leading to renal tubular acidosis?

Individual and family history questions
- What is the individual's height? What are the heights of the parents and sibling?
- Do any of the relatives have high blood pressure?
- Have other family members had testing, such as renal testing on the parents or siblings?

Does this individual or other relatives have other medical conditions, such as
- Learning or intellectual disabilities? If yes, see Section 4.5.
- Any unusual birth marks or skin findings? (Fabry disease, tuberous sclerosis complex, Birt-Hogg-Dubé)
- Anything unusual about the shape of the hands or feet or the nails? (periungual fibromas in tuberous sclerosis complex; nail hypoplasia in nail-patella syndrome)
- Hearing loss? (Commonly seen in many of the inherited renal syndromes; two of the more common syndromes with hearing loss and renal anomalies are branchio-oto-renal syndrome and Alport syndrome; see Section 4.3)
- Unusually shaped ears?
- Preauricular pits? (branchio-oto-renal syndrome)
- Ear tags?
- Eye/visual disorders? (see Section 4.4)
  - Retinal disease common? (e.g., Bardet-Biedel syndrome)
  - Aniridia? (absence of the iris is associated with Wilms tumor syndromes)
  - Coloboma? (seen in several of the chromosomal syndromes and multiple congenital anomaly syndromes)

(Continued)

TABLE 4.26   (Continued)

- Retinal angiomas? (von Hippel-Lindau disease)
- Early-onset cataracts? (galactosemia, Zellweger syndrome spectrum, rhizomelic chondrodysplasia, Smith-Lemli-Opitz syndrome, Wilson syndrome, Alport syndrome; see Tables 4.10 and 4.11)
- Lenticular opacities? (spoke-like, characteristic of Fabry disease)
- Amyloid deposits? (in some of the hereditary amyloidoses)
- Kaiser-Fleischer rings? (Wilson disease)
- Dark "cloverleaf" pigmentation at inner margin of iridses? (nail-patella syndrome)
- Cardiac disease, particularly cardiomyopathies? (see Section 4.13)
- Neurological disease, particularly seizures? (see Sections 4.8 and 4.9)
- Skeletal anomalies? (several skeletal dysplasias are associated with renal disorders; see Section 4.15
- Genital anomalies or ambiguous genitalia?
- Cancer? (particularly renal cell cancer, which can occur in tuberous sclerosis complex, von Hippel-Lindau disease, Birt-Hogg-Dubé; see Chapter 5)

General questions
- What is the family ethnic background? (this information can be particularly helpful in interpreting molecular genetic testing)
- Are the parents related as first cousins or closer? (suggests autosomal recessive inheritance)

[a]See Appendix A.7 for gene symbols, names, and patterns of inheritance.
Sources: Casas et al., 2007; Clarke, 2006; Lifton et al., 2009; Saudubray and Charpentier, 2001.

length, and sitting height rather than relying on a visual estimate; minor skeletal dysplasias such as hypochondroplasia are easy to miss (Graham and Rimoin, 2007).

The medical-family history questions to be asked when an individual has short stature are reviewed in Table 4.28. Medical-family history features of inherited metabolic disorders are reviewed in Table 4.12, and the features of chromosomal disorders, in Table 3.2. In taking a family history, do not use the antiquated terms *dwarf* in reference to an individual with disproportionate short stature) and *midget* (in reference to persons with proportionate short stature).

4.17   DIABETES

Diabetes mellitus is a term applied to a group of disorders that share glucose intolerance (Raffel et al., 2007). There are more than 75 syndromes associated with type 1 (insulin-dependent diabetes mellitus) and type 2 (non-insulin-dependent diabetes mellitus). Type 2 diabetes is distinguished by adult onset (usually after age 40 years), is associated with obesity, and is initially managed with oral medication and/or diet. Type 1 diabetes usually has onset in childhood or young adulthood, and individuals require insulin for survival.

There is a distinct form of non-insulin-dependent diabetes referred to as MODY (maturity onset diabetes of the young). MODY is the cause of glucose intolerance in 2–5% of people with type 2 diabetes (Raffel et al., 2007); it is not associated with

TABLE 4.27 Common Causes of Proportionate Short Stature[a]

Prenatal onset (intrauterine growth retardation IUGR)

Familial short stature (most common reason)
Constriction of fetal movement (i.e., from lack of amniotic fluid, multiple gestations, uterine
    anomalies)
Maternal infections (e.g., cytomegalovirus, rubella, varicella, syphilis, toxoplasmosis)
Placental insufficiency
Teratogenic exposures (e.g., alcohol, cocaine, heroin, hydantoin, trimethadione, warfarin)
Chromosomal anomalies (most common are Turner syndrome, trisomies 13 and 18, Down
    syndrome)
Dysmorphic genetic syndromes (many have cognitive delay or learning disabilities)

Examples[b]	*Inheritance Pattern*
Aarskog syndrome	XL
Bloom syndrome	AR
Cocakyne syndrome B (II)	AR
Dubowitz syndrome	AR
de Lange syndrome	AD, XL (mostly de novo)
Fanconi pancytopenia syndrome	multiple syndromes (AR)
Floating-Harbor syndrome	AD (usually new mutation)
Leri-Weill dyschondrosteosis	del, pseudoautosomal dominant
Noonan syndrome	AD
Opitz syndrome	AD
Pseudohypoparathyroidism (PHP1A)/ Albright hereditary osteodystrophy	AD, IMP mat
Pseudopseudohypoparathyroidism	AD, IMP pat
Rubinstein-Taybi syndromeb	AD, usually de novo del
Silver-Russell syndrome	usually sporadic, UPD chromosome 7, heterogeneous
Smith-Lemli-Opitz syndrome	AR
Williams syndrome	del
Xeroderma pigmentosum	AR, multiple loci

Postnatal onset

Familial short stature (most common reason)
Chronic malnutrition
Chronic childhood diseases (genetic and nongenetic)
    Cardiac (e.g., congenital heart disease)
    Gastrointestinal
    Renal
    Hematological (e.g., hemgloinopathies)
    Neurological
Chronic infections
Drug effects
Endocrine disorders
Psychosocial/emotional disturbances

Abbreviations: [a]XL = X-linked; AR = autosomal recessive; IM = imprinting; AD = autosomal dominant; del = microdeletion; UPD = uniparental disony.
[b]See Appendix A.7 for gene symbols and names.
Sources: Firth and Hurst, 2005; Graham and Rimoin, 2007.

TABLE 4.28 Medical-Family History Questions for Short Stature or Skeletal Dysplasias

Pregnancy history
- During her pregnancy, did this individual's mother have
  - Diabetes?
  - High fevers? If yes, at what stages in pregnancy?
  - Any infections? Explain.
  - Any prenatal testing particularly ultrasounds documenting fetal growth?

General family history questions
- What are the parental heights and the heights of the siblings? (Ideally, the parents should be examined for dysmorphic features and for anomalies, particularly of their hands and feet.)
- What is the family's country of origin?
- Are the parents related as first cousins, or more closely related?
- Is there a history of miscarriages, stillbirths, or babies who died?

Information on the individual
- Obtain documentation of a full set of skeletal X-rays (including skull, spine, limbs, pelvis, hands, feet, and bone age).
- Obtain the childhood growth charts.
- What is the individuals' present height? (Document upper to lower segment ratio, sitting height, and arm span.)
- What studies have been done? (e.g., skeletal survey, bone age, cytogenetics, CGH, growth hormone assays, thyroid studies, studies for inborn errors of metabolism)
- Is the person with short stature proportionate?
- If not, does the person with disproportionate short statue have
  - Short limbs?
  - Rhizomelic shortening? (proximal limb: humerus/femur)
  - Mesomelic shortening? (forelimb: radius and ulna; tibia and fibula)
  - Misshapen limbs? (bowing, talipes, Madelung deformity)
  - A short trunk?
- Was the short stature evident at birth? Or, did it develop during the 1st year of life, or later?
- Are there any prenatal ultrasounds documenting growth abnormalities?

Does the person or relatives have:
- Intellectual disability (mental retardation) or learning disabilities? If yes, is it progressive or nonprogressive? (see Section 4.5)
- A large or small head?
- An unusually shaped head?
- Unusual shape to face? (triangular in Silver-Russell syndrome)
- Dysmorphic facial features? With particular focus on:
  - Unusual placement/shape of eyes?
  - Synophrys? (common in mucopolysacchairde storage disorders, de Lange syndrome)
  - Unusual shape of nose?
  - Unusual shape/placement of ears?
  - Flat philtrum? (common in fetal alcohol syndrome, de Lange syndrome)
  - Coarsening of facial features? (common lysosomal storage disorders
- Problems with hearing loss? (See Section 4.3)
- Problems with vision? (See Section 4.4)

TABLE 4.28 *(Continued)*

- Congenital or juvenile cataracts? (e.g., Cocakyne syndrome, Smith-Lemli-Opitz syndrome; see Tables 4.10 and 4.11)
- Blue sclerae? (e.g., osteogenesis imperfecta, Hallerman-Streiff syndrome)
- Problems with the oral cavity? (mouth/dentition)
- Cleft lip/palate? (e.g., chondroectodermal dysplasia)
- Cleft plate? (common in Kniest dysplasia, spondyloepiphyseal dysplasia congenital, diastrophic dysplasia)
- Hair anomalies?
  - Hirsuitism? (common in de Lange syndrome, mucopolysaccharidoses, Rubinstein-Taybi syndrome)
  - Sparse? (seen in Dubowitz syndrome)
  - Low posterior hairline? (common in Noonan and Turner syndromes)
- Hand/nail anomalies?
  - Brachydactyly? (common in several short stature syndromes, including Aarskog syndrome)
  - Postaxial polydactyly? (common in chondroectrodermal dysplasia, lethal short-rib polydactyly syndromes, asphyxiating thoracic dysplasia)
  - Preaxial polydactyly? (maternal diabetes, atelosteogenesis)
  - Nail anomalies? (hypoplastic in chodroectodermal dysplasia; hypoplastic or absent in sclerosteosis/Van Buchem disease, and Fanconi pancytopenia syndrome; short/broad in cartilage-hair hypoplasia/McKusick type of metaphyseal dysplasia)
  - Broad thumbs? (e.g., Rubinstein-Taybi syndrome)
- Feet anomalies?
- Clubfeet? (e.g. spondyloepiphyseal dysplasia congenital, trisomy 18, diastrophic dysplasia)
- Skeletal involvement? (Obtain all skeletal films)
- Congenital dislocations or frequent posnatal dislocations?
- Multiple fractures? Note age at onset, and bones involved (e.g., osteogenesis imperfecta, congenital osteopetrosis, hypophsphastaisia; ostepetrotic syndrome in older individuals with fractures)
- Scoliosis?
- Pectus deformities?
- Limb anomalies? (common in many syndromes)
- Arthrogryposis (congenital contractures)? (seen in more than 120 syndromes, AD, AR, XL, and chromosomal and can also be attributed to maternal hyperthermia and infections)
- Unusual birth marks, rashes, or pigmentation? (common in Bloom syndrome, Fanconi pancytopenia syndrome)
- Congenital heart defects? (common in Turner syndrome, Noonan syndrome, William syndrome, chondroectodermal dysplasia)
- Genital anomalies?
- Cryptorchidism? (e.g., Smith-Lemli-Opitz syndrome)
- Hypospadias? (e.g., Smith-Lemli-Opitz syndrome, Opitz syndrome, Dubowitz syndrome, de Lange syndrome, Fanconi pancytopenia syndrome)
- Small genitalia? (e.g., Noonan syndrome, Robinow syndrome)
- "Shawl" scrotum? (common in Aarskog syndrome)

(Continued)

TABLE 4.28 *(Continued)*

- Infertility? (see Section 4.18)
- Seizures? (see Section 4.9)
- Renal anomalies? (see Section 4.15)
- Diabetes? (see Section 4.17)
- Obesity? (seen in pseudohypoparathyroidism and pseudopseudohypoparathyroidism)

[a]See Appendix A.7 for gene symbols, names, and patterns of inheritance.
Sources: Firth and Hurst, 2006; Graham and Rimoin, 2007.

obesity and usually has age of onset before age 25. There are at least six genes with mutations inherited in an autosomal dominant pattern associated with MODY (Firth and Hurst, 2005):

- MODY1 with mutations in *HNF4A* (accounts for a small proportion of families with MODY)
- MODY2 with mutations in glucokinase (*GCK*)
- MODY3 with mutations in *HNF1A*; over two thirds of persons with MODY have a mutation in this gene.
- MODY4 with mutations in *PDX1* (formerly called *IPF1*)
- MODY5 with mutations in *HNF1B*; associated with renal cysts that can occur in utero, early-onset type 2 diabetes, genital tract malformation/Müllerian aplasia, hyperuricaemia, and early-onset gout
- MODY6 with mutations in *NEUROD1* or *BETA2*

Homozygosity for *PDX1* results in nenonatal diabetes with pancreatic apalasia. Heterozygotes for glucokinase mutations usually have glucose intolerance or mild diabetes, but homozygotes have permanent nenonatal diabetes requiring insulin therapy (Raffel et al., 2007).

Currently, genetic counseling is provided from empirical risk tables. In a given family, the type of diabetes "runs true," meaning that the immediate family members are at increased risk for the specific type of diabetes that has already occurred in a relative. Raffel and colleagues (2007) review the many syndromes associated with diabetes mellitus. In most of these syndromes, diabetes is an important complication to be aware of for management purposes, but diabetes is seldom a presenting sign in the family history. Medical-family history questions for a family history of diabetes are given in Table 4.29.

4.18 MULTIPLE MISCARRIAGES, AND MALE AND FEMALE INFERTILITY

Approximately 10–15% of couples who wish to conceive experience infertility (Chandra and Stephen, 1998). Infertility is commonly defined as lack of conception after 1 year of unprotected intercourse. Infertility is a disease that affects a couple; both partners must be thoroughly evaluated because male and female factors

TABLE 4.29 Medical-Family History Questions for Diabetes Mellitus[a]

* What is the age of onset of diabetes? Are other family members affected?
* How is the diabetes managed? (e.g., with insulin injections; diet with or without oral medications)
* Is the person overweight? (obesity is a major risk factor for type 2 diabetes; severe obesity is associated with Prader-Willi syndrome, Alstrom syndrome, and Bardet-Biedl syndrome)
* Is there normal distribution of body fat? (lipodystrophy syndromes are associated with loss of subcutaneous adipose tissue and can be AD, AR, and nongenetic)
* Does the person have growth failure? (may be due to insulin resistance)
* Does the person use alcohol? How much and how often? (alcohol abuse is a risk factor for type 2 diabetes)
* Does the person have learning disabilities or intellectual disability? If so, are the intellectual ability progressive (regression in skills) or stable?
* Does this person have unusual facial features? (dysmorphic)

Does the person or any relatives have other diseases? Particularly:

* Visual disturbances? If yes, see Section 4.4.
  * Retinitis pigmentosa? (mitochondrial disorders)
  * Opthalmoplegia? (mitochondrial disorders)
  * Optic atrophy? (Wolfram syndrome)
* Ptosis? (can be a feature of muscle weakness and possible sign of myotonic dystrophy, mitochondrial myopathy)
* Hearing loss? If yes, see Section 4.3.
  * The AR Wolfram (DIDMOAD) syndrome is associated with juvenile onset diabetes, optic atrophy, and nerve deafness. It is thought to affect approximately 1 in 150 individuals with type 1 diabetes.
  * Kallmann syndrome is associated with anosmia, hypogonadotropic, hypogonadism, hearing loss, and sometimes cleft lip and palate, and glucose intolerance or type 1 diabetes.
  * Some of the mitochondrial myopathies are associated with diabetes and hearing loss, which usually precedes the diabetes.
* Pancreatic disease? (common in cystic fibrosis and hemochromatosis)
* Pulmonary disease? (e.g., cystic fibrosis, α-1-antitrypsin deficiency)
* Neurological problems? If yes, see Section 4.7.
  * Stroke-like episodes with mitochondrial disorders?
* Neuromuscular disease? (several of the hereditary ataxias, muscular dystrophies, myotonic dystrophy, and mitochondrial myopathies are associated with diabetes)

---

[a]Refer to Appendix A.7 for genetic disorders and patterns of inheritance.
Sources: Arnould-Devuyst et al., 2007; Firth and Hurst, 2005; Raffel et al., 2007; Wallace et al., 2007.

---

contribute almost equally (40% male, 40% female, and 20% both partners) (Layman, 2007). Infertility may also reflect early spontaneous abortion rather than inability to conceive. For as many as 25–30% of couples who undergo a comprehensive fertility evaluation, the cause of their infertility remains unknown. Genetic disorders represent only a small percentage of the causes of infertility. Family history features of multiple miscarriages, and male and female infertility are reviewed in Sections 4.18.1, 14.18.2, and 14.18.3, respectively.

4.18.1 Multiple miscarriages

The risk of miscarriage for any recognized pregnancy is at least 15% and may be at least 50% of all conceptions (Schreck and Silverman, 2007). The term *spontaneous abortion* is used for pregnancy loss up to 20 weeks, and *early pregnancy loss* often refers to pregnancies that are miscarried before 13 weeks. Pregnancy loss after 20 weeks is referred to as *intrauterine fetal death* or *premature delivery*.

A fetal chromosome anomaly is the single most common cause of pregnancy loss, particularly in the first trimester. Any couple who has experienced three or more miscarriages should be evaluated for a chromosome anomaly; the most common chromosome rearrangements are reciprocal or Robertsonian translocations (Schreck and Silverman, 2007). Women who are mosaic for Turner syndrome or who have deletions of the short arm of the X chromosome have an increased risk of miscarriage (Sybert, 2005).

Any maternal condition that decreases utero-placental flow may lead to fetal demise (e.g., hypertension, placental abruption from trauma, autoimmune disorders, diabetes mellitus). Miscarriages are also associated with a few maternal teratogenic agents (Shreck and Silverman, 2007), including:

- Coumarin derivatives (anticoagulants)
- Certain anticonvulsants
- Antineoplastic agents (such as aminopterin and methotrexate)
- Alcohol
- Possibly tobacco use
- Cocaine use
- Retinoids
- Misoprostol
- Organic solvents
- Mercury
- Lead

α-Thalassemia major (autosomal recessive) is an uncommon cause of pregnancy loss (although the carrier rate of α-thalassemia is high in many populations, particularly in Southeast Asia, Southern China, the equatorial belt of Africa, the Middle East, India, and the Mediterranean region). Other single-gene disorders associated with recurrent pregnancy loss are extremely rare. Most are X-linked with male lethality (X-linked dominant)—for example, aicardi syndrome, chondrodysplasia punctata, focal dermal hypoplasia, incontinentia pigmenti, orofacial digital syndrome, and Rett syndrome. With the exception of incontinentia pigmenti, most occur as a new mutation with little chance of recurrence in siblings; therefore, there is usually not a family history suggestive of the disorder.

Couples who have experienced one or more pregnancy losses often experience powerful feelings of grief, depression, shame guilt, anxiety, and distress (Laurino et al., 2005). It is important while taking the medical-family history to hear any theory that the woman or couple has for the cause of their miscarriage. This may be firmly rooted in cultural belief systems and may include notions about angering ancestral spirits, witchcraft, eating forbidden foods, breaking social or religious taboos, family conflicts, and misconduct by the woman or by her partner (Laurino et al., 2005). Being respectful of the client's belief systems while providing any medical explanation will help the client perceive the health professional as compassionate and supportive.

The medical-family history questions in association with a history of multiple miscarriages are reviewed in Table 4.30.

4.18.2 Female Infertility

There seem to be far fewer genetic causes of female infertility than male infertility (Layman, 2007). Causes of female infertility are primarily divided into problems of the hypothalamus, pituitary, gonad, and uterus/vagina (Layman, 2007). The most common causes of female infertility involve ovulatory dysfunction and fallopian tube disease. Müllerian duct anomalies are a rare cause of female infertility. Uterine fibroids may also play a role. Women with hand-foot-genital syndrome with mutations in *HOXA13* can have a bicornate uterus with our without two cervices (this is an extremely rare condition).

Women with structural chromosome anomalies may have difficulty conceiving, and testing for a chromosome rearrangement is a consideration for any woman with a history of infertility (Layman, 2007).

Turner syndrome (45,X) is a rare but important cause of female infertility and is characterized (in adult women) by proportionate short stature, mild dysmorphic features, primary amenorrhea, and failure of secondary sexual development. Women with triple X (47,XXX) may have menstrual irregularities and can have problems with fertility. Women with primary amenorrhea may also have male pseudohermaphroditism (strictly defined as an individual with a Y chromosome whose external genitalia fail to develop as usual for a male) (Simpson, 2007). These individual may be 45, X/46,XY mosaics. Individuals with X-linked androgen insensitivity formerly called testicular feminization (phenotypic females with a 46,XY karyotype) may also present with primary amenorrhea. Women with Kallmann syndrome (KS) can have primary amenorrhea, an arm span greater than height, and anosmia; mutations have been observed in three different autosomal dominant genes (KS2 with mutation in *FGFR1*, KS3 with mutation in *PROKR2*, and KS4 with mutation in *PROK2*). Males with infertility can have an X-linked form (mutations in *KAL1*).

There are rare autosomal recessive mutations known to affect pituitary development and function, but their contribution to female infertility remains unclear (Layman, 2007).

Premutation in the *FMR1* gene is being increasingly recognized as a cause of premature ovarian insufficiency (premature ovarian insufficiency is defined as menopause occurring before age 40) (Wittenberger et al., 2007). *FMR1* premutations have been identified in about 4% of women with sporadic idiopathic premature ovarian insufficiency but in about 12% of families in which there are two or more women with premature ovarian insufficiency (Layman, 2007). There are several other genes that are likely candidates for nonsyndromic premature ovarian insufficiency (Simpson et al., 2008; Zhao et al., 2008).

TABLE 4.30   Medical-Family History Questions Related to Recurrent Miscarriage

Questions specific to the fetal losses
- How many pregnancies have you had?
  - Document the outcome of each pregnancy (miscarriage, full-term live birth, stillbirth), and note if with current partner or with a different partner.
  - Note if partner has had miscarriages with another partner.
  - For miscarriages, note if the pregnancy was documented with a positive pregnancy test and/or fetal ultrasound.
- Were studies done on the fetal tissue? Obtain any chromosome studies/fetal pathology reports.
- Do you know whether the miscarriages were male or female?
  - X-linked male lethal conditions are a rare cause of multiple miscarriages, usually in the third trimester (e.g., incontinentia pigmenti).

Questions specific to the woman
- Do you know if you have any abnormalities of your uterus or cervix? (e.g., fibroids, structural defects)? More likely associated with second- and third-trimester miscarriages.
- Do you have any chronic illnesses?
  - Diabetes?
  - Anemia?
  - Polycystic ovary syndrome?
  - Immune disorders, such as systemic lupus erythematosus?
  - Thalassemia?
  - Thyroid disease? (more often associated with infertility)
- Have any thrombophilia studies been done?
  - Factor V Leiden?
  - Prothrombin G20210A?
  - Antithrombin III deficiency? (if personal or family history of venous thromboembolism)
  - Protein S deficiency? (if personal or family history of venous thromboembolism)
  - Protein C deficiency? (if personal or family history of venous thromboembolism)
- How much alcohol did you drink in the pregnancy? Note amount and timing in pregnancy.
- How much tobacco did you use in the pregnancy? Note number of packs per day (i.e., 20 cigarettes per pack) and timing in pregnancy.
- Did you take any drugs or medications during the pregnancy? (possible association with cocaine usage)
- How tall are you? Women with X chromosome anomalies (Turner syndrome mosaicism, distal deletions of the X chromosome) have a high risk of miscarriage.

Questions for the couple
- Do either of you have any learning disabilities or intellectual disability?
- Do any of your relatives have learning disabilities or intellectual disability?
- Do any close biological relatives (particularly siblings or parents) have a history of:
  - Infertility?
  - Recurrent miscarriage? Note gestation and fetal sex if known.
    - Were chromosome studies done on the fetal tissue?
  - Stillbirth/nenonatal death? Obtain autopsy reports, if available.
  - Deep vein thrombosis (DVT)? (suggests a hereditary thrombophilia)
  - Developmental delay?

TABLE 4.30 *(Continued)*

- Failure to thrive?
- Unusual facial features?
- Problems present at birth, particularly those requiring surgery? (e.g., cleft lip/palate, extra fingers/toes)
- Problems with skin blisters or unusual birth marks/skin pigmentation?
- Patchy or coarse hair?
- Dental anomalies?

General background questions
- What is your ethnic background? From what countries are your ancestors from? (consider evaluation for hemoglobinopathy particularly for clients of Southeast Asian and Mediterranean ancestry)
- Are you and your partner related as blood relatives? (e.g., cousins)
- Do you have any beliefs about why you have miscarried?

Sources: Laurino et al., 2005; Schreck and Silverman, 2007.

Blepharophimosis, ptosis, and epicanthus inversus type 1 (BPESI) with mutation in *FOXL2* is associated with premature ovarian dysfunction (De Bare, 2009).

4.18.3 Male Infertility

Infertility in men has been ascribed to multiple factors (Chandley, 1997), including:

- Radiation or chemical exposures (such as from chemotherapy)
- Infection (such as infection of the accessory gland)
- Anatomic causes (e.g., obstructive disorders, variocele)
- Cryptorchidism
- Endocrine causes
- Genetic disorders (Table 4.32), including syndromes with hypogonadism as a feature
- Immunologic causes (antisperm antibodies)
- Idiopathic

There may not be a single reason for infertility in the male being evaluated but rather a combination of genetic, hormonal, and environmental influences.

The first step in evaluating a man for infertility is semen analysis and physical examination (particularly looking for hypogonadism or variocele and some of the rare syndromic causes of infertility, as outlined in Table 4.32). Abnormalities in sperm motility, morphology, and concentration are particularly useful in assessing a genetic etiology for male infertility. There is overlap in terminology describing sperm in the ejaculate, but general usage is (Disteche, 2007; Firth and Hurst, 2005):

- Azoospermia: no sperm
- Oligozoospermia: <5–20×10^6 sperm/mL semen, with moderate being <1–5×10^6/mL, and severe $<1 \times 10^6$ mL

TABLE 4.31 Medical-Family History Questions Related to Female Infertility[a]

- How tall is the woman? (short stature can be seen in association with X chromosome anomalies such as Turner syndrome; single-gene mutations of hypothalamic and pituitary genes)
- Is she overweight? (obesity is linked to ovulatory dysfunction and seems to be linked to infertility in women with normal menses; extremely obese women who are hypogonadotropic may have a *LEP* gene mutation)
- What evaluations have been done? (such as serum gonadotropins, FSH and LH levels; ultrasounds, hysterosalpingogram; MRI for pituitary tumor)
- When did she first have her period? Is she still menstruating? (delayed puberty can be seen with X chromosome anomalies; premature ovarian insufficiency can be seen in women with *FMR1* gene premutations and in BPES1[b])
- When did she develop secondary sexual characteristics? (primary amenorrhea is a reason to consider chromosome studies; also can be seen in Kallmann syndrome)
- What is her pregnancy history and the outcome of each pregnancy? (for a history of miscarriages, see Table 4.30)
- Does the woman have learning disabilities or intellectual disabilities? (can be seen with chromosome anomalies, including Turner syndrome, fragile X mental retardation syndrome associated with *FMR1* gene mutations)
- Is there a family history of:
  - Learning disabilities or intellectual disabilities? (can be seen with chromosome anomalies and *FMR1* gene mutations)
  - Problems present from birth (such as congenital problems requiring surgery)? (can be seen with chromosome anomalies)
  - Infertility or multiple miscarriages? (can be seen with chromosome anomalies)
  - Eye anomalies? (ptosis, blepharophimosis, and epicanthus inversus in BPES)
  - Premature ovarian insufficiency? (can bee seen with FMR1, and with BPES)

[a]Refer to Appendix A.7 for list of genetic disorders and patterns of inheritance.
[b]BPES1 = blepharophimosis, ptosis, and epicanthus inversus syndrome.
Source: Layman, 2007.

- Asthenozoospermia: <50% of sperm having normal motility or <25% have any motility
- Teratozoospermia: <30% have normal morphology
- Globozoospermia: round-headed spermatozoa lacking an acrosome (the cap-like structure over the anterior head of the sperm)

Approximately 11% of men with infertility have azoospermia or oligospermia. Within this group of men there are several common genetic factors to consider:

1. *Chromosome anomalies*: Estimates are that between 4% and 7% of men with oligozoospermia and at least 13% of men with azoospermia have an abnormal karyotype (aneuploidy, sex chromosome mosaicism, ring chromosome, Robertsonian or reciprocal translocations, insertion, or inversion) (Van Assche et al., 2006). Klinefelter syndrome (47,XXY) is the most frequently observed chromosome anomaly in infertile men, affecting over 10% of men with non-obstructive azoospermia (Johnson, 1998). Autosomal structural chromosome anomalies are most commonly associated with oligospermia. Males with an isodicentric Y chromosome are phenotypically male

but have azoospermia because they do not have the AZF gene (Firth and Hurst, 2005). A phenotypic male with a 46,XX karyotype (XX-sex reversal) will be azoospermic because the gonads remain undifferentiated (Lissens et al., 2007).

2. *Cystic fibrosis transmembrane conductance (CFTR) mutations in men with congenital absence of the vas deferens (CAVD)*: Approximately 1–2% of men with azoospermia have CAVD (Foresta, 2005). Many (perhaps as high as 75%) of these men have *CFTR* mutations or mutations in disease-associated CFTR variants (such as the 5T allele) (Dork et al.,1997).

3. *Microscopic Yq-deletions*: The MSY (male-specific Y) region of the Y chromosome makes up 95% of the Y chromosome. It lies between the pseudoautosomal regions (regions of the Y that pair with like-regions on the X chromosome) at either end of the Y chromosome. Specific Y-deletions have been identified in 10–15% of men with nonobstructive azoospermia or severe oligospermia. Microdeletions of Yq in the MSY region are described by AZF (azoospermia factor) regions on the long arm of the Y chromosome and by the palindromes in the region. They include:

- AZFa (genes *DDX3Y, USP9Y*)
- AZFb (genes *RBMY1A1*, *HSFY1*)
- AZFc (*CDY1, DAZ1*)

Deletions in the AZFc region are the most common, and there is overlap in deletions that occur in the AZFb and AZFc regions of the gene (Disteche, 2007; Foresta et al., 2007). AZF region microdeletions are also found in men with oligozoospermia and solely men with azoospermia; therefore, the name AZF is a misnomer (Kremer et al., 1997). It is likely that additional deletion types will be discovered (Disteche, 2007). AZFc microdeletions are estimated to occur in about 13% of males with nonobstructive azoospermia and 6% of males with oligospermia (Oates, 2008), with an overall frequency of about 1 in 4,000. Men with microdeletions of the AZFa region are not likely to have sperm; therefore, testis sperm extraction (TESE) is unlikely to be successful (Oates, 2008).

4. Androgen receptor gene (*AR*) mutations on the X chromosome can cause testicular feminization that is complete or incomplete (traditionally referred to as 46,XY females) (Foresta et al., 2005; Lissens et al., 2007). The frequency of this condition is about 1 in 60,000 (Lissens et al., 2007).

5. Primary ciliary dyskinesias (PCD) make up a group of autosomal recessive disorders with defects in the motor apparatus (axoneme) of the ciliated cells of the respiratory tract and the tail of spermatozoa (Oates, 2008). There are multiple loci and together they have a frequency of about 1 in 25,000 (Lissens, 2007). Kartagener syndrome (sinusitis, brochiectasis, dextrocardia, and infertility) is the explanation for about 50% of PCD (Oates, 2008).

6. Mitochondrial mutations may be associated with asthenozoospermia (reduced sperm motility (Jensen et al., 2004; Lissen et al., 2007; St. John et al., 2007).

Suggestions for medical family history questions for male infertility are given in Table 4.32.

Infertile men with normal semen parameters may also have genetic mechanisms for infertility. Some etiologies proposed from mouse models suggest there may be

TABLE 4.32   Genetic Causes of Male Infertility Where Infertility May Be a Presenting Clinical Feature and Their Patterns of Inheritance[a]

Condition	Inheritance Pattern
Chromosomal	
Klinefelter syndrome (47, XXY)	Sporadic, chromosomal nondisjunction
Translocations of X or Y and an autosome	Sporadic or inherited
Autosomal translocations (Robertsonian and reciprocal)	Sporadic or inherited (test parent)
Chromosome inversions (pericentric)	Sporadic or inherited
Marker chromosome	Sporadic
Microscopic Y-Deletions	
AZF region (Yq11)	Sporadic
SRY region (Yp)	Sporadic
Single Gene[b]	
Androgen insensitivity resistance syndrome (testicular feminization)	XL
Congenital absence of vas deferens (CAVD)-cystic fibrosis (*CFTR*) mutations	AR
Ciliary dyskinesia, primary (multiple loci; includes kartagener syndrome and immotile cilia syndrome)	AR
Fibrous sheath dysplasias (affect the sperm flagella)	Unknown
5α-reductase deficiency	AR
Globozoospermia (rare)	Unknown, possibly AR with mutations in spermatogenesis-associated protein (*SPATA16*)
Hemochromatosis (possibly in association with transferrin receptor polymorphisms; impaired sperm motility)	AR
Kallmann syndrome	AD, XL
Luteinizing hormone deficiency	AR
Luteinizing (choriogonadotropin) hormone receptor defect (46,XY female or pseudohermarphrodite)	AR
Myotonic dystrophy	AD
Noonan syndrome (if cryptorchidism)	AD
Persistent müllerian duct syndrome (rare)	AR
Sickle cell disease (hypothalamic-pituitary dysfunction)	AR
Spinobulbular muscular atrophy (Kennedy disease)	XL
Steroid sulfatase deficiency (X-linked ichthyosis)	XL
Testosterone synthesis defects (several loci, but all rare)	AR
XX or XY-sex reversal (XY is rare) from *SRY* mutations	YL
Young syndrome (obstructive azoospermia, chronic sinopulmonary infections; sinusitis infertility syndrome)	AR

[a]Abbreviations: AD = autosomal dominant; AR = autosomal recessive; XL = X-linked; YL = Y-linked
[b]Disorders where infertility is a feature but not usually a presenting sign are excluded (e.g., Prader-Willi syndrome, Bardet-Biedl syndrome); see Appendix A.7 for gene symbols and names.
Sources: Buretić-Tomljanović et al., 2008; Dam et al., 2007; Foresta et al., 2005; Gunel-Ozcan et al., 2008; Lissens et al., 2007; Oates, 2008.

TABLE 4.33   Medical-Family History Questions Related to Male Infertility[a]

- What is the sperm count and sperm morphology? Obtain records.
- What is the man's height? (unusually tall stature seen in Klinefelter syndrome)
- At what age did the man go through puberty?
- Does the man have:
  - Anything unusual about the way he looks? (wide-spaced eyes and other dysmorphic features characteristic of Noonan syndrome)
  - A small penis? (seen in Klinefelter syndrome)
  - Small testes (cryptorchidism)? (seen in many infertile males)
  - Gynecomastia? (seen in Klinefelter syndrome)
  - Normal distribution of pubic hair?
  - Learning disabilities? (sometimes in Noonan, Kallmann, and Klinefelter syndromes, and myotonic dystrophy)
  - Any problems with his ability to smell (anosmia)? (seen in Kallmann syndrome)
  - Nasal polylps? (seen in cystic fibrosis, primary ciliary dyskinesia,Young syndrome)
  - Chronic infections, asthma, pulmonary disease, sinus infections? (seen in cystic fibrosis, primary ciliary dyskinesia, Young syndrome)
  - Any problems with muscle weakness? (seen in myotonic dystrophy, spinal bulbar muscular atrophy, possible mitochondrial disease)
  - Early cataracts? (myotonic dystrophy)
  - "Bronze" skin coloration? (possible hemochromatosis, untreated)
  - Any chronic diseases?
- Is there a family history of:
  - Miscarriages? (possible parental chromosomal rearrangement)
  - Learning disabilities or intellectual disability? (possible chromosomal disorder, myotonic dystrophy, Noonan syndrome, Kallmann syndrome)
  - Multiple birth defects? (possible chromosomal disorder)
  - Chronic infections, asthma, pulmonary disease, sinus infections? (see diseases as noted above)
  - Muscle disease? (myotonic dystrophy, spinal bulbar muscular atrophy; increased muscle mass can be seen in Kallmann syndrome)
  - Early cataracts? (seen in myotonic dystrophy)
- What is the man's ethnic background? (particularly useful to know for testing for cystic fibrosis mutations)
- Are the parents of the man related as cousins or more closely related? (possibility of autosomal recessive etiology)

[a]See Appendix A.7 for gene symbols, names and patterns of inheritance.
Sources: Buretić-Tomljanović et al., 2008; Dam et al., 2007; Foresta et al., 2005; Gunel-Ozcan et al., 2008; Lissens et al., 2007; Oates, 2008.

hereditary factors involved with the ability of sperm to bind with the zona pellucida or with the later steps of sperm maturation (Okabe, 1998).

The potential heritability of infertility is an important topic to discuss with men with male-factor infertility undergoing various assisted reproductive techniques (such as epididymal sperm aspiration to conceive a pregnancy with ICSI (intracytoplasmic sperm injection) and IVF (in vitro fertilization) (Bhasin, 2007; Johnson, 1998; Kremer et al., 1997). From my observations, couples with male-factor infertility whom I have counseled before ICSI are sometimes more concerned about passing on infertility to a future child than about possibly having a child with cystic fibrosis, even though a child with CF might be perceived as having more health burdens. Such couples undergo considerable emotional and financial expense to arrive at a decision to undergo treatment for infertility and ART; they usually consider carefully the potential to place future offspring at-risk to experience similar emotional heartache and frustrations. Preimplantation diagnosis can be done for embryos with Y-microdeletions; all male embryos will carry the paternal Y-microdeletion, and thus the parents might request transfer of only female embryos (Oates, 2008). The reproductive impact on the children conceived by ICSI will not be known for another 20 or more years from when these individuals begin to have children.

4.19 SUDDEN INFANT DEATH SYNDROME (SIDS)

Strictly defined, SIDS is the unexpected death of a well child over 1 month of age for which no explanation can be found despite postmortem examination. The greatest risk is from 2 to 4 months of life, and the risk of SIDS decreases after age 6 months. There is association with increase risk of SIDS with prone sleeping, soft bedding, tobacco exposure, in utero exposure to maternal substance abuse (particularly opiates), premature birth and multiple births, and having a sibling with SIDS (Opdal and Rognum, 2004; Weese-Mayer et al., 2007). The "Back to Sleep" campaign to encourage supine sleeping has been the most effective intervention to reduce the incidence of SIDS in the United States (Ackerman et al., 2007; National Institute of Child Health and Development, 2008).

There are multiple genetic and environmental factors contributing to SIDS. The strongest single-gene association is with channelopathies (disorders of cardiac rhythm with defects in the cardiac ion channels) most of which are autosomal dominant with variable expression and reduced penetrance (Tester and Ackerman, 2008).

The long-QT syndrome (LQTS) with mutations in SCN5A (LQTS3) and other channelopathies that result in rhythm disturbances can explain the etiology of 10–15% of SIDS (Arnstead et al., 2007; Lenhart et al., 2007; Weese-Mayer et al., 2007). Not only does making the diagnosis of LQTS post-mortem help identify recurrence risks for the parents but at-risk relatives can also be identified. There are various interventions that can be considered to help prevent arrhythmias and sudden death in probands and their relatives identified with LQTS (Lenhart et al., 2007). In fact, there is a movement in Europe and the United States to consider screening all newborns for cardiac rhythm disturbances to help prevent sudden death (Berul and Perry, 2007).

Gene alterations resulting in dysregulation of the autonomic nervous system are a possible contributor to SIDS (Weese-Mayer et al., 2007). There are also likely genetic polymorphisms that predispose infants to death in critical situations such as infection (Opdal and Rognum., 2004; Weese-Mayer et al., 2007).

There are multiple inborn errors of metabolism (IEM) that are candidate causes of SIDS, but as a group these are rare causes of SIDS. Any IEM that is associated with life-threatening complications (particularly when the infant is fasting or has an infection) is a possible explanation for SIDS. To date, the most common IEM but still rare causes of SIDS are the fatty-acid-metabolism disorders such as from defects in medium chain acyl-coenzyme A dehydrogenase (MCAD) (accounting for less than 1% of SIDS) (Opdal and Rognum, 2004; Yange et al., 2007). These conditions should be considered if autopsy shows hepatic steatosis (Yange et al., 2007). Genetic deficiencies in the hepatic glucose-6-phosphatase system (in the enzyme glucose-6-phosphatase or the glucose-6-phosphate transporter) associated with fasting hypoglycemia may also be linked with SIDS (Forsyth et al., 2007).

To identify an IEM it is useful to obtain autopsy reports on the child, particularly looking for fatty changes in the liver, and pathological changes of skeletal and heart muscle. A history of illness before death (such as diarrhea, vomiting, poor feeding and failure to thrive) might suggest a metabolic etiology. Consanguinity in the parents might increase the suspicion of an inherited etiology of SIDS because of an increased likelihood that the child had a condition inherited as an autosomal recessive disorder. A careful family history should be taken to look for clues of an IEM (refer to Table 4.12). A family history of sudden death at age 65 or younger could suggest a familial cardiac rhythm disturbance such as mutations in *SCN5A* (Ackerman et al., 2001; Lenhart et al., 2007).

4.20 SUMMARY

A targeted family history based on a person's history of their present illness or conditions in the family history is a first step in identifying persons at risk for various inherited disorders. With most conditions there is genetic heterogeneity. Information gathered from the family history can help the clinician target genetic testing so that it is cost-effective and likely to be informative, based on the clinical presentation and variables such as the patient's ethnicity.

4.21 REFERENCES

Abudul-Rahman O, Hudgins L. (2006). The diagnostic utility of a genetics evaluation in children with pervasive developmental disorders. *Genet Med* 8:50–54.

Ackerman MJ, Siu BL, Stumer WQ, et al. (2001). Postmortem molecular analysis of *SCN5A* defects in sudden infant death syndrome. *JAMA* 286(18):2264–2269.

Arnestad M, Crotti L, Rognum TO, et al. (2007). Prevalence of Long-QT syndrome gene variants in sudden infant death syndrome. *Circulation* 115:361–367.

Arnould-Devuyst V, Maumenee IH, Korf BR (2007). Optic atrophy and congenital blindness. In: Rimoin DL, Connor JM Pyeritz RE, Korf BR, eds., *Emery & Rimoin's Principles and Practices of Medical Genetics*, 5th ed. Philadelphia: Elsevier, pp. 3115–3132.

Ballabio F, Bersano A, Bresolin N, Candelise L. (2007). Monogenic vessel diseases related to ischemic stroke: A clinical approach. *J Cereb Blood Flow Metab* 27(10):1649–1662.

Ballana E, Ventayol M, Rabionet R, Gasparini P, Estivill X. (2009). Connexins and Deafness. January 23, 2009. Available at http://davinci.crg.es.deafness. Accessed January 24, 2009.

Bashour M. (2008). Cataract, Congenital, Emedicine from WebMD. Available at www.emedicine.com/oph/topic45.htm. October 22, 2008. Accessed November 20, 2008.

Benacerraf BR. (2007). *Ultrasound of Fetal Syndromes*, 2nd ed. New York: Churchill Livingstone.

Berry GC, Bennett MJ. (1998). A focused approach to diagnosing inborn errors of metabolism. *Contem Ped* 15:79–102.

Bérubé M. (1996). *Life As We Know It: a Father, a Family and an Exceptional Child*. New York: Pantheon Books.

Berul CI, Perry JC. (2007). Contribution of long-QT syndrome genes to sudden death syndrome: Is it time to consider newborn electrocardiographic screening. *Circulation* 115(3):294–296.

Bevans S, Markus H. (2004). The genetics of stroke. *ACNR* 4(4):8–11.

Bhasin S. (2007). Approach to the infertile man. *J Clin Endocrinol Metab* 92(6):1995–2004.

Bilek BJ, Steegers-Theunissen RP, Blok LJ, et al. (2008). Genome-wide pathway analysis of folate-responsive genes to unravel the pathogenesis of orofacial clefting in man. *Birth Defects Res A Clin Mol Teratol* 82(9):627–635.

Buretić-Tomljanović A, Vlastelić I, Radojčić Badovinac A, et al. (2008). The impact of hemochromatosis mutations and transferrin genotype on gonadotropin serum levels in infertile men. *Fertil Steril* (2008; epub ahead of print).

Burn J, Goodship J. (2007). Congenital heart disease. In: Rimoin DL, Connor JM, Pyeritz RE, Korf BR, eds., *Emery & Rimoin's Principles and Practices of Medical Genetics*, 5th ed. Philadelphia, Elsevier, pp. 1083–1159.

Buxbaum JD, Cai G, Caste P, et al. (2007). Mutation screening of the PTEN gene in patients with autism spectrum disorders and macrocephaly. *Am J Med Get B Neuropsychiatr Genet* 144(4):484–491.

Casas KA, Kamil ES, Rimoin DL. (2007). Congenital disorders of the urinary tract. In: Rimoin DL, Connor JM Pyeritz RE, Korf BR, eds., *Emery & Rimoin's Principles and Practices of Medical Genetics*, 5th ed. Philadelphia: Elsevier, pp. 1445–1477.

Chandley AC. (1997). Infertility. In: Rimoin DL, Connor JM, Pyeritz RE, eds., *Emery & Rimoin's Principles and Practice of Medical Genetics*, 3rd ed. New York: Churchill Livingstone, pp. 667–675.

Chandra A, Stephen EH. (1998). Impaired fecundity in the United States: 1982–1996. *Fam Plann Perspect* 30:34–42.

Chang E, Kolln KA, Nishimura C, et al. Pendred/BOR Homepage. Available at www.healthcare.uiowa.edu/labs/pendredandbor. Accessed January 24, 2009.

Clarke JTR. (2006). *A Clinical Guide to Inherited Metabolic Diseases*, 3rd ed. New York: Cambridge University Press.

Cohen MM. (1997). *The Child with Multiple Birth Defects*, 2nd ed. Oxford: Oxford University Press.

Cohen MM. (2007). Craniofacial disorders. In: Rimoin DL, Connor JM, Pyeritz RE, Korf BR, eds., *Emery & Rimoin's Principles and Practice of Medical Genetics*, 5th ed. New York: Elsevier, pp. 3303–3348.

Cowan J, Morales A, Dagua J. Hershberger RE. (2008). Genetic testing and genetic counseling in cardiovascular genetic medicine: Overview and preliminary recommendations. *Congest Heart Fail* 14(2):97–105.

Czeizel AE, T'oth M, Rockenbauer M. (1996). Population-based case control study of folic acid supplementation during pregnancy. *Teratology* 53:345–351.

Dam AH, Koscinski I, Kremer JA, et al. (2007). Homozygous mutation in *SPATA16* is associated with male infertility in human globozoospermia. *Am J Hum Genet* 81:813–820.

De Baere E. (2009). Blepharophimosis, ptosis, and epicanthus inversus. Gene Reviews. November 12, 2009. Available at www.ncbi.nlm.nih.gov. Accessed November 28, 2009.

Detera-Wadleigh S, Goldin LR. (2002). Affective disorders. In: King RA, Rotter JI, Motulsky AG, eds., *The Genetic Basis of Common Diseases*, 2nd ed. New York: Oxford University Press, pp. 831–849.

Deterding R, Fan LL. (2005). Surfactant dysfunction mutations in children's interstitial lung disease and beyond. *Am J Resp Critical Care Med* 171:940–941.

Disteche CM. Y chromosome infertility. Gene Reviews. March 19, 2007. Available at www.ncbi.nlm.nih.gov. Accessed November 28, 2009.

Dork T, Dworniczak B, Aulehla–Scholz C, et al. (1997). Distinct spectrum of *CFTR* gene mutations in congenital absence of vas deferens. *Hum Genet* 100:365–377.

Elkind MSV, Brown D, Burke Worrall B. (2006) Genetic and inflammatory mechanisms in stroke. June 14, 2006. Available at emedicine.medscape.com/article/1163331-overview. Accessed January 24, 2009.

Elmslie F, Gardiner M. (1997). The epilepsies. In: Rimoin DL, Connor JM, Pyeritz RE, eds., *Emery & Rimoin's Principles and Practice of Medical Genetics*, 3rd ed. New York: Churchill Livingstone, pp. 2177–2196.

Evans WF, Wapner RT. (2005). Invasive prenatal diagnostic procedures 2005. *Semin Perinatol* 4:215–218.

Falk RE, Honrubia D, Fischel-Ghodsian N. (2007). Hereditary hearing loss and deafness. In: Rimoin DL, Connor JM, Pyeritz RE, Korf BR, eds., *Emery and Rimoin's Principles and Practice of Medical Genetics*, 5th ed. Philadelphia: Elsevier, pp. 3265–3302.

Fernandez M, Bird TD. (2002). In: King RA, Rotter JI, Motulsky AG, eds., *Genetic Basis of Common Disease*, 2nd ed. New York: Oxford University Press, pp. 779–804.

Finnell RH, Mitchell LE. (2007). Neural tube defects. In: Rimoin DL, Connor JM, Pyeritz RE, Korf BR, eds., *Emery & Rimoin's Principles and Practice of Medical Genetics*, 5th ed. Philadelphia: Elsevier, pp. 2648–2660.

Finucane B. (1998) *Working with Women Who Have Mental Retardation: A Genetic Counselor's Guide*. Pennsylvania: Elwyn.

Firth HV, Hurst JA. (2005). *Oxford Desk Reference Clinical Genetics*. Oxford, New York: Oxford University Press.

Foresta C, Garolla A, Bartoloni L, et al. (2005). Genetic abnormalities among severely oligospermic men who are candidates for intracytoplasmic sperm injection. *J Clin Endorinol Metab* 90(1):152–156.

Forsyth L, Scott HM, Howatson A, et al. (2007). Genetic variation in hepatic glucose-6-phosphatase system genes in cases of sudden infant death syndrome. *J Pathol* 212(1):112–120.

Francis J, Raghunathan S, Khanna P. (2007). The role of genetics in stroke. *Postgrad Med J* 83(983):590–595.

Gallagher CL. (2005). Neurogenetics Review. Hospital Physician, Neurology Board Review Manual. Available at www.turner-white.com/pdg/brm_Neur_V9P1.pdf. Accessed November 30, 2008.

Gene Reviews. (2009). Welcome to Gene Tests. Available at www.ncbi.nlm.nih.gov/sites/GeneTests/?db-GeneTests. Accessed November 28, 2009.

Golden CM, Ryan LM, Holmes LB. (2003). Chorionic villus sampling: A distinctive teratogenic effect on fingers. *Birth Defects Res A Clin Mol Teratol* 67(8):557–562.

Graham JM, Rimoin DL. (2007). Abnormal body size and proportion. In: Rimoin DL, Connor JM, Pyeritz RE, Korf BR, eds., *Emery & Rimoin's Principles and Practice of Medical Genetics*, 5th ed. Philadelphia: Elsevier, pp. 948–963.

Greenwood Genetic Center (2008). XLMR Update, Greenwood Genetic Center. January 2009. Available at www.ggc.org/xlmr.htm. Accessed January 24, 2009.

Gunel-Ozcan A, Basar MM, Kisa U, Ankarali HC. (2008). Hereditary haemochromatosis gene (HFE) H63D mutation shows an association with abnormal sperm motility. *Mol Biol Rep* (2008; ePub ahead of print).

Heckenlively JR, Daiger SP. (2007). Hereditary retinal and choroidal degenerations. In: Rimoin DL, Connor JM, Pyeritz RE, Korf BR, eds., *Emery & Rimoin's Principles and Practice of Medical Genetics*, 5th ed. Philadelphia: Elsevier, pp. 3197–3227.

Herman GE, Butter E, Enrile B, et al. (2007). Increasing knowledge of *PTEN* germline mutations: Two additional patients with autism and macrocephaly. *Am J Med Get* 143(6):589–593.

Hershberger RE, Kushner JD, Parks SB. (2008). Dilated cardiomyopathy overview. July 10, 2008. Available at www.genereviews.org. Accessed December 5, 2008.

Holm IE, Brown JM, Isaacs AM. (2007). *CHMP2B*-Related Frontotemporal Dementia. August 23, 2007. Available at www.genereviews.org, Accessed January 24, 2009.

Honein MA, Rasmussen SA, Reefhuis J, et al. (2007). Maternal smoking and environmental tobacco smoke exposure and the risk of orofacial clefts. *Epidemiology* 18(2):226–233.

Israel J, Cunningham M, Thumann H, Arnos KS. (1996). Deaf culture. In: Fisher NL, ed., *Cultural and Ethnic Diversity: A Guide for Genetics Professionals*. Baltimore: Johns Hopkins Univeristy Press, pp. 220–239.

Jensen M, Leffers H, Petersen JH, et al. (2004). Frequent polymorphism of the mitochondrial DNA polymerase gamma gene (POLG) in patients with normal spermiograms and unexplained subfertility. *Hum Reprod* 19:65–70.

Jezewski PA, Vieira AR, Nishimura C, et al. (2003). Complete sequencing shows a role for *MSX1* in non-syndromic cleft lip and palate. *J Med Genet* 40(6):399–407.

Johnson MD. (1998). Genetic risk of intracytoplasmic sperm injection in the treatment of male infertility recommendations for genetic counseling and screening. *Fertil Steril* 70:397–411.

Jones, KL. (2005). *Smith's Recognizable Patterns of Human Malformation*, 6th ed. Philadelphia: Saunders.

Jorde LB, Hasstedt SJ, Ritvo ER, et al. (1991). Complex segregation analysis of autism. *Am J Hum Genet* 49:932–938.

Kalter H, Warkany J. (1983). Congenital malformations—Etiologic factors and their role in prevention. *N Engl J Med.* 308:424–431, 491–297 (2 parts).

Kendler KS. (1997). The genetic epidemiology of psychiatric disorders: A current perspective. *Soc Psychiatry Psychiatr Epidemiol* 32:5–11.

Kendler KS, Silberg JL, Neale MC, et al. (1991). The family history method: Whose psychiatric history is measured? *Am J Psychiatry* 148:1501–1504.

Khoury MJ, Oliney RS, Rickson JD. (1997). *Epidemiology.* In: Tewfik TL, Der Kaloustian VM, eds., *Congenital Anomalies of the Ear, Nose, and Throat*. New York: Oxford University Press, pp. 47–56.

Kinney DK. (2007). Schizophrenia. In: Rimoin DL, Connor JM, Pyeritz RE, Korf BR, eds., *Emery & Rimoin's Principles and Practice of Medical Genetics*, 5th ed. Philadelphia: Elsevier, pp. 2602–2614.

Kochar A, Hildebrand MS, Smith RJH. (2007). Clinical aspects of hereditary hearing loss. *Genet Med* 9:393–408.

Kremer J, Tuerlings J, Meueleman E, et al. (1997). Microdeletions of the Y chromosome and intracytoplasmic sperm injection: From gene to clinic. *Hum Repr* 12(4):687–791.

Lachman R. (2006). Taybi and Lachman's Radiology of Syndromes, *Metabolic Disorders and Skeletal Dysplasias*, 5th ed. Philadelphia: Mosby.

Laurino MY, Bennett RL, Saraiya DS, et al., (2005). Genetic evaluation and counseling of couples with recurrent miscarriage: Recommendations of the National Society of Genetic Counselors. *J Genet Couns* 14(3):165–181.

Layman LC. (2007). The genetic basis of human infertility. In: Rimoin DL, Connor JM, Pyeritz RE, Korf BR, eds., *Emery & Rimoin's Principles and Practice of Medical Genetics*, 5th ed. Philadelphia: Elsevier, pp. 841–855.

Lehnart SE, Ackerman MJ, Benson W, et al. (2007). Inherited Arrhythmias. A National Heart, Lung, and Blood Institute and Office of Rare Diseases Workshop Consensus Report. *Circulation* 116:2325–2345.

Lifton RP, Somlo S, Giebisch G, Seldin DW, eds., (2009). *Genetic Diseases of the Kidney*. Burlington: Academic Press.

Lissens W, Liebaers I, Van Steirteghem AV. (2007). Male infertility. In: Rimoin DL, Connor JM, Pyeritz RE, Korf BR, eds., *Emery & Rimoin's Principles and Practice of Medical Genetics*, 5th ed. Philadelphia: Elsevier, pp. 856–874.

Little J, Cardy A, Arslan MT, et al. (2004). Smoking and orofacial clefts: A United Kingdom-based case-control study. *Cleft Palate Craniofac J* 41(4):381–386.

Lynch DR. (2006). *Neurogenetics, Scientific and Clinical Advances*. New York: Taylor and Francis.

McInnis MG, Burmeister M, DePaulo JR. (2007). Major Mood Disorders. In: Rimoin DL, Connor JM, Pyeritz RE, Korf BR, eds., *Emery & Rimoin's Principles and Practice of Medical Genetics*, 5th ed. Philadelphia: Elsevier, pp. 2615–2628.

Middleton A, Hewison J, Mueller RF. (1998). Attitudes of deaf adults toward genetic testing for hereditary deafness. *Am J Hum Genet* 63:1175–1180.

Milne BJ, Caspi A, Crump R, et al. (2008). The validity of the family history screen for assessing family history of mental disorders. *Am J Med Genet B Neuropychatri Genet* 150B(1):41–49.

Moser HW, Moser AB, Steinberg SJ, Raymond GV. (2006). X-linked adrenoleukodystrophy. Available at www.genereviews.org. July 27, 2006. Accessed January 24, 2009.

Munshi A, Kaul S. (2008). Stroke genetics—Focus on PDE4D gene. *Int J Stroke* 3(3):188–192.

Murray JC, Schutte BC. (2004). Cleft palate; players, pathways, and pursuits. *J Clin Invest* 113(12):1676–1678.

National Institute of Child Health and Development. (2008). SIDS: "Back to Sleep" Campaign, 10/16/2008. Available at www.nichd.nih.gov/sids. Accessed January 24, 2009.

Nauman D, Morales A, Cown J, et al. (2008). The family history as a tool to identify patients at risk for dilated cardiomyopathy, *Prog Cardiovasc Nurs* 23(1):41–44.

Oates RD. (2008). The genetic basis of male reproductive failure. *Urol Clinic N Am* 35(2):257–270.

Okabe M, Ikawa M, Ashkenas J. (1998). Gametogenesis '98. Male infertility and the genetics of spermatogenesis. *Am J Hum Genet* 62:1274–1281.

Opdal SH, Rognum TO. (2004). The sudden infant death syndrome gene: Does it exist? *Pediatrics* 114(4):e506-e512.

Orrico A, Galli L, Orsi A, et al. (2008). Novel PTEN mutations in neurodevelopmental disorders and microcephaly. *Clin Genet* (2008; ePub ahead of print).

Paladini D, Volpe P. (2007). *Ultrasound of Congenital Fetal Anomalies*. Boca Raton, PL: Taylor & Francis.

Pericak-Vance MA, Haines JL. (2002). Alzheimer's disease. In: King RA, Rotter JI, Motulsky AG, eds., *The Genetic Basis of Common Diseases*, 2nd ed. New York: Oxford University Press, pp. 818–830.

Pollen DA. (1993). *Hannah's Heirs. The Quest for the Genetic Origins of Alzheimer's Disease*. New York: Oxford University Press.

Potash JB. (2006). Carving chaos: Genetics and the classification of mood and psychotic syndromes. *Harv Rev Psychiatry* 14(2):47–63.

Prasad AN, Prasad C. (2007). Genetic aspects of human epilepsy. In Rimoin DL, Connor JM Pyeritz RE, Korf BR, eds., *Emery & Rimoin's Principles and Practice of Medical Genetics*, 5th ed. Philadelphia: Elsevier, pp. 2676–2702.

Prentice A, Goldberg G. (1996). Maternal obesity increases congenital malformations. *Nutr Rev* 54:146–150.

Rabinowitz YS, Cotlier E, Bergwerk KL. (2007). Anomalies of the lens. In: Rimoin DL, Connor JM, Pyeritz RE, Korf BR, eds., *Emery & Rimoin's Principles and Practice of Medical Genetics*, 5th ed. Philadelphia: Elsevier, pp. 3175–3196.

Raffel LJ, Goodarzi MO, Rotter JI. (2007). In: Rimoin DL, Connor JM, Pyeritz RE, Korf BR, eds., *Emery & Rimoin's Principles and Practice of Medical Genetics*, 5th ed. Philadelphia: Elsevier, pp. 1980–2022.

Raymond GV. (2007). Abnormal mental development. In: Rimoin DL, Connor JM, Pyeritz RE, Korf BR, eds., *Emery and Rimoin's Principles and Practice of Medical Genetics*, 5th ed. Philadelphia: Elsevier, pp. 931–947.

Reardon W, Toriello HV, Downs CA. Gorlin RJ. (2004). Epidemiology, etiology, genetic counseling and genetic patterns. In: Toriello, HV, Reardon W, Gorlin RJ, eds., *Hereditary Hearing Loss and Its Syndromes*. Oxford: Oxford University Press, pp. 8–16.

Resta, RG. (1997). Carolyn's feet. *Am J Med Genet* 72:1–2.

Robinson A, Linden MG. (1993). *Clinical Genetics Handbook*, 2nd ed. Boston: Blackwell Scientific.

Romitti PA, Sun L, Honein MA, et al. (2007). Maternal periconceptional alcohol consumption and risk of orofacial clefts. *J Epidemiol* 166(7):775–785.

Rosenberg RN, Di Mauro S, Paulson HC, Ptacek L, Nester EJ, eds., (2007). *The Molecular and Genetic Basis of Neurologic and Psychiatric Disease*, 4th ed. Philadelphia: Lippincott Williams and Wilkins.

Roveland N, Zielhuis GA, Gabreels F. (1997). The prevalence of mental retardation: A critical review of recent literature. *Dev Med Child Neurol* 39:125–132.

Rubenstein WS. (1997). A "normal" practice. *JAMA* 278:216.

Rutter M, Simonoff E. (2007). Autism spectrum disorders (including Rett syndrome). In Rimoin DL, Connor JM, Pyeritz RE, Korf BR, eds., *Emery & Rimoin's Principles and Practice of Medical Genetics*, 5th ed. Philadelphia: Elsevier, 2576–2584.

St. John JC, Bowles EJ, Amaral A. (2007). Sperm mitochondria and fertilisation. *Soc Reprod Fertil Suppl* 65:399–416.

St. John JC, Cook ID, Barratt CL. (1997). Mitochondrial mutations and male infertility. *Nat Med* 3:124–125.

Sagoo GS, Butterworth AS, Sauders S, et al. (2009). Array CGH in patients with learning disability (mental retardation) and congenital anomalies: updated systematic review and meta–analysis of 19 studies and 13,926 subjects. *Genet Med* 11(3):134–146.

Sanders RC, Blackmon LR, Hogge WA, Wulfsberg EA, eds., (2002). *Structural Fetal Abnormalities: The Total Picture*, 2nd ed. St Louis: Mosby.

Saudubray JM, Charpentier C. (2001). Clinical phenotypes: Diagnosis/algorithims. In: Scriver CR, Beaudet AL, Sly WS, et al. eds., *The Metabolic and Molecular Bases of Inherited Disease*, 8th ed. New York: McGraw-Hill, pp. 1327–1403.

Savoia A, Balduini CL. (2008). MYH9-Related disorders. Available at http://genereviews.org. November 20, 2008. Accessed December 22, 2008.

Schaefer GB, Mendelsohn NJ. (2008). Genetics evaluation for the etiologic diagnosis of autism spectrum disorders. *Genet Med*: 10(1):4–12.

Schalock RL, Luckasson RA, Shogren KA, et al. (2007). The renaming of mental retardation: Understanding the change to the term intellectual disability. *Intellect Dev Disabil* 45(2):116–124.

Schreck R, Silverman NS. (2007). Fetal loss. In: Rimoin DL, Connor JM, Pyeritz RE, Korf BR, eds., *Emery & Rimoin's Principles and Practice of Medical Genetics*, 5th ed. Philadelphia: Elsevier, pp. 875–888.

Sedel F, Baumann N, Turpin JC, et al. (2007). Psychiatric manifestations revealing inborn errors of metabolism in adolescents and adults. *J Inherit Metab Dis* 30:631–641.

Shprintzen RJ, Wang F, Goldberg R, Marion R. (1985). The expanded velo–cardio–facial syndrome (VCF): additional features of the most common clefting syndrome. *Am J Hum Genet* 37:A77.

Sikich L, Wassink TH, Pelphrey KA, Piven J. (2006). Austism and related disorders. In Runge MS, Patterson C, eds., *Principles of Molecular Medicine*, 2nd ed. Totowa, NJ: Humana Press, pp. 1228–1236.

Sikora DM, Pettit-Kekek K, Penfield J, et al. (2006). The near universal presence of autism spectrum disorders in children with Smith-Lemli-Opitz syndrome. *Am J Med Genet A* 140(14):1511–1518.

Simpson JL. (2007). Disorders of the gonads, genital tract, and genitalia. In: Rimoin DL, Connor JM, Pyeritz RE, Korf BR, eds., *Emery & Rimoin's Principles and Practice of Medical Genetics*, 5th ed. Philadelphia: Elsevier, pp. 2055–2092.

Simpson JL. (2008). Genetic and phenotypic heterogeneity in ovarian failure: Overview of selected candidate genes. *Ann N Y Acad Sci* 1135:146–154.

Stevenson RE, Scwartz CE, Schroer RJ. (2000). X-Linked Mental Retardation. New York: Oxford University Press.

Sutherland GR, Gécz J, Mulley JC. (2007). Fragile X syndrome and other causes of X-linked mental handicap. In: Rimoin DL, Connor JM, Pyeritz RE, Korf BR, eds., *Emery & Rimoin's Principles and Practice of Medical Genetics*, 5th ed. Philadelphia: Elsevier, pp. 2523–2547.

Sybert VP. (2010). *Genetic Skin Disorders*. New York: Oxford University Press

Sybert VP. (2005). Turner syndrome. In: Cassidy SB, Allanson JE, eds., *Management of Genetic Syndromes*, 2nd ed. New York: Wiley-Liss, pp. 459–484.

Tester DJ, Ackerman M. (2008). Cardiomyopathic and chaennelopathic causes of sudden, unexpected death in infants and children. *Annu Rev Med* (2008; ePub ahead of print).

Tewfix TL,Teebi AS, Der Kaloustian VM. (1997). Syndromes and conditions associated with genetic deafness. In Tewfik TL, Der Kalustian VM, eds., *Congenital Anomalies of the Ear, Nose, and Throat*. New York: Oxford University Press.

Toriello HV, Reardon W, Gorlin RJ. (2004). *Hereditary Hearing Loss and Its Syndromes*, 2nd ed. Oxford Monographs on Medical Genetics. Oxford University Press, New York.

United States Food and Drug Administration, Office of Public Affairs. (1996). Folic Acid Fact Sheet, February 29, 1996. Available at www.cfsan.fda.gov/~dms/wh-folic.html. Accessed November 1, 2008.

Van Assche E, Bonduelle M, Tournaye H, et al. (2006). Cytogenetics of infertile men. *Hum Reprod* 11 (Suppl 4):1–26.

Van Camp G, Smith RJH. (2009). Hereditary Hearing Loss Homepage. Available at http://webh01.ua.ac.be/hhh. Accessed January 24, 2009.

Wallace DC, Lott MT, Procaccio. (2007). Mitochondrial genes in degenerative disease, cancer, and aging. In: Rimoin DL, Connor JM, Pyeritz RE, Korf BR, eds., *Emery & Rimoin's Principles and Practice of Medical Genetics*, 5th ed. Philadelphia: Elsevier, pp. 194–298.

Watkins ML, Rasmussen SA, Honein, MA, et al. (2003). Maternal obesity and risk for birth defects. *Pediatrics* 111:1152–1158.

Weese-Mayer DE, Ackerman MJ, Marazita ML, Berry-Kravis EM. (2007). Sudden infant death syndrome: A review of implicated genetic factors. *Am J Med Genet A* 143A(8):771–788.

Wheeler VC, Persichetti F, McNeil SM, et al. (2007). Factors associated with HD CAG repeat instability in Huntington disease. *J Med Genet* 44(11):694–701.

Wilcox AJ, Lie RT, Solvoll K, et al. (2007). Folic acid supplements and risk of facial clefts: a national population based case-control study. *BMJ* 334(7591):464.

Wilson GN, Cooley WC. (2006). *Preventive Health Care for Children with Genetic Conditions*. New York: Cambridge University Press.

Winter RM, Knowles SAS, Biever FR, Baraitser M. (1988). *The Malformed Fetus and Stillbirth*. New York: Wiley.

Winter–Baraitser Dysmorphology Database. (2006). London Medical Databases. Available at http://lmdatabases.com. Accessed November 28, 2009.

Wise AL, Scwartz DA. (2007). Pulmonary fibrosis, familial. October 2, 2007. Available at www.genereviews.org. Accessed January 24, 2009.

Wittenberger MD, Hagerman RJ, Sherman SL, et al. (2007). The *FMR1* premutation and reproduction. *Fertility Sterility* 87(3):456–465.

World Health Organization, Food and Agriculture Organization of the United Nations. (2004). Vitamin and Mineral Requirements in Human Nutrition: Report of a Joint FAO/WHO Expert Consultation, Bangkok, Thailand, 21–30 September 1998. Geneva, Switzerland: World Health Organization.

Yange Z, Lantez PE, Ibdah JA. (2007). Post-mortem analysis for prevalent beta-oxidation mutations in sudden infant death. *Pediatr Int* 49(6):883–887.

Zariwala M, Knowles MR, Leigh MW. (2008). Primary ciliary dyskinesia. February 1, 2008. Available at www.genereviews.org. Accessed January 4, 2009.

Zhao H, Chen ZJ, Qin Y, et al. (2008). Transcription factor FIGLA is mutated in patients with premature ovarian failure. *Am J Hum Genet* 82(6):1342–1348.

Zhu L, Belmont JW, Ware SM. (2006). Genetics of human heterotaxias. *Eur J Hum Genet* 14:17–25.

Chapter *5*

Using a Pedigree to Recognize Individuals with an Increased Susceptibility to Cancer

I just returned home from the hospital, having a small cyst removed from my right breast. Second time. It was benign. . . . My scars portend my lineage, I look at Mother and I see myself. Is cancer my path too? . . . I belong to a Clan of One-Breasted Women. My mother, my grandmothers, and six aunts have all had mastectomies. Seven are dead. . . .This is my family history.
—*Terry Tempest Williams (1991)*

5.1 USING MEDICAL FAMILY HISTORY TO IDENTIFY PERSONS AT-RISK FOR AN INHERITED CANCER SYNDROME

Every cancer is due to genetic mechanisms that have gone awry in the normal life cycle of cells, but most cancer is not inherited. Of all cancers, 5–10% are thought to be due to hereditary syndromes in which a single gene is mutated. In comparison, approximately 30% of all cancers are associated with tobacco exposure (National Institute for Environmental Health Services, 2003; Offit, 1998). It is likely that an array of modifying genes and environmental factors influence each individual's risk for developing cancer. With inherited cancer syndromes there are usually specific subtypes of cancer for which a person is predisposed.

The Practical Guide to the Genetic Family History, Second Edition, by Robin L. Bennett
Copyright © 2010 John Wiley & Sons, Inc.

TABLE 5.1   Medical-Family History Features Suggesting a Hereditary Cancer Syndrome or a Site-Specific Inherited Cancer Susceptibility

- Multiple closely related individuals with cancer (of any type)
- Persons affected in each generation (autosomal dominant pattern)
- Early age of onset of cancer, such as:
  - Premenopausal breast cancer
  - Colon cancer <age 50
  - Uterine cancer <age 50
  - Prostate cancer <age 60
  - Childhood cancer
- Bilateral disease in paired organs, such as:
  - Retinoblastoma
  - Retinal angioma
  - Kidney cancer
  - Breast cancer
- Gastric polyps or multiple colon polyps (10 or more seen on one screening or over time)
- More than one primary tumor
  - Metachronous (diagnosed at different times)
  - Synchronous (diagnosed at the same time)
- Rare cancers or tumors, such as:
  - Lung cancer in a nonsmoker
  - Male breast cancer
  - Ovarian cancer
  - Pheochromocytoma
  - Paraganglioma
  - Adrenal cortical cancer (particularly in children)
  - Pancreatic cancer (particularly < age 50, non–smoker)
  - Diffuse gastric cancer (linitis plastica)
  - Cerebellar gangliocytoma (Lhermitte-Duclos disease)
  - Choroid plexus tumor (particularly in children)
  - SCTAT (sex cord tumor with annular tubules)
  - Sebaceous adenocarcinoma
  - Transitional carcinoma ureter and renal pelvis (particularly if non–smoker)
- Clusters of rare cancers in multiple individuals in a family
- Absence of occupational or environmental risk factors

A pedigree is an effective tool for identifying individuals who, because of genetic factors, may have a higher susceptibility to cancer than their age-related background risk. Inherited cancer syndromes have several key medical-family history features as shown in Table 5.1. No single factor indicates the certainty of an inherited cancer syndrome, but taken together the factors in Table 5.1 can help the practitioner estimate the likelihood that a person or family has an inherited cancer syndrome. Because taking a pedigree can be time-consuming, a brief cancer family history screening form (such as the one in Appendix A.3) is helpful for screening seemingly low-risk persons. A more extensive history in the form of a pedigree can be obtained

TABLE 5.2   Medical-Family History Queries for Cancer[a]

Questions related to person with cancer
- Type of cancer(s)? (document with pathology reports)
- Age at diagnosis of cancer?
- If more than one cancer, document if new primary or metastasis. (obtain pathology reports)
- Bilateral or multifocal cancer?
- Treatment or management? (e.g., chemotherapy, radiation, mastectomy, oophorectomy, hysterectomy, colectomy)
- Age of menarche and menopause? (for women with breast cancer)
- Presence of colonic or gastric polyps?
    - How many polyps and their location?
    - Confirm with pathology and endoscopy reports.
    - Endoscopy screening interval.
    - If gastric polyps, determine if history of treatment with chronic acid suppression therapy.
- Childhood cancers.
- Potential occupational exposures? (see Table 5.7)
- Potential environmental exposures? (including alcohol, obesity, tobacco use, radiation treatment; see Table 5.7)
- Developmental delays/cognitive impairment?

General family history questions
Information on consultand and living and deceased relatives. Ideally include relatives two generations back from consultand and two generations forward (four generations):
- Current age or age at death and cause of death?
- Biopsies? (confirm with pathology reports)
- Surgical procedures? (e.g., mastectomy, oophorectomy, hysterectomy, colectomy)
    - Review pathology reports.
- Chronic diseases? (particularly gastrointestinal disorders such as ulcers, Crohn disease, or ulcerative colitis)
- Use of oral contraceptives? (particularly for the consultand and for women with breast cancer or colon cancer)
- Ethnicity/countries of family origin? (ask specifically if eastern European Jewish)
- Consanguinity?

Targeted medical system review
- Blindness or eye tumors? (RB, TSC, VHL, WTS)
- Hearing loss? (NF2, VHL)
- Lumps, bumps, birthmarks, or other skin changes?
    - Acral keratoses, palms and soles and sometimes on the proximal extremities and trunk (flesh-colored or slightly pigmented, flat-topped or smooth; CS)
    - Adenoma sebaceum? (perivascular fibromata/angiofibroma; MEN1, TSC)
    - Brown/black macules around the mouths and lips, buccal mucosa, palms and fingers, penis, anal region? (PJS, CNC; usually not on oral mucosa but often on border of lips, conjunctiva and ocular canthi)
    - Basal cell carcinomas? (multiple dome-shaped skin-colored to tan papules; NBCCS)
    - Café au lait spots, axillary, and inguinal freckling? (NF1, CNC, CMMR-D; biallelic mutations in Lynch syndrome)
    - Confetti lesions? (TSC)

(Continued)

TABLE 5.2   (Continued)

- Collagenomas? (MEN1)
- Epidermoid cysts? (FAP, NBCCS)
- Fibrofolliculomas? (raised skin lesion with a central hair; BHD)
- Fibromas?
  - Cutaneous? (CS, FAP, NF1, CMMR-D)
  - Gingival? (TSC)
  - Periungal? (TSC)
- Keratoacanthomas? (Lynch)
- Leiomyomas, cutaneous? (flesh-colored or light brown firm papules and nodules; HLRCC)
- Lipomas? (BHD, CS, FAP, MEN1)
- Multiple moles? (dysplastic nevi; in melanoma susceptibility syndromes)
- Papillomas? (CS)
- Palmoplantar keratoses? (translucent, hard papules on the palms and soles; CS)
- Pitting in palms of the hands and feet? (CS, NBCCS)
- Sebaceous adenomas? (Lynch)
- Shagreen patches and ashleaf hypopigmented macules? (TSC)
- Skin tags? (achrochordons; BHD, CS)
- Telangiectasias? (possible association with hereditary hemorrhagic telangiectasia, HHT; and juvenile polyposis, JP; with *ENG* mutations and *SMAD4*)
- Trichilemmomas? (facial, tan-yellow verrucous papules; CS)
- Trichodiscoma? (hamartoma of the mesodemal portion of the of the hair disk; BHD)
- "Lumps" on tongue? (mucosal neuromas in MEN2, papillomas in CS)
- Myxomas, penduculated? (CNC; often on eyelid, external ear, nipple)
- Bronzing or graying of skin? (history of hepatocellular carcinoma secondary to untreated hemochromatosis)
- Lips "full or blubbery"? (MEN2B)
- Dental enamel pits? (TSC)
- Jaw cysts? (osteomas in FAP, odontogenic keratocysts in NBCCS)
- Macrocephaly? (large head; NBCCS; sometimes CS, CMMR-D, NF1)
- Other health problems?
  - Autism? (CS, TSC, CMMR-D, possible NF1)
  - Ataxia? (TSC)
  - Broad ligament adenoma? (VHL)
  - Diabetes mellitus, insulin dependent? (associated with pancreatic cancer)
  - Epididymal adenoma? (VHL)
  - Leukemia? (LFS)
  - Intellectual disability (formerly called mental retardation) or learning disabilities, with or without dysmorphic features? (CMMR-D, CS, NBCCS, NF1, TSC, WTS)
  - Ovarian fibromas? (NBCCS)
  - Peptic ulcers? (MEN1)
  - Seizures? (possible CNS tumor)
  - Spontaneous pneumothorax? (BHD; secondary to lymphangiomyomatosis in females with TSC type 2)

TABLE 5.2   (*Continued*)

- Thyroid disease? (adenoma, multinodular goiter) or cancer? (CS, FAP, FMTC, MEN2)
- Uterine fibroids? (leiomyomas; CS, HLRCC)
- Vascular anomalies? (venous angioma,/developmental venous anomaly, DVA, and macrocephaly associated with CS)

Abbreviations: [a]BHD = Birt-Hogg-Dube; CMMR-D = constitutional mismatch repair deficiency (associated with biallelic Lynch syndrome mutations); CNC = Carney complex; CS = Cowden syndrome; ENG = endoglin; FAP = familial adenomatous polyposis; FMTC = familial medullary thyroid cancer; HLRCC = Hereditary leiomyomatosis and renal cell cancer; LFS = Li-Fraumeni syndrome; MEN = multiple endocrine neoplasia; NBCCS = nevoid basal cell carcinoma syndrome (Gorlin syndrome); NF = neurofibromatosis; PJS = Peutz-Jeghers syndrome; RB = retinoblastoma, TSC = tuberous sclerosis complex; VHL = von Hippel-Lindau syndrome, WTS = Wilms tumor syndrome; see Appendix A.7 for genes and patterns of inheritance.

on individuals with positive responses on the screening questionnaires that raise suspicion of a familial cancer syndrome. Table 5.2 reviews the screening questions for individuals with a family history of cancer.

The approach to genetic testing and recommendations for cancer surveillance are based on the patient's placement in the pedigree in relation to relatives affected with cancer. Information gleaned from a patient's medical history and pedigree analysis (with or without genetic testing) provides the clinician with the opportunity to discuss multiple health issues with the patient. Individuals who may benefit from cancer genetic counseling include healthy persons with a family history of cancer and those with cancer who are concerned about their risks of having another primary malignancy or the chances their offspring may develop cancer. Recommendations can be made regarding age of initiation (and method) of cancer screening, encouraging healthy lifestyle choices (i.e., healthy diet, regular exercise, limit use of alcohol, refrain from use of tobacco products), contraceptive choices (e.g., use of oral contraceptives to reduce ovarian cancer risk), hormone therapies, surgical interventions, and possibly even occupational choices (NCCN, 2009; NCI, 2009).

The focus of this chapter is to identify the clues in the medical-family history that can identify the growing number of single-gene familial cancer susceptibility syndromes (Table 5.3). The majority of these cancer syndromes follow an autosomal dominant inheritance pattern. Many of these cancer susceptibility syndromes include more than one site of malignancy. For example, Lynch syndrome (formerly called hereditary non-polyposis coli, HNPCC) is primarily associated with cancer of the colon, stomach, uterus, and ovary. Some cancer susceptibility syndromes involve other medical features besides neoplasm. Cowden syndrome is associated with breast and thyroid carcinoma, thyroid disease, benign hamartomas, and specific dermatologic findings. Table 5.4a and b correlate the type of cancer, benign tumors, and other physical features that are associated with many of the autosomal dominant cancer susceptibility syndromes listed in Table 5.3. Tables 5.4a and b are resources for helping recognize a potential hereditary cancer syndrome when a cluster of cancers is found in a family history.

Increased risk for malignancy is a secondary characteristic of more than 100 single-gene and chromosomal disorders (Friedman, 1997; Schneider, 2002). For most

TABLE 5.3 Highly Penetrant Autosomal Dominant Cancer Predisposition Syndromes with High Rates of Penetrance and Their Gene Locations

Autosomal Dominant Cancer Predisposition Syndromes and Common Abbreviation	Gene(s)
Birt-Hogg-Dubé (BHD)	FLCN
Carney complex (CNC), (NAME: nevi, atrial myxoma, myxoid neurofibromas, ephelides; LAMB: lentigenes, atrial myxomas, mucocutaneous myxoma, blue nevi)	PKAR1A, 2p16, Possible 3rd locus
Cowden syndrome (CS), Bannayan-Riley-Ruvalcaba (BRR)	PTEN
Familial adenomatous polyposis coli (FAP), Gardner syndrome, attenuated APC	APC
Familial atypical multiple mole-melanoma (FAMM), dysplastic nevus syndrome	CDKN2A/p16, CDK4, CMM
Familial medullary thyroid carcinoma (FMTC)	RET
Familial prostate cancer (FPC)	Probably multiple loci
Hereditary breast-ovarian cancer syndrome (HBOC)	BRCA1, BRCA2
Hereditary clear-cell renal carcinoma (HCRC)	Unknown
Hereditary diffuse gastric cancer (HDGC)	CDH1/E-cadherin
Hereditary leiomyomatosis and renal cell carcinoma (HLRCC)	Fumarate hydratase (FH)
Hereditary mixed-polyposis syndrome (HMPS)	CRAC1, Unknown
Lynch syndrome (formerly hereditary non-polyposis colon cancer or HNPCC)	MSH2, MLH1, MSH6, PMS2, TACTD1, Possibly MSH3
Hereditary papillary renal cell cancer type 1 (HPRC1)	MET
Juvenile polyposis (JPS)	SMAD4/MADH4, BMPR1A/ALK3, Unknown
Li-Fraumeni syndrome (LFS)	TP53
Muir-Torre syndrome	MSH2, MLH1, MSH6, PMS2, TACSTD1
Multiple endocrine neoplasia 1 (MEN1)	MEN1
Multiple endocrine neoplasia 2 (MEN2A, MEN2B)	RET
Neuroblastoma	NB (multiple loci and associated with single-gene syndromes)
Neurofibromatosis 2 (NF2)	NF2
Nevoid basal cell carcinoma syndrome (NBCCS), Gorlin syndrome	PTCH
Papillary thyroid carcinoma (cribriform-morular type can be associated with APC mutations)	Unknown
Hereditary paraganglioma syndromes (PGL)	SDHB, SDHC, SDHD (maternal imprinting), SDHAF2
Peutz-Jeghers syndrome (PJS)	LKB1/STK11
Retinoblastoma (RB)	RB1
Tuberous sclerosis complex (types 1 and 2)	TSC1, TSC2
Turcot-FAP variant	APC
Turcot-Lynch (HNPCC) variant	MLH1, MSH2, MSH6, PMS2, TACSTD1
Von Hippel-Lindau syndrome (VHL)	VHL
Wilms tumor (WT) syndromes, Denys-Drash syndrome, WAGR syndrome (Wilms tumor, anridia, genital abnormalities and intellectual delay)	WT1, WT2

Sources: Eeles et al. 2004; Evans and Farndon 2002; Firth and Hurst 2005; Gonzalez et al. 2009; Howe et al. 2007; Kovacs et al. 2009; Landi et al., 2006; Lindor et al. 2008; OMIM, 2009; Schneider, 2002; Sweet et al. 2005; van Hattem et al. 2008; Wei et al. 2005; Young and Abboud 2006.

TABLE 5.4 Autosomal Dominant Cancer Syndromes and Their Associations with Solid Tumors (Benign and Neoplastic) Part a.

Benign tumors and malignancies	HBOC1 (BRCA1)	HBOC2 (BRCA2)	LFS	Lynch	CMMR-D	FAP	CS	PJS	JPS	HDGC
Ocular										
CHRPE						X				
Ocular melanoma		?								
Brain/CNS tumors										
Brain tumors/all types			X		X					
Astrocytoma			X		X					
Cerebellar gangliocytoma							X			
Choroid plexus			X[b]							
Glioblastoma			X	X[b]	X					
Glioma			?				X			
Meningioma			?				?			
Medulloblastoma			X		X	X[b]				
Neuroblastoma			?							
Endocrine										
Adrenal cortical tumors			X							
Thyroid adenomas/goiter							X			
Follicular thyroid adenocarcinoma							X			
Papillary thyroid carcinoma						X[b]	X			
Respiratory										
Nasal polyps								X		
Laryngeal carcinoma			?							
Lung adenocarcinoma			X					?		
Reproductive										
Breast fibroadenomas							?			
Breast cancer (female)	X[c]	X[d]	X				X	X		X[e]
Breast cancer (male)	X[b]	X[b]					?	?		

(Continued)

183

TABLE 5.4 (Continued)

Benign tumors and malignancies	Syndromes[a]									
	HBOC1 (BRCA1)	HBOC2 (BRCA2)	LFS	Lynch	CMMR-D	FAP	CS	PJS	JPS	HDGC
Breast, phyllodes tumor			X[b]							
Ovarian cancer	X[f]	X[f]	?	X			?			
Fibrosarcoma			X							
SCTAT								X		
Uterine cancer	X[b]			X[g]			X[b]	?		
Uterine leiomyoma							?			
Cervical cancer			?	?			?	X		
Cervical adenoma malignum								X		
Sertoli cell tumors								X		
Gastrointestinal										
Glycogenic acanthosis, esophagus							X			
Gastric cancer			?	X		X	?	X		X[h]
Gastric polyps						X		X	X	
Fundic gland polyps						X				
Small bowel cancer				X		X	?	X		
Small bowel polyps								X		
Colorectal Cancer—polyposis						X		X		
Colorectal cancer—non-polyposis			X	X[i]	X (can have multiple polyps)				X	
Colonic hamartomas							X	X[j]	X	
Prostate cancer	?	X	?				X	X		
Desmoid tumors						X				
Liver (Heptaoblastoma)						X				
Pancreatic	X[b]	X[b]	?	X[b]		?		X[b]	?	
Genitourinary										
Transitional cell tumors of renal pelvis or ureter				X						

184

	HBOC1	HBOC2	LFS	Lynch	CMMR-D	FAP	CS	PJS	JPS	HDGC
Wilms tumor			X							
Renal cell cancer			?				?			
Connective tissue										
Osteosarcoma			X							
Soft tissue sarcomas			X							
Osteomas						X				
Arteriovenous malformation and hemangiomas							X[b]			
Hematologic and lymphatic										
Hematologic malignancy			X[b]		X					
Skin										
Melanoma		X[b]	X				?			
Sebaceous adenocarcinoma				X						
Keratoacanthoma				X						
Cutaneous findings (see Table 5.2)				X	X	X	X	X		
Other										
Macrocephaly					X		X			
Learning disabilities/ cognitive impairment					X		X[b]			

[a] Abbreviations: HBOC1 = Hereditary breast-ovarian cancer syndrome 1 (*BRCA1*); HBOC2 = Hereditary breast-ovarian cancer syndrome 2 (*BRCA2*); LFS = Li-Fraumeni syndrome; Lynch syndrome (HNPCC or hereditary non-polyposis colon cancer); CMMR-D = constitutional mismatch repair deficiency (biallelic or homozygous Lynch mismatch-repair genes); FAP = Familial adenomatous polyposis (*APC*); CS = Cowden syndrome; PJS = Peutz-Jeghers syndrome; JPS = Juvenile polyposis syndrome; HDGC = hereditary diffuse gastric cancer; CHRPE = congenital hypertrophy of the retinal pigment epithelium; SCTAT = sex cord tumor with annular tubules; ? = associations that are not well characterized or are controversial.

[b] Recognized but uncommon manifestation.

[c] Association with high-grade tumors with high mitotic rates, high proliferative fractions, "triple negative" histology with estrogen receptor negative and HER2/neu negative.

[d] Association with high-grade tumors, estrogen receptor positive, luminal phenotype, less likely to express basal keratin or overexpress HER2/neu protein.

[e] Lobular breast cancer.

[f] Usually papillary serous/epithelial, rarely mucinous or borderline.

[g] Often poorly differentiated, FIGO stage II, tumor infiltrating lymphocytes, higher mitotic rates.

[h] Diffuse gastric (linitis plasticus).

[i] Often right sided, poorly differentiated, mucinous/signet-ring cell differentiation, and densely infiltrated by lymphocytes.

[j] PJS-type polyps have mucosa with interdigitating smooth muscle bundles in a branched-tree pattern, which sometimes displaces the underlying epithelium with pseudocarcinomatous invasion of muscularis mucosa; most common in jejunum.

Source: Refer to Table 5.3 for the sources for this table.

TABLE 5.4 Part b (Continued)

Benign Tumors/Growths and Malignancies	Syndromes[a]										
	MEN1	MEN2	NF2	CNC	PGL	NBCCS	TSC	VHL	BHD	FAMM	HLRCC
Ocular											
Retinal angioma								X			
Retinal hamartoma			X				X				
Oral											
Jaw cysts						X					
Oropharynx myxoma				X							
Mucosal neuromas		X									
Fibromas/papules	X[b]					X			X		
Head and Neck											
Parasympathetic paragangliomas					X						
Squamous cell head and neck										X[b]	
Brain/CNS tumors											
Endolymphatic sac tumor								X			
Vestibular scwannomas—bilateral			X								
Psammomatous melanotic schwannoma				X							
Astrocytoma				X			X				
Ependymoma	?		X				X				
Glioma			X		?						
Hemangioblastoma								X			
Meningioma	?		X			X[b]					
Medulloblastoma						X[c]					

Endocrine

	MEN1	MEN2	NF2	CNC	PGL	NBCCS	TSC	VHL	BHD	FAMM	HLRCC
Adrenal cortical, carcinoma	?			X							
Adrenal cortical, adenoma	X										
Primary pigmented nodular adrenocortical disease				X							
Carcinoid	X										
Parathyroid adenoma	X	X (only in 2A)									
Pituitary adenoma	X (often prolacti-nomas)			X							
Thyroid adenoma-follicular				X							
Thyroid cancer—medullary		X									
Thyroid cancer—papillary				X	X[b]						
Thyroid cancer—follicular				X							
Pancreatic adenoma	X										
Pheochromocytoma		X			X (*SDHB, SDHD*)			X			
Paraganglioma		X			X (multifocal, abdominal-*SDHD*)			X			
Neuroectodermal tumor (psammomatous melanotic schwannoma)				X							

Respiratory

	MEN1	MEN2	NF2	CNC	PGL	NBCCS	TSC	VHL	BHD	FAMM	HLRCC
Lung cysts									X (also spontaneous pneumothorax)		

(Continued)

TABLE 5.4 (Continued)

Benign Tumors/Growths and Malignancies	Syndromes[a]										
	MEN1	MEN2	NF2	CNC	PGL	NBCCS	TSC	VHL	BHD	FAMM	HLRCC
Cardiovascular											
Cardiac myxoma				X							
Cardiac rhabdomyoma							X				
Reproductive											
Breast myxoma				X							
Ovarian fibroma						X					
Cystadenoma—epididymal or broad ligament								X			
Uterine fibroma(s) (leiomyomas)											X often numerous and large
Myxoma (uterus, cervix, vagina)				X							
Genitourinary											
Carcinoid	X[b]	X[b]	X[b]	X				X[b]			
Large-cell calcifying sertoli cell tumors				X							
Epididymal or papillary cystadenoma				X				X			
Renal cell carcinoma—clear cell					?		X	X	X		X
Renal cell carcinoma, papillary									X		
Renal cell carcinoma, chromophobe									X		
Oncocytoma									X		
Angiomyolipoma								X			
Pancreatic islet cell tumors	X							X[b]			
Pancreatic cancer	X[b]			?				X[b]		X[b]	

Manifestation	MEN1[a]	MEN2	NF2	CNC	PGL	NBCCS	TSC	VHL	BHD	FAMM	HLRCC
Gastrointestinal											
Stromal tumors (GIST)					X						
Connective tissue											
Cardiac fibroma						X[b]					
Osteochondromyxoma				X							
Skin											
Basal cell carcinoma						X					
Café au lait				X							
Melanoma										X	
Multiple nevi/dysplastic nevi										X	
Cutaneous findings				X (myxoma)		X			X	X	Leiomyomas
Skeletal anomalies											
Calcification of falx; wedge shaped vertebrae; rib anomalies (bifid ribs)						X					
Other											
Macrocephaly						X					
Learning disabilities/cognitive impairment						X[b]	X				
Dental anomalies						X	X				

Abbreviations: [a]MEN1 = multiple endocrine neoplasia 1; MEN2 = multiple endocrine neoplasia 2; NF2 = neurofibromatosis 2; CNC = Carney complex PGL = paraganglioma syndromes; NBCCS = nevoid basal cell carcinoma syndrome (Gorlin syndrome); TSC = tuberous sclerosis complex; VHL = von Hippel-Lindau; BHD = Birt-Hogg-Dubé; FAMM = familial malignant melanoma; HLRCC = hereditary leiomyomatosis with renal cell carcinoma.

[b]Recognized but uncommon manifestation.

[c]Primitive neuroectodermal tumors (PNET), usually before age 7 years.

Source: Refer to Table 5.3.

TABLE 5.5 Selected Medical Genetic Syndromes with Increased Risk for Neoplasms and Their Inheritance Patterns

Inheritance Pattern	Neoplasm	Syndrome
Autosomal dominant	Breast cancer	Mutation in *CHEK2* and *PALB2* seem to confer increased breast cancer risk with cancer risks varying; clinical utility of testing being determined
	Esophageal cancer (squamous cell)	Focal palmoplantar keratoderma (tylosis) type A (thickening of the skin on the soles and palms)
	Hepatocellular carcinoma	α-1-Antitrypsin deficiency (chronic lung disease, juvenile cirrhosis and liver disease); co-dominant inheritance with expression of both alleles
	Neural crest tumors	Congenital central hypoventilation syndrome (hypoventilation with normal respiratory rates during sleep, 20% with Hirschsprung disease); usually new-dominant mutation
	Optic glioma, glomus tumors of the fingers	Neurofibromatosis 1 (neurofibromas on skin, subcutaneous tissue, cranial nerves and spinal root nerves, café au lait spots, axillary freckling, some with DD)[a]
	Osteochondroma	Multiple exostoses (bony growths primarily on long bones, pelvis, and shoulders)
	Pancreatic cancer	Hereditary pancreatitis with gene muations in *PRSS1* or *SPINK*
	Pheochromocytoma	Neurofibromatosis 1 (see above)
	Retinoblastoma, osteosarcoma, sarcomas, pinealoma, melanoma	Hereditary retinoblastoma (childhood cancer arising from immature retinal cells)
	Schwannomas, rhabdoid tumor	Schwannomatosis (non–vestibular tumors, rhabdoid tumors); associated with *SMARCB*
	Wilms tumor	Hereditary Wilms tumor syndrome
Autosomal recessive	Multiple neoplasms (including non-Hodgkin's lymphoma, acute leukemia, carcinomas of the mouth, stomach, larynx, esophagus, colon, skin, breast and cervix)	Bloom syndrome (growth deficiency, DD, erythema with telangiectasias on face and neck, characteristic facies, hypogonadism, innunodeficiency); risk of developing cancer about 20%, with approximately half before age 20; about 1 in 200 carrier frequency in Ashkenazi population
	Leukemia and lymphoma	Ataxia telangiectasia (AT; progressive ataxia with choreoathetosis, dystonia, dysarthria, multiple telangiectasia, immunodeficiency, DD); other cancers include melanoma, breast, stomach, pancreas, and ovary; *ATM* and a few families with mutation in *MRE11*

TABLE 5.5 (*Continued*)

Inheritance Pattern	Neoplasm	Syndrome
	Breast cancer	Women biallelic for ATM have a higher incidence of breast cancer; carrier women seem also have an increased risk of breast cancer
	Leukemia (acute myelogenous leukemia), myelodysplastic syndrome, in childhood; hepatocellular carcinoma; head and neck cancers (squamous cell); esophagus; vulva; uterus; cervix	Fanconi anaemia syndrome (pancytopenia, radial ray defects with multiple congenital anomalies, DD, deafness); general heterozygote frequency ~1 in 200 with estimates of 1 in 90 in South African Afrikaners and Ashkenazism; risk of squamous cell carcinoma of the neck is 21% by age 40, and onset can be as early as age 10; 8 different genes; *FANCD1* is the same as *BRCA2*)
	Multiple cutaneous malignancies in childhood	Xeroderma pigmentosum (XP; acute hypersensitivity to sun with invariable cutaneous malignancy); other cancers include leukemias and cancers of the brain, lung, stomach, breast, uterus, and testes; incidence 1 in 250,000, and 1 in 40,000 in Japan; 8 different genes
	Basal and squamous cell carcinoma	Albinism I and II (congenital absence of pigment production)
	Squamous cell carcinoma of the head and neck	Fanconi anemia (see above)
	Ileum adenocarcinoma	Cystic fibrosis (chronic lung infections, pancreatic insufficiency)
	Sarcomas, melanoma, thyroid cancer, hematological malignancies	Werner syndrome (multisystem problems related to premature aging)
	Hepatocellular carcinoma	Hemochromatosis, untreated (iron storage disorder)
		Tyrosinemia 1 (fumarylacetoacetate hydrolases deficiency), untreated
	Colon cancer, multiple polyposis	MYH-associated polyposis (MAP)
	Osteogenic syndrome	Rothmund-Thomson syndrome (skin atrophy, marbleized pigmentation, telangiectasia, cataracts, short stature; rare with only several hundred cases reported worldwide)
X-linked	Lymphoma	X-linked lymphoproliferative syndrome
	Squamous cell cancers and pancreatic adenocarcinoma	Dyskeratosis congenita (leucoplakia, nail dystrophy, DD, pigmentation)
Chromosomal	Leukemia (acute megakaryocytic leukemia)	Down syndrome (trisomy 21)
	Gonadoblastoma	45,X/46,XY

(*Continued*)

TABLE 5.5 (Continued)

Inheritance Pattern	Neoplasm	Syndrome
	Breast and testicular cancer; extragonadal germ cell tumors	Klinefelter syndrome (47,XXY; tall, female body habitus, small testes, infertility)
	Chondrosarcoma	Langer-Gideon syndrome (deletion 8q24.13; DD, microcephaly, characteristic facial features with scant fragile hair, multiple exostoses, and other skeletal anomalies)
	Uterine, leukemia and gonadal tumors	Turner syndrome (45,X or abnormalities in the structure of the X chromosome; short stature, web neck, learning disabilities, infertility)
	Wilms tumor	WAGR (Wilms tumor, aniridia, genital abnormalities and mental retardation; deletion 11p13)

[a]DD = developmental delay.
Sources: Aguirre et al., 2006; Ahmed & Rahman, 2005; Brems et al., 2009; Eeles et al., 2004; Firth & Hurst, 2005; Friedman,1997; Gorlin et al., 2001; Hadfield et al., 2008; Lindor et al., 2008; NCI, 2007; Offit, 1998; Renwick et al., 2006; Sahlin et al., 2007; Schneider, 2002; Swensen et al., 2009.

of these conditions, knowledge about increased risk for neoplasm is important for the lifelong health management of these individuals, but cancer is unlikely to be the presenting diagnostic feature (e.g., leukemia in Down syndrome or adenocarcinoma of the ileum in cystic fibrosis). Listed in Table 5.5 are examples of some of the more well known genetic syndromes associated with neoplasms and their modes inheritance. Most of the syndromes in Table 5.5 are diagnosed in childhood.

Knowledge about the phenotypes of the familial cancer syndromes is in constant flux as the tools of molecular genetics continue to define the germline mutations associated with particular cancer syndromes. For example, Turcot syndrome (a rare inherited condition associated with susceptibility to brain tumors and colon cancer) is known to be associated with germline mutations in at least five separate genes—the adenomatous polyposis coli (*APC*) gene and the Lynch syndrome associated genes, *MLH1, MSH2, MSH6, TACSTD1,* and *PMS2* (Lebrun et al., 2007; Kovacs et al., 2009). The brain tumors associated with mutations in the APC gene are typically medulloblastomas, and those associated with Lynch syndrome gene mutations are glioblastomas (Offit, 1998). Until recently, mutations in the *PTEN* gene were thought to be responsible for three rare disorders—juvenile polyposis syndrome, Cowden syndrome, and Bannayan-Zonana or Bannayan-Ruvalcaba-Riley syndrome—that have intestinal hamartomas, lipomas, macrocephaly, and other features (Eng, 2003; Jacoby et al., 1997; Liaw et al., 1997; Lynch, et al., 1997; Marsh et al., 1997). Upon further molecular analysis, juvenile polyposis syndrome has been identified as a separate identity due to mutations in *SMAD4* and *BMPR1/ALK3* (Merg and Howe, 2004; Wirtzfeld et al., 2001; Zhou, 2001), and the clinical spectrum for *PTEN* has been expanded to include a subset of individuals with macrocephaly and autism-spectrum disorder (Buxbaum et al., 2007; Herman et al., 2007; Orrico et al., 2008). It has been proposed that this collection of syndromes defined by *PTEN* mutations be referred to as PTEN hamartoma tumor syndrome, or PHTS (Eng, 2000).

There are a number of genetic conditions that can be associated with various polyposis histologies: adenomatous, hamartomatous, Peutz-Jeghers, juvenile, hyperplastic, and mixed polyposis. Careful review of polyp histology is required as is physical examination of the patient to look for dermatologic findings that can be associated with some of these conditions. The spectrum of the phenotype in the polyposis syndromes is wide and may be quite subtle; a thorough family history is particularly essential when exploring the etiology of these syndromes (Jass, 2000; Sweet et al., 2005).

5.2 INFORMATION TO RECORD IN A CANCER FAMILY HISTORY

The traditional concept of a three-generation pedigree is likely inadequate for most cancer risk assessment. Instead, it is most useful to take a pedigree that includes the consultand's siblings and half-siblings and then extends two generations forward (to include children and grandchildren) and two generations back (to include parents, aunts and uncles, and grandparents). For the patient interested in cancer genetic counseling a family pedigree can be quite expansive, often extending *five* generations!

On the pedigree it is just as important to note which family members are *unaffected* as it is to record information on relatives who have had cancer. When a relative with cancer is identified, the medical-family history should extend as far back in prior generations as possible. Information about the health of the children and grandchildren of affected relatives is also significant. Remember to inquire about any family history of cancer in the *spouse or partner* of an affected relative and his or her family; a significant family history of cancer may actually extend from a family member who has no biological relationship to the person seeking cancer risk assessment. Also keep in mind that hereditary breast-ovarian cancer syndromes can be inherited through a male relative, just as a predisposition to prostate cancer can be inherited through a female relative.

5.3 CANCER RISK ASSESSMENT REQUIRES ACCURATE INFORMATION ON CANCER DIAGNOSES

Paramount to accurate genetic risk assessment is the correct notation of the age of onset of cancer(s) and the type of primary cancer(s). Douglas and colleagues (1999) found that medical management of 11% of families was changed by information obtained with confirmation of cancer diagnoses. In families with identified *TP53* mutations associated with Li-Fraumeni syndrome, relying on verbal histories of cancers would have led to genetic testing in fewer than half of these families (Schneider et al., 2004).

Families with relatives who died young of cancer may be particularly vulnerable to incomplete or distorted knowledge of the family history of cancer (Patenaude, 2005). Remarriage of the surviving parent may further distance the child from access to relatives with information about cancer in the family.

The medical information relayed by the consultand regarding cancers in family members can be alarmingly inaccurate, particularly when recalling information about deceased relatives and family members who are related as second-degree relatives or beyond (Breuer et al., 1993; Kerber and Slattery, 1997; Schneider, 2002; Schneider et al., 2004; Theis et al., 1994). In a study by Love and colleagues (1985), the tumor histology verified the reported medical history of cancer in 83% of first-degree relatives (i.e., parents, siblings, children), but only 60% of second-degree relatives (i.e., grandparents, aunts and uncles, half-siblings, nieces and nephews, grandchildren), and 67% of third-degree relatives (i.e., cousins). A Utah study observed higher sensitivity for the subjects' reports of breast (83%), colorectal (73%), and prostate (70%) cancer but less recall of ovarian (60%) and uterine (30%) cancers (Kerber and Slattery, 1997); similar findings were found in a literature review by Murf and colleagues (2004). In a California registry study of 1,111 probands there was generally high accuracy of reporting for breast (~95%), colorectal (~90%), ovarian (~83%), and prostate cancers (~79%) (Ziogas and Anton Culver, 2003). In a study of 143 men evaluated in Houston, Texas, with prostate cancer, King and colleagues (2002) found an overall accuracy of reporting of cancer in first-degree relatives of 81% with the high rates of concordance for breast (95%), colon (~92%), pancreatic (100%), lung (93%), and prostate (86%) cancers but lower accuracy for cancers of the stomach (~50%), cervix (50%), and uterus (40%). Douglas and colleagues (1999) found similar accuracies in self-reporting for cancer, with 95% of breast cancer and 80% of abdominal and gynecological cancers reported correctly. They also observed that stomach cancer was a frequent description of any type of abdominal cancer, and that "womb cancer" included cervical as well as endometrial cancer. A 14% error corroborating family history information with clinical data was found in a study of ovarian cancer in Alberta, Canada (Kock et al., 1989). Errors included missed malignancies, benign lesions graded as malignancies, and incorrect cancer site as well as inaccurate dates of birth, diagnosis, and death.

In a comparison study of the accuracy of verbal family history reporting when compared to medical records in families with hereditary breast-ovarian cancer syndrome (HBOCS) or Li-Fraumeni syndrome (LFS), 74% of participants reported a correct history of ovarian cancer and 55% of the LFS associated cancers (Schneider et al., 2004). The verbal report of age at breast cancer diagnosis was accurate within 5 years in 60% of families with LFS and 53% in families with HBOCS. This study found correlations with increased accuracy of reporting of information if there was a known *BRCA1* gene mutation in the family, the historian was female, the historian was well educated, and there were fewer than five first-degree or second-degree relatives with cancer.

Overall, studies that have measured the accuracy of self-report of cancer family history demonstrate low instances (in the range of 2–6%) of overreporting of cancer diagnosis (false-positives) (Airewele et al., 1998; Ziogas and Anton-Culver, 2003).

Studies have focused on confirming the type of cancer but not the age at diagnosis. Few studies have focused on confirming the absence of cancer in relatives reported as unaffected.

Kerr and associates (1998) described five families seen in a family cancer clinic where a factitious family or personal history led to erroneous risk estimation. Signs indicating that the family history was false included separate clinic staff obtaining different family cancer diagnoses and age at diagnosis of relatives, unrealistic length of survival based on clinical features reported, and lack of detailed knowledge of the illness in close relatives. A person may give a false family history in hopes of qualifying with the necessary family history parameters for gaining access to insurance coverage for expensive genetic testing or because the person has high cancer worry and is seeking more extensive cancer screening or even prophylactic surgery. If a cancer history is found to be false or significantly embellished, involvement of a mental health professional is important; such behavior often indicates a need for psychological treatment of the underlying insecurities, fears, and anxiety (Patenaude, 2005).

Some common errors made in recalling details of cancer in a family history include:

- The relative who provides family history information may not make a distinction between multiple sites of primary and metastatic disease. For example, the brain is a common site of metastasis for breast, melanoma, lung, kidney, and gastrointestinal cancers (Ries et al., 2006). The preferential metastatic sites of human tumors are listed in Table 5.6. Note that liver cancer is almost always a metastatic site, and bone cancer is rarely a primary site.
- Family members may be embarrassed to discuss gender-specific cancers. Ovarian, uterine, or cervical cancer may be referred to as "female cancer," or the historian may fail to make a distinction between testicular cancer and prostate cancer. "Womb cancer" may be used to describe cervical or uterine cancer (Douglas et al., 1999).

TABLE 5.6   Preferential Metastatic Sites of Some Human Tumors

Primary Tumor	Common Metastatic Site(s)
Breast adenocarcinoma	Bone, brain, lung, liver, adrenal, ovary
Prostate adenocarcinoma	Bone
Lung small cell carcinoma	Bone, brain, liver
Colon carcinoma	Liver
Rectal carcinoma	Lung, liver
Stomach	Ovary
Skin, cutaneous melanoma	Brain, liver, bowel
Thyroid adenocarcinoma	Bone
Kidney, clear cell carcinoma	Bone, liver, thyroid
Testis carcinoma	Liver
Bladder carcinoma	Brain
Neuroblastoma	Liver, adrenal

Source: Reprinted with permission from Moghaddam and Bicknell (1995), p. 48.

- Women with several affected relatives with breast cancer may overreport the number of people with breast cancer (Parent et al., 1997). For example, the historian may believe a relative had breast cancer when actually a biopsy was benign.
- Melanoma is easily confused with basal and squamous cell carcinomas (Aitken et al., 1996).
- Medical information on common cancers (such as breast and colon) is more likely to be correct than on rare cancers (e.g., osteosarcomas) (Schneider et al., 2004).
- Stomach cancer may be used to describe any abdominal cancer (Douglas et al., 1999).
- Benign prostatic hyperplasia may be confused with prostate cancer (King et al., 2002).

Suggestions for strategies to assist families in obtaining medical documentation of tumor pathology are discussed in Chapter 6. Information on death certificates can be useful as a way of determining the types of cancer affecting relatives (see Chapter 6). There are common metastatic sites of tumors as noted in Table 5.6. In taking a family history, if you are unable to obtain a report of tumor pathology, an awareness of these preferential metastatic sites may sway your index of suspicion in the direction of a metastatic process in contrast to concluding that a person had multiple primary cancers. If medical documentation is not available, asking about how the cancer was diagnosed and treated can help with verification of the type of cancer.

5.4   YOUNG AGE OF ONSET IS TYPICAL OF INHERITED CANCER SYNDROMES

Age is the most important risk factor for familial cancer, with earlier age of cancer onset associated with higher risk for cancer in first-degree relatives. The cancers in familial cancer syndromes tend to occur at an earlier age than usual. In the inherited breast cancer syndromes, breast cancer is often diagnosed before menopause. The age of onset of colon cancer in familial adenomatosus polyposis (FAP) and Lynch syndrome is often before age 50. Li-Fraumeni syndrome is characterized by childhood cancers, particularly brain cancers, sarcomas, and adrenocortical carcinoma. Several studies have found that when adrenal cortical cancer is diagnosed in a child before age 18 years, there is a greater than 80% likelihood of identifying a *TP53* mutation (Ribeiro et al., 2001; Varley, 2003). Early studies on hereditary prostate cancer suggest that the age of onset of hereditary forms are more likely to be before the age of 50–60 years (Gronberg et al., 1997). It is important to document on the pedigree the age (and ideally the year of birth) of both affected and unaffected relatives and the age at diagnosis of cancer. The age of onset of cancer in relatives is one of the most important factors for developing an approach to genetic testing and implementing plans for cancer surveillance and risk reduction for a person and their relatives.

5.5 RARE CANCERS CAN BE A CLUE TO AN INHERITED CANCER SYNDROME

Cancer is common in most family histories. When a cancer occurs in a person or family that rarely occurs in the general population, this can be a clue to a hereditary cancer syndrome. For example, it is estimated that 80% of childhood adrenal cortical cancers are associated with Li-Fraumeni syndrome and mutation in *TP53* (see Section 5.4). Pheochromocytomas are often seen with the hereditary paraganglioma syndromes, von Hippel-Lindau syndrome, *RET* mutations, or neurofibromatosis type 1 (Bertherat and Gimenez-Roqueplo, 2005). Gastric cancer can be diffuse or intestinal; if a family has the diffuse gastric type, sometimes including a history of lobular breast cancer, there is a high probability of a gene mutation in E-Cadherin (*CDH1*) (Kaurah et al., 2007). Cervical adenoma malignum is found in Peutz-Jeghers syndrome.

Refer to Section 5.8 and Tables 5.1, 5.2, 5.4a, 5.4b, and 5.8 for clues for when to consider genetic testing for persons with rare cancers or cancers occurring at a young age.

5.6 SEX-LIMITED, SEX-INFLUENCED, AND PARENT OF ORIGIN EFFECTS (PARENTAL IMPRINTING AND UNIPARENTAL DISOMY)

Noting the sex of all individuals on the pedigree, both affected with cancer and unaffected is essential for cancer risk assessment. A tumor site may be *sex-limited* (such as ovarian cancer) or *sex-influenced* (such as breast cancer), potentially masking or hiding the familial pattern of disease expression. It is unusual for a man to have breast cancer, thus it is not uncommon for a healthy father to pass the gene alteration for HBOCS (*BRCA1* or *BRCA2*) to his children. If a woman has a history of premenopausal breast cancer, it is just as critical to document how many female relatives did *not* have breast cancer as it is to document the relatives with cancer in the family. If such a woman has multiple sisters and aunts who live to be elderly, there may be less suspicion for an inherited cancer syndrome. A hereditary prostate cancer may be difficult to recognize if a man has several sisters and no brothers. If a man with prostate cancer has many healthy brothers there may be fewer concerns that he has inherited prostate cancer susceptibility.

There are several cancer syndromes in which the expression of disease is different depending on whether the gene mutation is inherited from the mother or the father (*parental imprinting*). In families with hereditary paraganglioma and mutations in SDHD, maternal imprinting affects disease expression of this autosomal dominant condition; the disease is not manifested when the mutation is inherited from the mother, but is highly penetrant when inherited from the father (Young and Abboud, 2006). Beckwith-Wiedemann syndrome (BWS) with hemihypertrophy (HH) (characterized by excessive intrauterine and postnatal growth, organomegaly, several specific congenital anomalies, and hemihypertrophy—overgrowth of one side of the limb or face) is associated with Wilms tumor. In some children with BWS and HH there is a duplication of 11p15 that occurs on the chromosome inherited from the unaffected father. Less commonly, a child with BWS inherits both copies of chromosome 11 from his or her father (*uniparental disomy*) (Santiago et al., 2008).

5.7   ENVIRONMENTAL AND OCCUPATIONAL RISK FACTORS FOR CANCER

Potential environmental and occupational risk factors should be recorded in a cancer family history (Table 5.7). For example, lung cancer in a 70-year-old person with a 50 pack-year history of smoking is not surprising, but lung cancer in a 30-year-old nonsmoker is remarkable. Pack years are calculated by dividing the number of cigarettes smoked per day by 20 (the number of cigarettes in a pack) and multiplying this figure by the number of years a person has smoked. For example, a person who smokes 40 cigarettes a day and has smoked for 10 years would have a 20 pack-year smoking history (40 cigarettes per day ÷ 20 cigarettes per pack = 2; 2 × 10 years of smoking = 20 pack-year history). Excessive tobacco and alcohol use remain the most common environmental exposures linked to increase risk for cancer (National Institute Environment Health Services, 2003).

Increasingly, viruses and bacterial infections are being linked to human cancer (Goon et al., 2009; National Institute Environment Health Services, 2003):

- Human papilloma virus with cervical, anal, and head and neck carcinomas
- Hepatitis B and C with liver carcinoma
- HTLV (human lymphotrophic virus 1) with adult T-cell leukemia, non-Hodgkin lymphoma
- Epstein Barr virus with nasopharyngeal carcinoma, Burkitt lymphoma, and posttransplantation polycolonal lymphomas, Kaposi sarcoma, and lymphomas
- HIV infection with Kaposi sarcoma and non-Hodgkin lymphoma
- Kaposi sarcoma–associated herpesvirus (KSHV)/human herpesvirus 8 (HHV-8) and Kaposi sarcoma
- *Helicobacter pylori* infection and stomach carcinoma
- Possible association with *H. pylori* infection with MALT lymphoma and pancreatic cancer
- Schistosomiasis (parasitic infection) and bladder, liver and intestinal carcinoma

In persons with relatives from Asia, particularly Korea and Japan, there is an epidemic of stomach cancer related to *H. pylori* infections. A family history that suggests a dominantly inherited gastric cancer may be primarily environmental.

It is interesting that there may be an emerging "epidemic" of gastric fundic gland polypsis related to treatment of acid reflux with chronic acid suppression therapy with proton pump inhibitors (Freeman, 2008). Traditionally fundic gland polyposis has been considered a possible manifestation of familial adenomatous polyposis coli

TABLE 5.7 Lifestyle and Occupational Risk Factors for Cancer

Exposures	Related Cancer
Tobacco (cigarettes, pipe smoking, cigar)	Mouth, throat, nasal cavity, larynx, lung, esophagus, stomach, pancreas, kidney, colon, lip, bladder, cervix, liver, leukemia, vulva
Secondhand smoke	Lung
Alcohol (2 drinks daily, particularly with tobacco use)	Breast, mouth, pharynx, larynx, esophagus, liver, possibly colon
Dietary fats	Possible association with colon, prostate, lung, breast
Obesity	Breast, endometrial, kidney, gallbladder, colon, esophagus
Red meat consumption	Colon, possibly endometrial
Betel nut chewing	Colon
Beryllium (aerospace and defense industries, X-ray tubes, nuclear weapons, aircraft, brakes, rocket fuel, ceramic manufacturing)	Lung
Diethylstilbestrol (DES) exposure in utero	Cervix, vagina (clear-cell)
Estrogen replacement	Uterus, breast
Alkylating agents (chemotherapy)	Leukemia
Sun exposure, tanning beds	Skin
Multiple sexual partners (risk of human papilloma virus)	Cervix
Daily perineal talcum powder use (from silicate particles)	Possible ovarian
Arsenic (mining, copper smelting, pesticides, glass making, wood preservatives)	Lung, liver, skin, bladder, kidney
Asbestos (shipyard, mining, cement, millers, textile, pipe insulation, building demolition)	Lung, larynx, mesothelioma
Aromatic amines (dyes)	Bladder
Benzene (varnishes, other industrial uses)	Leukemia
Bis-ether	Lung
Shoe (manufacturing)	Nasal cavity
Chromium (metal plating)	Lung
Hardwood manufacturing	Nasal cavity
Hermatite mining	Lung
Isopropyl alcohol manufacturing	Para-nasal sinuses
Mustard gas	Lung, pharynx, larynx
Pesticides (high doses)	Lymphoma, leukemia, lip, stomach, lung, brain, prostate, melanoma, skin, kidney
Nickel refining	Lung, nasal sinuses
Rubber industry (benzidine, napathylamine)	Leukemia, bladder
Silica dust (coal mines, mills, granite quarry, sandblasting)	Lung
Soot, tars, oils	Skin, lung, bladder
Vinyl chloride (PVC)	Liver (angiosarcoma)
Wood dust (sanding, furniture manufacture)	Nasal cavities and sinuses

TABLE 5.7   *(Continued)*

Exposures	Related Cancer
Uranium	Lung
Radon (uranium mining, natural exposures)	Lung
Radiation (atomic bomb fallout, nuclear accident)	Oral cavity, esophagus, stomach, colon, liver, lung, non-melanoma skin, breast, ovary, bladder, nervous system, and thyroid (papillary)
Ionizing radiation (used to treat acne, ring worm)	Thyroid

Sources: Bravi et al. 2008; Hamatani et al. 2008; Muscat and Huncharek 2008; National Cancer Institute 2008; National Institute Environment Health Services 2003; Pelucci et al. 2006; Preston et al. 2007.

(FAP); therefore, a medication history has growing importance when considering candidates for genetic testing and consideration of further screening for gastrointestinal cancers.

5.8   BE CAUTIOUS IN ASSUMING A CANCER IS SPORADIC OR A NEW MUTATION IF THE CANCER IS DIAGNOSED AT A YOUNG AGE OR IS UNCOMMON

When cancer is diagnosed at a young age or at a younger age than typical, the family history is more likely to be unremarkable for a history of cancer because the person's first- and second-degree relatives are also young and are less likely to have developed cancer. For example, a person diagnosed with colon cancer in his or her 20s and 30s may have siblings and parents who are all under the age of 50. A small family size may also hide a familial cancer syndrome (Weitzel et al., 2007). In these situations it is better to err on the side of caution and offer genetic testing then to miss a diagnosis of an inherited cancer syndrome. This approach is important for the person with cancer who is being evaluated because many inherited cancer syndromes are associated with risks for other cancers, and thus the person would have different cancer surveillance than typical. Also, close relatives (i.e., first- or second-degree relatives) might be offered cancer surveillance at a younger age than usual.

Most cancer genetic testing does not identify all of the possible mutations in a gene, so a negative genetic test in the proband will reduce, but not entirely eliminate, the possibility of an inherited cancer syndrome. Table 5.8 lists some of the cancers for which it is reasonable to consider genetic testing in the setting of a noncontributory family history of cancer based on the age at diagnosis and particularly if the type of cancer is uncommon. Further clinical evaluation may also be warranted preceeding or in conjunction with gene mutation analysis. For example, a diagnosis of cribriform-morular variant of papillary thyroid cancer may be a sign of familial adenomatous polyposis (FAP) (Tomoda et al., 2004), and endometrial cancer diagnosed before age 50 suggests the possibility of Lynch syndrome (Walsh et al., 2008); in both cases, colonoscopy screening should be considered. (Walsh et al., 2008).

TABLE 5.8 Examples of Solid Tumors and Tumor Sites Where Genetic Testing Should Be Considered Even if the Family History of Cancer Seems Unremarkable

Tumors, Tumor Site and Clues from Age at Diagnosis	Gene/Syndrome[a]	Estimate of Likelihood of Finding a Mutation, in Absence of Family history[b]	Pathology Clues	References
Choroid plexus carcinoma (childhood)	*TP53*/LFS	Rare cancer, but several reports in LFS; study by Gonzalez et al., suggests likelihood of identifying mutation may approach 100%		Gonzalez et al. (2009); Krutilokova et al., (2005); Russell-Swetek et al. (2008)
Primitive neuroectodermal tumors (PNET) (< age 3 y)	*PTCH*/NBCCS	Unknown, examine for clinical features	Generally desmoplastic subtype	Evans and Farndon (2008)
	Biallelic and homozygosity for Lynch mutations CCMR–D	Unknown but high yield if suggestive IHC	Consider MSI and IHC for *MLH1*, *MSH2*, *MSH6*, and *PMS2*	Wimmer and Etzler (2008)
Dysplastic gangliocytoma of the cerebellum (Lhermitte-Duclos disease or LDD)	*PTEN*/Cowden	Considered pathognomonic in adults		Pilarski (2009)
Breast cancer, female (premenopausal)[c]	*BRCA1*/HBOC1	7–13% (higher if ancestry is associated with founder mutations such as Ashkenazi)	Triple negative (estrogen receptor neg/progesterone receptor and neg./Her2/Neu neg)	Diaz et al. (2007); Lakhani et al. (2005)
	BRCA2/HBOC2	Similar to *BRCA1*	More likely to be high grade, estrogen receptor positive	
	PTEN/CS	Unknown	Consider if concurrent macrocephaly	Buxbaum et al. (2007); Lachlan et al. (2007); Pilarski (2009)

(Continued)

TABLE 5.8 *(Continued)*

Tumors, Tumor Site and Clues from Age at Diagnosis	Gene/Syndrome[a]	Estimate of Likelihood of Finding a Mutation, in Absence of Family history[b]	Pathology Clues	References
Breast cancer, male	BRCA1/HBOC1 BRCA2/HBOC2	3–11% (founder mutations in BRCA2: 40% likelihood of identifying 995del5 if affected male Icelandic; ~13% if affected male Ashkenazi)		Thorlacius et al. (2007); Chodick et al. (2008)
	PTEN/Cowden	Case reports in Cowden syndrome; look for dermatological findings, and might consider if macrocephaly		Pilarski, (2009)
Ovarian cancer (any age)	BRCA1/HBOC1 BRCA2/HBOC2	10–15% if Northern Europeans, ~30% if Ashkenazi	Primarily papillary serous	Brozek et al. (2008); Chetrit et al. (2008)
Primary peritoneal cancer	BRCA1/HBOC1 BRCA2/HBOC2	Similar frequency to those with ovarian cancer		Menczer et al. (2003)
Fallopian tube cancer (any age)	BRCA1/HBOC1 BRCA2/HBOC2	Slightly higher frequency than observed with ovarian cancer	Often distal/fibria	Medeiros et al. (2006)
Endometrial cancer (<50 y)	MLH1, MSH2, MSH6, PMS2, TACSTD1/ Lynch	9–20% in unselected families (do MSI/IHC on uterine tissue if available before germline testing)	Often poorly differentiated, FIGO stage II, tumor-infiltrating lymphocytes, higher mitotic rates; if possible do MSI and IHC on tumor tissue before germline testing	Hampel et al. (2006); Kovacs et al. (2009); Lu et al. (2007); Umar et al. (2004); Walsh et al. (2008)

Colon cancer (<50 y)	*MLH1, MSH2, MSH6, PMS2, TACSTD1/* Lynch	Unknown	Often right sided, poorly differentiated, mucinous/signet-ring cell differentiation and densely infiltrated by lymphocytes; if possible do MSI and IHC on tumor tissue before germline testing	Jass (2000; 2008); Kovacs et al., (2009); Umar et al. (2004)
Colon cancer, synchronous or metachronous Lynch syndrome related tumors[c] (any age)	*MLH1, MSH2, MSH6, PMS2, TACSTD1/* Lynch	Unknown	If possible, do MSI and IHC on tumor tissue before germline testing	Umar et al. (2004)[c]
Polyposis, >10 adenomatous polyps	*MYH/*MAP, *APC/*FAP	Unknown		Jass (2000); Lefevre et al. (2006)
Hyperplastic polyps/mixed polyposis	*PTEN/*CS, *STK11/*PJS	Unknown		Sweet et al. (2005)
Diffuse gastric cancer (DGC) (<35 y)	*CDH1/*HDGC	Unknown; the incidence of gastric cancer varies widely in different populations. Threshold for testing would be lower in populations where gastric cancer rare; may even consider in persons < 50 with DGC if from low-risk population		Suriano et al. (2005)

(Continued)

TABLE 5.8 *(Continued)*

Tumors, Tumor Site and Clues from Age at Diagnosis	Gene/Syndrome[a]	Estimate of Likelihood of Finding a Mutation, in Absence of Family history[b]	Pathology Clues	References
Diffuse gastric cancer, synchronous/metachronous lobular breast cancer (any age)	*CDH1*/HDGC	Unknown		Suriano et al. (2005)
Clear cell renal cancer, bilateral	*VHL*	Unknown		
Renal tumors, more than one morphology	*FLCN*/BHD	Unknown	Particularly chromosome and oncocytoma	
Papillary thyroid cancer (cribriform-morular variant or CMV)	*APC*/FAP	May be as high as 25%	Predominantly females and young age at diagnosis; consider screening for polyposis	Tomoda et al. (2004)
Medullary thyroid cancer	*RET*/MEN2A, MEN2B, FMTC	May be as high as 25%		Richards (2009)
Adrenal cortical cancer <18 y	*TP53*/LFS	>80%		Gonzalez et al. (2009); Varley et al. (2003)
Primary pigmented nodular adrenocortical dysplasia (PPNAD)	*PKAR1A*/CNC	Unknown		Lindor et al. (2008)
Hepatoblastoma, <15 y (usually 6 mo.– 3 y)	*APC*/FAP	10%		Aretz et al. (2006)
Pheochromocytoma Paraganglioma	*VHL, SDHB, RET, SDHD*/PGL1, *SDHAF2*/PGL2, *SDHC*/PGL3, *SDHB*/PGL4	22–30% ~30% of head and neck paragangliomas		Dahia (2006) Boedeker et al. (2007); Dahia (2006)

Pathology	Gene/Syndrome	Likelihood/Comment	Reference
Thymic neuroendocrine carcinoma (carcinoid)	MEN1/MEN1	Unknown	Ferolla et al. (2007)
Sebaceous adenoma/carcinoma	MLH1, MSH2, MSH6, PMS2, TACSTD1/ Lynch	Unclear how often Lynch syndrome would be identified by this pathology without other clinical features of Lynch,[c] but at least make sure a good family history is taken and consider IHC and MSI	Consider MSI and IHC for MLH1, MSH2, MSH6 and PMS2; more likely on trunk (as compared to head/neck); more often adenoma than carcinoma; keratoacanthomalike	Chhibber et al. (2008); Singh et al. (2008)
Trichilemmomas	PTEN/Cowden	Pathognomonic for Cowden syndrome	Pilarski (2009)
Sertoli-cell tumors	STK11/PJS	Unknown	Calcifying sertoli tumor (LCCSCT)[d]	Amos et al. (2007)
	PRKAR1A/Carney complex	Unknown	Calcifying sertoli tumor (LCCSCT)	Stratakis et al. (2001)
Ovarian SCTAT (sex cord tumors with annular tubules)	STK11 (LKB1)/PJS	50% or higher	Bilateral, multifocal, small	Young (2005)
Adenoma malignum of the cervix	STK11 (LKB1)/ PJS	Unknown but probably high yield to testing		Amos et al. (2007)

[a]Refer to Table 5.4a and b for syndrome abbreviations.

[b]Few large studies are available to estimate the likelihood of finding a mutation in association with a particularly pathology. Disorders are included in this table where the likelihood of a mutation-positive test is reasonable, particularly given the importance of identification of the familial cancer syndrome and the opportunity to provide cancer screening and cancer risk reduction to the identified individual.

[c]Lynch syndrome or hereditary nonpolyposis colorectal cancer (HNPCC) related cancers include colorectal, small bowel, endometrial, stomach, ovarian, pancreas, ureter and renal pelvis, biliary tract, brain tumors (usually glioblastoma as seen in Turcot syndrome), sebaceous gland adenomas, and keratoacanthomas in Muir–Torre syndrome.

[d]LCCSCT = large cell calcifying Sertoli cell tumors.

5.9   FAMILY ANCESTRY IS IMPORTANT FOR CANCER RISK ASSESSMENT

It is important to record the ethnicity of each grandparent because a number of founder mutations have been identified for various cancer syndromes. For example, the 999del5 mutation in *BRCA2* accounts for 40% of inherited breast cancer risk in Iceland (Thorlacius, 1997), and in individuals of Ashkenazi Jewish ancestry the founder mutations in *BRCA1* (185delAG and 5382insC) and *BRCA2* (6174delT) are common. The likelihood of identifying a *BRCA1* or *BRCA2* mutation in a man or woman of Ashkenazi ancestry with a family history of breast and/or ovarian cancer is higher than for a non-Ashkenazi person with a similar family history. For example, a Caucasian woman with ovarian cancer and no family history of breast or ovarian cancer has about a 13% probability of having a *BRCA1* or *BRCA2* mutation as compared to a 22–35% likelihood of testing positive for a mutation if the woman is Ashkenazi Jewish (Myriad Genetics Laboratories, 2006). Also, the son or daughter of a parent with one of the *BRCA* Ashkenazi Jewish founder mutations is offered screening for all three *BRCA* mutations if the other parent is Ashkenazi Jewish, given the high frequency of these BRCA founder mutations in that population (Berliner and Fay, 2007; Rubenstein, 2004)

Another example of the importance of noting a client's ethnicity in cancer risk assessment is in genetic evaluation of the hereditary polyposis syndromes. The auto-somal recessive MYH-associated polyposis or MAP syndrome is associated with two common *MYH* mutations in the northern European population, Y16C and G282D; therefore, targeted genetic testing is often the approach; gene sequencing would be required for a person of non-European ancestry as there are other mutations that could be responsible (Lefevre et al., 2006).

The likelihood of identifying a genetic sequence variant of uncertain significance varies in different populations. For example, the probability of finding a variant of unknown significance of the *BRCA1* or *BRCA2* gene is about 7% in a person of northern or central European ancestry, but 21% in a person of African American ancestry, 14% in person of Asian ancestry, and 8% in a person of Native American ancestry (Myriad Genetics, personal correspondence, July 2006). Persons undergoing cancer genetic counseling should be advised of this possibility before they undergo genetic testing (Trepanier et al., 2004).

5.10   CONSANGUINITY AND CANCER RISK ASSESSMENT

The offspring of closely related individuals are at higher risk to have inherited the same autosomal recessive gene mutations from a common ancestor (autozygosity) (Bennett et al., 2002). Some of the autosomal recessive conditions associated with cancer are listed in Table 5.6. *MYH*-associated polyposis or MAP is a fairly common cause of increased risk for colon cancer and is inherited in an autosomal recessive pattern. For individuals with MAP, evaluation of the partner would be particularly important if the couple is consanguineous because the partner may be heterozygous for the same recessive mutation. Therefore their children would be at 50% risk to be homozygous for the *MYH* mutation, and thus at potential risk to be affected with multiple adenomatous colon polyps associated with increased risk for colon cancer.

Fumaric aciduria (fumarase deficiency) is a severe inborn error of metabolism in homozygous or compound heterozygotes for mutations in *FH*; monoallelic carriers of mutations in *FH* may have manifestations HLRCC (hereditary leiomyomatosis with multiple cutaneous and uterine leiomyomas and renal cell carcinoma) (Alam et al., 2005; Wei et al., 2006). Although this is a rare condition, it is a condition to consider in relation to consanguinity if the diagnosis is made in a heterozygous adult with leiomyomatosis and/or renal cell cancer, or in a child with fumarase deficiency.

The role of consanguinity in relation to autosomal dominant cancer syndromes has not been well studied (Bennett et al., 2002). There is the potential risk of inheriting the mutant allele from both parents related through a common ancestor. Having two *BRCA1* gene mutations (*biallelic*) is considered an embryonic lethal, whereas individuals who have two parents who each have a *BRCA2* mutation are at 25% risk to be biallelic for the *BRCA2* mutation that causes Fanconi anemia group D1 (Alter et al., 2007). There is a suggestion of embryonic lethality inheritance with certain biallelic *BRCA2* mutations as well (Rahman and Scott, 2007).

Having two mutations (homozygosity or compound heterozygosity) in the Lynch syndrome mismatch repair genes (*MLH1, MSH2, MSH6, PMS2, TACSTD1*) is associated with a condition called constitutional mismatch repair deficiency (CMMR-D), which first appeared in the literature as the syndrome CoLoN: colon tumors or/and leukemia/lymphoma or/and neurofibromatosis type 1 features (Bandipalliam, 2005; Gallinger et al., 2004; Hedge et al., 2005; Will et al., 2007). The cancers have been primarily identified in childhood, with the predominance of cancers being brain, colon, and hematological, and the children have neurofibromatosis features (such as café au lait spots, axillary freckling, macrocephaly). Although each parent carries a mutation in one of the Lynch syndrome genes, the child may not have a family history of the typical cancers seen in Lynch syndrome (Senter et al., 2008; Wimmer and Etzler 2008). This may be particularly true with *PMS2* mutations for which the penetrance of cancer seems to be significantly lower than with the other Lynch syndrome mutations (Senter et al., 2008, Wimmer and Etzler, 2008). Many of the children affected with CMMR-D have had consanguineous parents (Poley et al., 2007; Wimmer and Etzler, 2008).

Traditionally, genetic counseling for couples who are consanguineous has focused on risks that their offspring will have severe autosomal recessive disorders that present in the first few years of life; hence forward, more attention should be paid to noting a family history of common adult-onset disorders, particularly cancer.

Biallelic mutations in the cancer susceptibility gemes *PALB2/FACN* and *BR1P1* also cause Fanconi anemia (Seal et al., 2006; Schindler et al., 2007).

5.11 CANCER WORRY: THE PEDIGREE AS A PSYCHOSOCIAL TOOL

Coyote's Call

For Ron, July 30, 2002

We are sitting on top of the porch stairs side by side, Chaco and I listening to the quiet,
Watching the small wind-driven waves slowly make their way across the clear plate
glass, until reflections ripple—each in our own private worlds.

I am thinking of you,
80 miles south in your bed,
Connected to all those lines
With "Your Paddy" spending the night—a one of a kind sleep over.

It starts—one, two and then a serenade of strange, wild yips
Inspired by the last days of the full moon.
Chaco startles and heads down the stairs.

I summon him back
"Those are just your ancestors calling," I reassure.
Then it occurs to me that ours have voices not yet audible
And they are calling you.

I don't want either of you to leave me . . . even to join them.
I can hold onto Chaco, I cannot do that for you.
There is a call—stronger, more powerful than mine.
It wants you there;
I, and we, want you here.
Please, turn off your silent voices!

It is morning now, the moon is fading;
We hold on for another day.

Coda:

2004

Now they are calling me too.
I do not want to go. I know you did not either.
I intend to fight as long as I possibly can.
Then I too will join you.

2005

Now it is time.

—**Dona Boyd-MacDonald (1944–2006, printed with permission of Steve Boyd,
Seattle)**

Reviewing a pedigree is not only the major tool for providing cancer risk assessment but is also an obvious reference to the experience of cancer in the family. Have
people in the family survived their cancer? Were several people in the family diagnosed with cancer over a short time span? Did available cancer surveillance methods

such as mammography reliably identify cancer in relatives? A person who is undergoing cancer risk assessment needs to be able to tell his or her family story (Schneider, 2002). Taking time to listen to worries about developing cancer can help the clinician understand the patient's concerns about the effectiveness of cancer screening and treatment.

The clinician can also be alerted to significant correlations between the patient's feelings and actions and his or her family history. For example, the patient may seek aggressive prevention strategies such as prophylactic mastectomy or colectomy because a parent or sibling did not survive their cancer. The patient may be more anxious about participating in cancer screening as he or she approaches the age at which a relative developed cancer, or even become more complacent about cancer screening because he or she has passed the age at which the relative developed cancer and thus has "escaped" the disease. A woman may fear becoming pregnant because a relative was diagnosed with cancer in her pregnancy. If multiple relatives have developed cancer, the patient may feel that cancer is the norm rather than the exception (Patenaude, 2005).

Almost everyone who has a relative with cancer worries that the cancer in that person may be inherited, placing them at risk for cancer as well. Overestimation of cancer risk is common in both people who have a hereditary risk and those for whom there is little evidence that there is high risk for cancer (Patenaude, 2005). A pedigree can be used as a tool to educate the patient about cancer risks, as well as relieve anxieties about risk for cancer in the absence of significant family history factors.

5.12 MODELS FOR PREDICTING THE RISK OF DEVELOPING CANCER OR THE PROBABILITY OF TESTING MUTATION-POSITIVE FOR AN INHERITED CANCER SYNDROME

The development of models that factor family history into the likelihood of developing cancer or the likelihood of having a positive test for a cancer genetic syndrome are becoming readily available (NCI, 2009). Most of the models factor in the age at cancer diagnosis of the consultand and in closely related relatives. The models predicting breast cancer risk or the likelihood of having a *BRCA1* or *BRCA2* mutation are more advanced as compared to other cancer syndromes. Each model has it flaws, but certainly they each can be useful in a clinical setting (Barcenas et al., 2006; Jacobi et al., 2008; Kang et al., 2006). The Claus model is useful for predicting breast cancer risk for women with one or two first- or second-degree relatives with breast cancer (Claus et al., 1994). This model considers the current age of the woman and the ages at which her first- and second-degree relatives developed cancer. It does not consider ovarian cancer, male breast cancer, or bilateral breast cancer. Figure 5.1 illustrates how significantly a younger age at breast cancer diagnosis positively influences a first- or second-degree relative's likelihood of developing breast cancer (with the risks being higher for breast cancer diagnosed before menopause). The Gail model has been used primarily for postmenopausal women who have a limited family history of breast cancer. This model does not factor in the age that the relatives developed breast cancer,

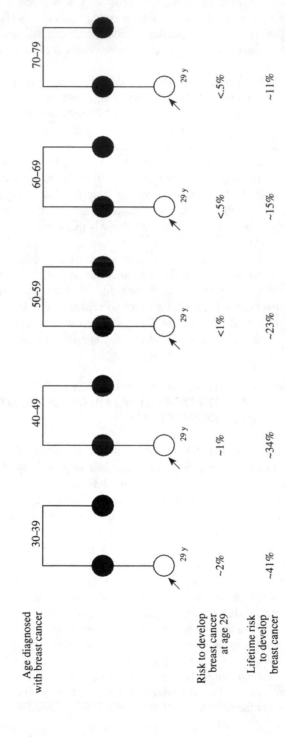

Figure 5.1 The empirical risk to develop breast cancer based on the age of onset of breast cancer in a mother and a maternal aunt. Note that if the consultand's mother and aunt develop breast cancer between the ages of 70 and 79 years, the consultand's lifetime risk to develop breast cancer is similar to the background risk to develop cancer by age 80. Risk figures derived from Claus et al. (1994).

only the number of first-degree relatives with breast cancer. Other personal factors such as the age of the women, age at first live birth, ethnicity, and breast biopsies are also factored into the model. This model can underestimate hereditary risk. The Myriad-Frank model is derived from the family history information regarding the age and types of cancer in the consultand and his or her first- and second-degree relatives listed on requisition forms from persons undergoing the commercial test for *BRCA1* and *BRCA2* through Myriad Genetics Laboratory (www.myriadtests.com), and they have developed a similar model in relation to persons undergoing genetic testing for Lynch syndrome.

The National Cancer Institute website (at http://riskfactor.cancer.gov/cancer_risk_prediction) is a comprehensive resource with links to summaries of many of the cancer risk assessment models and related bibliographies. Another essential resource is the BayesMendel Lab (2009) (http://astor.som.jhmi.edu/BayesMendel/index.html), which includes references on cancer susceptibility and links to models for predicting who may carry a cancer susceptibility gene (all open source software). Models such as these are likely to play a growing role in determining which persons are the best candidates for genetic testing and for whom increased cancer surveillance is indicated based on family history alone when the available genetic tests do not identify all of the possible mutations. Although the models' predicting the likelihood of identifying a cancer susceptibility mutation or for predicting the risk for cancer can be useful in aggregate, the models give widely varying predictions (Jacobi et al., 2008). Therefore, an understanding of the assumptions used in creating each model and the appropriate clinical application is essential.

5.13 SUMMARY

The instruments of molecular genetics, in concert with a precise genetic family history, provide clinicians with powerful investigative tools to identify individuals with an increased risk to develop various cancers. Corroborating verbal history of cancer with medical records is key so that accurate cancer risk assessment and a plan for genetic testing and cancer screening and prevention can be implemented. Verbal recall of cancer diagnoses is less likely to be accurate on distant relatives and for female cancers and rare cancers.

For most men and women with a personal or family history of cancer, counseling about cancer screening and prevention will rely on a through assessment of the family history rather than a genetic test result. With the ever-expanding palette of commercially available tests that predict cancer susceptibility, medical professionals must be prepared to offer accurate counseling about the meaning of a positive, negative, or ambiguous test result. Testing, if performed, must be interpreted in the context of the family history. It is irresponsible to order a cancer genetic test without taking a medical family history. Such testing, done poorly, can cause more harm than benefit. Test results have profound reverberations for an individual's psychological and physical health, insurability, and family and social functioning (Greely, 1997; McKinnon et al., 1997; Patenaude, 2005; Schneider, 2002; Trepanier, 2004).

Cautions Dr. Kenneth Offit (1998), former chair of the American Society of Clinical Oncology's Subcommittee on Genetic Testing for Cancer Susceptibility, "A genetic test of outstanding scientific interest is of little clinical value if the clinician is unable to interpret it, the patient afraid or unsure how to act on it, and the national health-care system unable to provide it without penalty or discrimination."

A dramatic example of the power of pedigree analysis is shown in Figure 5.1. A healthy 29-year-old woman is concerned about her risk of developing breast cancer given a history of breast cancer in her mother and maternal aunt, with no other family history of breast or other cancers. The occurrence of postmenopausal breast cancer in her aunt and mother does not significantly change her risk to develop breast cancer from that of other women her age. In contrast, the consultand's lifetime risk to develop breast cancer (based on empirical risk figures from the Claus model) approaches that of an autosomal dominant syndrome if her mother and aunt have breast cancer diagnosed in their 30s (Claus et al., 1994). For many individuals with fears about a family history of cancer, careful pedigree analysis can reassure them that their lifetime risk to develop cancer is not significantly different from other people their age.

5.14   REFERENCES

Aguirre D, Nieto K, Lazos M, et al. (2006). Extragonadal germ cell tumors are often associated with Klinefelter syndrome. *Hum Path* 37(4):477–480.

Ahmen M, Rahman N. (2006). ATM and breast cancer susceptibility. *Oncogene* 25:5906–5911.

Aitken JF, Youl P, Green A, et al. (1996). Accuracy of case-reported family history of melanoma in Queensland, Australia. *Melanoma Res* 6:313–317.

Airewele G, Adatto P. Cunninham J, et al. (1998). Family history of cancer in patients with glioma: A validation study of accuracy. *J Natl Cancer Inst.* 90(7):543–544.

Alam NA, Olpin S, Rowan A, et al. (2005). Missense mutations in fumarate hydratase in multiple cutaneous and uterine leiomyomas and renal cell cancer. *J Mol Diagn* 7(4):437–443.

Alter BP, Rosenberg PS, Brody LC. (2007). Clinical and molecular features associated with biallelic mutations in FANCD1/BRCA2. *J Med Genet* 44:1–9.

Amos CI, Frazier ML, McGarrity TJ. (2007). Peutz-Jeghers Syndrome. May 15, 2007. Available at www.genereviews.org. Accessed January 24, 2009.

Aretz S, Koch A, Uhlhass S, et al. (2006). Should children at risk for familial adenomatous polyposis be screened for hepatoblastoma and children with apparently sporadic hepatoblastoma be screened for APC germline mutations? *Pediatr Blood Cancer* 47:811–818.

Bandipalliam P. (2005). Syndrome of early onset colon cancers, hematologic malignancies and features of neurofibromatosis in HNPCC families with homozygous mismatch repair gene mutations. *Fam Cancer* 4:323–333.

Barcenas CH, Hosain GM, Arun B, et al. (2006). Assessing BRCA carrier probabilities in extended families. *J Clin Oncol* 24(3):354–360.

BayesMendel Lab (2009). BayesMendel Lab Home. Available at http://astor. som.jhmi.edu/BayesMendel/index.html. Accessed November 22, 2009.

Bennett RL, Motulsky AG, Bittles A, et al. (2002). Genetic evaluation of consanguineous couples and their offspring: Recommendation of the National Society of Genetic Counselors. *J Genet Couns* 11(2):97–119.

Berliner JL, Fay AM. (2007). Risk assessment and genetic counseling for hereditary breast ovarian cancer: Recommendations of the National Society of Genetic Counselors. *J Genet Couns* 16(3):241–260.

Bertherat J, Gimenez-Roqueplo AP. (2005). New insights in the genetics of adrenocortical tumors, pheochromocytomas and paragangliomas. *Horm Metab Res* 37(6):384–390.

Birch JM, Alston RD, McNally RJ, et al. (2001). Relative frequency and morphology of cancers in carriers of germline TP53 mutations. *Oncogene* 20:4621–4628.

Boedeker CC, Neumann HP, Maier W, et al., (2007). Malignant head and neck paragangliomas in SDHB mutation carriers. *Otolaryngol Head Neck Surg* 137:126–129.

Bonne AC, Bodmer D, Schoenmakers EF, et al. (2004). Chromosome 3 translocations and familial renal cell cancer. *Curr Mol Med.* 4:849–854.

Bravi F, Scotti L, Bosetti C, et al. (2008). Food groups and endometrial cancer risk: A case control study from Italy. *Am J Obstet Gynecol* (2003; ePub ahead of print).

Brems H, Park C, Maertens O, et al. (2009). Glomus tumors in Neurofibromatosis type 1: genetic, functional, and clinical evidence of a novel association. *Cancer Res* 69(18):7393–7401.

Breuer B, Kash KM, Rosenthal G, et al. (1993). Accuracy of case-reported family history of melanoma in Queensland, Australia. *Melanoma Res* 6:313–317.

Brozek I, Ochman K, Debniak J, et al. (2008). *Gynecol Oncol* 108(2):433–437.

Buxbaum JD, Cai G, Chaste P, et al. (2007). Mutation screening of the PTEN gene in patients with autism spectrum disorders and macrocephaly. *Am J Med Genet B Neuropsychiatr Genet.* 144(4):484–491.

Chetrit A, Hirsh-Yechezkel G, Ben-David Y, et al. (2008). Effect of BRCA1/2 mutations on long-term survival of patients with invasive ovarian cancer: the national Israeli study of ovarian cancer. *J Clin Oncol* 26(1):20–25.

Chhibber V, Dresser K, Mahalingam M. (2008). *MSH6*: Extending the reliability of immuno-histochemistry as a screening tool in Muir-Torre syndrome. *Mod Pathol* 21(2):159–164.

Chodick G, Struewing JP, Ron E, et al. (2008). Similar prevalence of founder *BRCA1* and *BRCA2* mutations among Ashkenazi and non-Ashkenazi men with breast cancer: Evidence from 261 cases in Israel, 1976–1999. *Eur J Med Genet* 51(2):141–147.

Claus EB, Risch N. Thompson WD. (1994). Autosomal dominant inheritance of early-onset breast cancer. Implications for risk prediction. *Cancer* 73:643–651.

Cowgill SM, Muscarella P (2003). Genetics of pancreatic cancer. *Am J Surg* 186:279–286.

Dahia P. (2006). Evolving concepts in pheochromocytoma and paraganglioma. *Curr Opinions Onc* 18:1–8.

Diaz LK, Cryris VL, Symmans WZF, Sneige N. (2007). Triple negative breast carcinoma and the basal phenotype: From expression profiling to clinical practice. *Adv Anat Pathol.* 14(6):419–430.

Douglas FS, O'Dair LC, Robinson M, et al. (1999). The accuracy of diagnoses as reported in families with cancer: a retrospective study. *J Med Genet.* 36:309–312.

Eeles RA, Easton DF, Ponder BAJ, Eng C, eds. (2004). *Genetic Predisposition to Cancer,* 2nd ed. Arnold: London.

Eng C. (2003). Invited mutation update. *PTEN*: One gene, many syndromes. *Hum Mutat* 22:183–198.

Eng C. (2000). Will the real Cowden syndrome please stand up: Revised diagnostic criteria. *J Med Genet* 37:828–830.

Evans DG, Farndon PA. (2008). Nevoid basal cell carcinoma syndrome. January 25, 2008. Available at www.genereviews.org. Accessed November 20, 2009.

Ferolla P, Falchetti A, Filosso P. et al. (2007). Thymic neuroendocrine carcinoma (carcinoid) in multiple endocrine neoplasia type 1 syndrome: The Italian series. *J Clin Encrinol Metab*. 90(5):2603–2609.

Firth HV, Hurst JA. (2005). *Oxford Desk Reference—Clinical Genetics*. New York: Oxford University Press.

Foulkes WD, Thiffault I, Gruber SB, et al. (2002). The founder mutation *MSH2*∗1906G C is an important cause of hereditary nonpolyposis colorectal cancer in the Ashkenazi Jewish population. *Am J Hum Genet* 71(6):1395–1412.

Freeman HJ. (2008). Proton pump inhibitors and an emerging epidemic of gastric fundic gland polyposis. *World J Gastroenterol* 14(9):1318–1320.

Friedman JM. (1997). Genetics and epidemiology, congenital anomalies and cancer. *Am J Hum Genet* 60:469–473.

Gallinger S, Aronson M, Shayan K, et al. (2004). Gastrointestinal cancer and neurofibromatosis type 1 features in children with germline homozygous *MLH1* mutation. *Gastroenterology* 26:576–585.

Gonzalez KD, Noltner KA, Buzin CH, et al. (2009). Beyond Li-Fraumeni syndrome: clinical characteristics of families with p53 germline mutations. *J Clin Oncol* (2009; ePub ahead of print).

Goon PK, Stanley MA, Ebmeyer J, et al. (2009). HPV and head and neck cancer: a descriptive update. *Head Neck Oncol* 1(1): 1–36.

Gorlin RJ, Cohen MM, Levin LS. (2001). *Syndromes of the Head and Neck*. New York: Oxford University Press.

Greely HT. (1997). Genetic testing for cancer susceptibility: Challenges for creators of practice guidelines. *Oncology* 11:171–176.

Gronberg H, Issacs SD, Smith JR, et al., (1997). Characteristics of prostate cancer in families potentially linked to the hereditary prostate cancer 1 (*HPC1*) locus. *JAMA* 278:1251–1255.

Hadfield KD, Newman WG, Bowers NL, et al. (2008). Molecular characterisation of *SMARCB1* and *NF2* in familial and sporadic schwannomatosis. *J Med Genet* 45(6): 332–339.

Hamataini K, Eguchi H, Ito R, et al. (2008). *RET/PTC* rearrangements preferentially occurred in papillary thyroid cancer among atomic bomb survivors. *Cancer Res* 68(17):7176–7182.

Hampel H, Frankel W, Panescu J, et al. (2006). Screening for Lynch syndrome (hereditary nonpolyposis colorectal cancer) among endometrial cancer patients. *Cancer Res* 66(15):7810–7817.

Hedge MR, Chong B, Blazo ME, et al. (2005). A homozygous mutation in *MSH6* causes Turcot syndrome. *Clin Cancer Res* 11:4689–4693.

Herman GE, Henninger N, Ratliff-Schaub K, et al. (2007). Genetic testing in autism: How much is enough? *Genet Med*. 9(5):268–274.

Howe JR, Haidle JL, Lal G, et al., (2007). ENG mutations in *MADH4/BMPR1A* mutation negative patients with juvenile polyposis. *Clinical Genet* 71:91–92.

Jacobi CE, De Bock GH, Siegerink B, van Asperen CJ. (2008). Differences and similarities in breast cancer risk assessment models in clinical practice: which model to choose? *Breast Cancer Res Treat* (2008; ePub ahead of print).

Jacoby RF, Schlack S, Sekhon G, Laxova R. (1997). Del (10)(q22.3q24.1) associated with juvenile polyposis. *Am J Med Genet* 70:361–364.

Jass JR. (2008). Colorectal polyposis: From phenotype to diagnosis. *Pathol Res Pract* 204(7):431–447.

Jass JR. (2000). Pathology of hereditary non-polyposis colorectal cancer. *Ann N Y Aead Sci* 910:62–73.

Kang HH, Williams R, Leary J, et al. (2006). Evaluation of models to predict BRCA germline mutations. *Br J Cancer* 95:914–920.

Kaurah P, MacMillan A, Boyd N, et al. (2007). Founder and recurrent *CDH1* mutation in families with hereditary diffuse gastric cancer. *JAMA* 297(21):2360–2372.

Kerber RA, Slattery ML. (1997). Comparison of self-reported and database-linked family history of cancer data in case-control study. *Am J Epidemiol* 146:244–248.

Kerr B, Foulkes WD, Cade D et al. (1998). False family history in the family cancer clinic. *Euro J Surg Onc* 24:275–279.

King TM, Ton L, Pack RT, et al. (2002). Accuracy of history of cancer as reported by men with prostate cancer. *Urology* 59(4):546–550.

Kock M, Gaedke H, Jenkins H. (1989). Family history of ovarian cancer patients: A case-control study. *Int J Epidemiol* 18:275–279.

Kovacs ME, Papp J, Szentirmay Z, et al. (2009). Deletions removing the last exon of *TACSTD1* constitute a distinct class of mutations predisposing to Lynch syndrome. *Hum Mut* 30(2):197–203.

Krutilkova V, Trkova M, Fleitz J, et al. (2005). Identification of 5 new families strengthens link between child choroid plexus carcinoma and germline *TP53* mutations. *Eur J Canc* 41:1597–1602.

Lachlan KL, Lucassen AM, Bunyan D, Temple IK. (2007). Cowden syndrome and Bannayan Riley Ruvalcaba syndrome represent one condition with variable expression and age-related penetrance: Results of a clinical study of *PTEN* mutation carriers. *J Med Genet* 44(9):579–585.

Lakhani SR, Reis-Filno JS, Fulford L. (2005). Prediction of *BRCA1* status in patients with breast cancer using estrogen receptor and basal phenotype. *Clin Canc Res* 11: 5175–5180.

Landi MT, Bauer J, Pfeiffer RM, et al. (2006). *MCIR* germline variants confer risk for *BRAF*-mutant melanoma. *Science* online.

Lebrun C, Olschwan S, Jeannin S, et al. (2007). Turcot syndrome confirmed with molecular analysis. *Eur J Neurol* 14(4):470–472.

Lefevre JH, Rodrigue CM, Mourra N, et al., (2006). Implication of *MYH* in colorectal polyposis. *Ann Surg* 244(6):874–880.

Levy-Lahad E, Friedman E. (2007). Cancer risks among *BRCA1* and *BRCA2* mutation carriers. *British J Canc* 96:11–15.

Liaw D, Marsh DJ, Li J, et al. (1997). Germline mutations of the *PTEN* gene in Cowden disease, an inherited breast and thyroid cancer syndrome. *Nature Genet* 17: 79–83.

Lindor M, McMaster ML, Lindor CJ, Greene MH. (2008). Concise Handbook of Familial Cancer Susceptibility Syndromes. 2nd ed. *J Natl Cancer Instit Monogr* (38): 1–93.

Love R, Evans AM, Josten DM. (1985). The accuracy of patient reports of a family history of cancer. *J Chron Dis* 38:289–293.

Lu KH, Schorge JO, Rodabaugh K, et al. (2007). Prospective determination of prevalence of lynch syndrome in young women with endometrial cancer. *J Clin Oncol* 25(33):5143–5146.

Lynch ED, Ostermeyer EA, Lee MK, et al. (1997). Inherited mutations that are associated with breast cancer, Cowden disease, and juvenile polyposis. *Am J Hum Genet* 61:1254–1260.

Marsh DJ, Dahia PLM, Zheng Z, et al. (1997). Germline mutations in *PTEN* are present in Bannayan-Zonana syndrome. *Nature Genet* 16:333–334.

McKinnon WC, Baty B, Bennett RL, et al. (1997). Predisposition genetic testing for late-onset disorders in adults: A points to consider document of the National Society of Genetic Counselors. *JAMA* 278:1217–1220.

Medeiros F, Muto MG, Lee Y, et al. (2006). The tubal fimbria is a preferred site for early adeno-carcinoma in women with familial ovarian caner syndrome. *Am J Surg Pathol* 3(2):230–236.

Menczer J, Chetrit A, Barda G, et al. (2003). Frequency of *BRCA* mutations in primary peritoneal carcinoma in Israeli Jewish women. *Gynecol Oncol* 88(1):58–61.

Merg A, Howe JR. (2004). Genetic conditions associated with intestinal juvenile polyps [Seminar]. *Am J Med Genet* 129C:44–55.

Mizusawa N, Uchino S, Iwata T, et al. (2006). Genetic analyses in patients with familial isolated hyperparathyroidism and hyperparathyroidism-jaw tumour syndrome. *Clin Encorinol* (Oxf) 65(1):9–16.

Moghaddam A, Bicknell R. (1995). The organ preference of metastasis—The journey from the circulation to secondary site. In: Vile RG, ed., *Cancer Metastasis: From Mechanisms to Therapies*. New York: J Wiley, p. 48.

Murff HJ, Spigel DR, Syngal S. (2004). Does this patient have a family history of cancer? An evidence-based analysis of the accuracy of family cancer history. *JAMA* 292(12):1480–1489.

Muscat JE, Huncharek MS. (2008). Perineal talc use and ovarian cancer: A critical review. *Eur J Cancer Prev* 17(2):139–146.

Myriad Genetic Laboratories. (2006). Mutation prevalence tables. Spring 2006. Available at www.myriadtests.com. Accessed February 1, 2009.

National Cancer Institute. (2008). Prevention, genetics, causes. December 4, 2008. Available at www.cancer. gov/cancertopics/prevention-genetics-causes. Accessed November 20, 2009.

National Cancer Institute (2009b). Cancer risk prediction resources. October 2, 2009. Available at http://riskfactor. cancer.gov/cancer_risk_prediction. Accessed November 20, 2009.

National Comprehensive Cancer Network. (2009). NCCN clinical practice guidelines in on-cology. Genetic/familial high-risk assessment: Breast and ovarian. May 4, 2009. Available at www.nccn.org/professionals/physician_gls/PDF/genetics_screening.pdf. Accessed November 20, 2009.

National Institute for Environment and Health Services, U. S. Department of Health and Human Services. (2003). Cancer and the environment. Available at www.niehs.nih.gov/health/scied/documents/CancerEnvironment.pdf. August 2003. Accessed February 1, 2009.

Offit K. (1998). *Clinical Cancer Genetics: Risk Counseling and Management*. New York: Wiley.

OMIM (Online Mendelian Inheritance in Man). Available at http://www.ncbi. nlm.nih.gov/omim. Accessed November 22, 2009.

Oricco A, Galli L, Orsi A, et al. (2008). Novel *PTEN* mutations in neurodevelopmental disorders and microcephaly. *Clin Genet* (2008; ePub ahead of print).

Parent ME, Ghadirian P, Lacroix A, Perret C. (1997). The reliability of recollections of family history: Implications for the medical provider. *J Cancer Edu* 12(2):114–120.

Patenaude AF. (2005). *Genetic Testing for Cancer: Psychological Approaches for Helping Patients and Families*. Washington, DC: American Psychological Association.

Pelucchi C, Gallus S, Garavello W, et al. (2006). Cancer risk associated with alcohol and to-bacco use: Focus on upper aero-digestive tract and liver. *Alcohol Res Health* 29(3):193–198.

Pilarski R. (2009). Cowden syndrome: A critical review of the clinical literature. *J Genet Couns* 18:13–27.

Poley JW, Wagner A, Hoogmans MM, et al. (2007). Biallelic germline mutations of mismatch-repair genes: A possible cause for multiple pediatric malignancies. *Cancer* 207 109(11):2349–2356.

Preston DL, Ron E, Tokuoka S, et al. (2007). Solid cancer incidence in atomic bomb survivors: 1958–1998. *Radiat Res* 168(1):1–64.

Rahman N, Scott RH. (2007). Cancer genes associated with phenotypes in monoallelic and biallelic mutation carriers: new lessons from old players. *Hum Molec Genet* 16: R60–R66.

Renwick A, Thompson D, Seal S, et al. (2006). *ATM* mutations that cause ataxia-telangiectasia are breast cancer susceptibility genes. *Nat Genet* 38:873–875.

Ribeiro RC, Sandrini F, Figueiredo B, et al. (2001). An inherited *p53* mutation contributes in a tissue-specific manner to pediatric adrenal cortical carcinoma. *Proc Natl Acad Sci* 98:933–9335.

Richards ML. (2009). Thyroid cancer genetics: multiple endocrine neoplasia type 2, non-midullary familial thyroid cancer, and familial syndromes associated with thyroid cancer. *Surg Oncol Clin N Am* 18(1): 39–52.

Ries LAG, Harkins D, Krapcho M, et al., eds. (2006). *SEER cancer statistics review, 1975–2003*, Bethesda, MD: National Cancer Institute. Available at http://seer.cancer.gov/csr/1975_2003. Accessed September 6, 2007.

Risch HA, McLaughoin JR, Cole DE, et al. (2006). Population *BRCA1* and *BRCA2* mutation frequencies and cancer penetrances: A kin-cohort study in Ontario, Canada: *J Natl Cancer Inst* 98:1694–1706.

Rubenstein WS. (2004). Hereditary breast cancer in Jews. *Familial Cancer* 3:249–257.

Russell-Swetek A, West AN, Mintern JE, et al. (2008). Identification of a novel *TP53* germline mutation E285V in a rare case of paediatric adrenocortical carcinoma and choroids plexus carcinoma. *J Med Genet* 45(9):603–606.

Santiago J, Muszlak M, Samson C, et al. (2008). Malignancy risk and Wiedemann-Beckwith syndrome: What follow-up to provide? *[French]. Arch Pediatr* 15(9):1498–1502.

Schindler RS, Hanenberg H, Barker K. (2007). Biallelic mutations in *PALB2* cause Fanconi anemia subtype FA–N and predispose to childhood cancer. *Nat Genet* 39(2): 162–164.

Schneider KA. (2002). *Counseling about Cancer 2nd ed*. New York: Wiley-Liss.

Schneider KA, DiGianni LM, Patenaude AF, et al. (2004). Accuracy of cancer family histories: Comparison of two breast cancer syndromes. *Genet Testing* 8:222–228.

Seal S, Thompson D, Renwick A, et al. (2006). Truncating mutations in the Fanconi anemia J gene *BRIP1* are low penetrance breast cancer susceptibility alleles. *Nat Genet* 38:1239–1241.

Senter L, Clendenning M, Sotamaa K, et al. (2008). The clinical phenotype of Lynch syndrome due to germ-line *PMS2* mutations. *Gastroenterology* 135(2):419–428.

Shattuck TM, Välimäki S, Obara T, et al. (2003). Somatic and germ-line mutation of the *HRPT2* gene in sporadic parathyroid carcinoma. *N Engl J Med* 349(18):1722–1729.

Singh RS, Grayson W, Redston M, et al. (2008). Site and tumor type predicts DNA mismatch repair status in cutaneous sebaceous neoplasia. *Am J Surg Pathol* 32(6):936–942.

Stratakis CA, Kirschner LS, Carney JA. (2001). Clinical and molecular features of the Carney complex: Diagnostic criteria and recommendations for patient evaluation. *J Clin Endocr Metabo* 86:4041–4046.

Suriano G, Yew S, Ferreira P, et al. (2005). Characterization of a recurrent germ line mutation of the e-cadherin gene: Implications for genetic testing and clinical management. *Clin Cancer Res* 11:5401–5409.

Sweet K, Willis J, Zhou XP, et al. (2005). Molecular classification of patients with unexplained hamartomatous and hyperplastic polyposis. *JAMA* 294:2498–2500.

Swensen JJ, Keyser J, Coffin CM, et al. (2009). Familial occurrence of schwannomas and malignant rhabdoid tumor associated with a duplication in *SMARCB1*. *J Med Genet* 46:68–72.

Tan WH, Baris HN, Burrows PE, et al. (2007). The spectrum of vascular anomalies n patients with *PTEN* mutations: implications for diagnosis and management. *J Med Genet* 44(9):594–602.

Theis B, Boyd N, Lockwood G, Tritchler D (1994). Accuracy of family cancer history in breast cancer patients. *Eur J Cancer Prev* 3:321–327.

Thorlacius S, Sigurdsson S, Bjarnadottir H, et al. (1997). Study of a single *BRCA2* mutation with high carrier frequency in a small population. *Am J Hum Genet* 60:1079–1084.

Tomoda C, Miyauchi A, Uruno T, et al. (2004). Cribriform-morular variant of papillary thyroid carcinoma: Clue to early detection of familial adenomatous polyposis-associated colon cancer. *World J Surg* 28(9):886–889.

Trepanier A, Ahrens M, McKinnon W, et al. (2004). Genetic cancer risk assessment and counseling: recommendations of the National Society of Genetic Counselors. *J Genet Couns* 13(2):83–114.

Umar A, Boland CR, Terdiman J, et al., (2004). Revised Bethesda guidelines for HNPCC (Lynch syndrome) and MSI. *J Natl Cancer Inst* 96:261–267.

van Hattem WA, Brosens LA, deLeng WW, et al. (2008). Large genomic deletions of *SMAD4*, *BMPR1A* and *PTEN* in juvenile polyposis. *Gut* 57(5):623–627.

Varley JM. (2003). Germline p53 mutations and Li-Fraumeni syndrome. *Hum Mut* 21:313–320.

Walsh MD, Cummings MC, Buchanan DD, et al. (2008). Molecular, pathologic, and clinical features of early-onset endometrial cancer: Identifying presumptive lynch syndrome patients. *Clini Cancer* 14(6):1692–1700.

Wei M-H, Toure O, Glenn GM, et al. (2006). Novel mutations in *FH* and expression of the spectrum of phenotypes expressed in families with hereditary leiomyomatosis and renal cell cancer. *J Med Genet* 43:18–27.

Weitzel JN, Lagos VI, Cullinane CA, et al. (2007). Limited family structure and *BRCA* gene mutation in single cases of breast cancer. *JAMA* 297(23):2587–2595.

Will O, Carvajal-Carmona LG, Gorman P et al. (2007). Homozygous *PMS2* deletion causes a severe colorectal cancer and multiple adenoma phenotype without extraintestinal cancer. *Gastroenterology* 132:527–530.

Williams TT. (1991). *Refuge, An Unnatural History of Family and Place.* New York: Vintage Books.

Wimmer K, Etzler J. (2008). Constitutional mismatch repair-deficiency syndrome: Have we so far seen only the tip of an iceberg? *Hum Genet* 124(2):105–122.

Wirtzfeld DA, Petrelli NJ, Rodriguez-Bigas MA. (2001). Hamartomatous polyposis syndromes: Molecular genetics neoplastic risk and surveillance recommendations. *Ann Surg Oncol* 8:319–327.

Young RH. (2005). Sex cord-stromal tumors of the ovary and testis: Their similarities and differences with consideration of selected problems. *Mod Pathol Suppl* 2:S81–S98

Young WF, Abooud AL. (2006). Editorial: Paraganglioma—All in the family. *J Clin Endocrinol Metab* 91:790–792.

Zhou X-P, Woodford-Richens K, Lehtonen R, et al. (2001). Germline mutations in *BMPR1A/ALK3* cause a subset of cases of juvenile polyposis syndrome and of Cowden and Bannayan-Riley-Ruvalcaba syndromes. *Am J Hum Genet* 69(4):704–711.

Ziogas A, Anton-Culver H. (2003). Validation of family history data in cancer family registries. *Am J Preven Med* 24(2):190–198.

Chapter 6

Medical Verification of Family History, and Resources for Patients to Record Their Genetic Family Histories

There is a moral and philosophical respect for our ancestors which elevates the character
and improves the heart
—Honorable Daniel Webster (1863)

6.1 VALIDATION OF FAMILY MEDICAL INFORMATION IS A NECESSITY

Genetic diseases are unique in that a whole family is in essence your patient. Confirming family lore by obtaining medical records is time-consuming but essential. Two clear illustrations from my own practice emphasize the need to corroborate oral reports of family-medical history information with formal medical documentation.

1. Elizabeth, a healthy 40-year-old woman, requested presymptomatic testing for Huntington disease (an autosomal dominant, adult-onset, neurodegenerative condition). It was her belief that her father and sister died of complications from

The Practical Guide to the Genetic Family History, Second Edition, by Robin L. Bennett
Copyright © 2010 John Wiley & Sons, Inc.

Huntington disease. Even though accurate DNA testing is available to identify the gene mutation in Huntington disease, we insisted that Elizabeth obtain both her father's and sister's medical records in order to confirm their diagnoses. Our review of their medical records indicated that her father and sister had a similar neurodegenerative illness, and that their symptoms were not typical of Huntington disease. Based on this information, we arranged for additional neuropathology studies on the stored brain tissue from her sister's autopsy, and from the results we diagnosed a form of autosomal dominant cerebellar ataxia. If Elizabeth had proceeded with DNA testing for Huntington disease, her testing would have been negative (normal). Elizabeth would have been falsely reassured that she was no longer at risk for her family's devastating neurodegenerative illness, when in fact she remained at 50:50 risk to develop the same disease that affected her father and sister. Given this new information we were able to offer Elizabeth accurate genetic testing and appropriate genetic counseling.

2. Diane, a healthy 30-year-old woman, was interested in information about her chance of developing ovarian cancer; 8 years earlier her mother died of ovarian cancer at age 50 years. With the exception that Diane's 70-year-old maternal uncle died of stomach cancer, there was no other family history of cancer. We obtained pathology reports on the tumors in both of these individuals; Diane's mother did not have ovarian cancer but a metastatic cancer of her abdomen of unknown primary origin (but not believed to be ovarian), and Diane's uncle had metastatic melanoma but not stomach cancer. Diane was planning to have a prophylactic oophorectomy because of her overwhelming fear of ovarian cancer. We were able to reassure Diane that we did not recognize an obvious hereditary cancer syndrome in her family, and that she should be screened for cancer in the same manner as any other woman of her age. She cancelled her surgery.

Your patient may know that his father and paternal grandfather died of colon cancer, but he is unlikely to know the details from the pathology reports. Most people have limited information about the details of the medical health of their extended family, and the facts they do know may be inaccurate. Even the family genealogist, or kin-keeper, may have limited medical details about family members. The traditions of genealogy focus on recording dates and locations of significant kinship alliances (such as births, deaths, and marriages), not documenting family illness. The purpose of early pedigrees was to document kinships for creating alliances of land and wealth as well as to prove relationship to aristocracy (Hey, 1993).

Although the onus is on your patient to obtain medical and family history information, your patient may be at a total loss as to where and how to begin. Such a task may seem especially daunting if the patient is geographically or emotionally distanced from the family. This chapter contains several resources for people to help them approach family members to obtain further medical history information. I have also included resources for patients to learn how to record their own family health history. This information is meant to encourage people to be partners in their health care with their health professionals.

6.2 HOW TO APPROACH FAMILY MEMBERS

Often the most effective means of approaching family members about obtaining medical and family history data is in person, at a family gathering. Family members may have different comfort levels with forms of communication (for example some would rather share information by telephone or in person, others in writing by letter or e-mail). Currently, there is a wondrous array of methods for communication. A patient may choose to initiate contact with family members by telephone, letter, fax, e-mail, text message, instant messaging, social networking sites such as MySpace and FaceBook, or even blogs. Several Internet search engines can comb the Internet for phone numbers and contact information of forgotten relatives. There are free tools, like yellowbook.com, that search directories through the United States. There are many sophisticated people search engines available; peoplefinders.com is a particularly useful website for this purpose. Unfortunately, there do not seem to be any free services for advanced people searching, although the subscription costs for services seem fairly reasonable (such as $30 for a monthly access, and increased costs to access vital records).

Many of the Internet sites discussed in Section 6.6 review hints for people to use when approaching relatives to request family health information. Usually beginning with general questions about the family and then discussing more personal and sensitive health information is a successful strategy.

6.3 THE PRIVACY OF A PERSON'S LIFE

Family members who fear an invasion of privacy may feel better about sharing the intimate details of their medical lives if only specific information is requested as compared to a blanket request to browse their medical records. Aunt Martha may be willing to share the pathology report from her breast surgery, but not the entire account of her painful emotional and physical recovery from a radical mastectomy and chemotherapy.

Medical records contain more than just medical facts. The records may reveal family secrets such as adoption, conception by gamete donation, discrepant paternity, mental instability, sexual orientation, or drug and alcohol abuse. Records, which seem dry to a health professional, may spark a plethora of charged emotions for the relative who reads them. It is not just the specifics of the family member's illness, but an adult may be reminded of the trauma of losing a mother to breast cancer (Matloff, 1997), or the records may chronicle the short, medically involved life of a much-desired child who died of a severe chromosome unbalance. While researching my own medical-family history I obtained the account of my grandfather's tumultuous death from pancreatic cancer. Although he died years before my birth, it felt awkward knowing the intimacies of the last breaths of life of this man I never met. When a patient requests sensitive family medical records, I recommend that this mail be opened at a time when there is an opportunity for reflection.

6.4 REQUESTING MEDICAL DOCUMENTATION

The most efficacious way to obtain medical records is to provide your patient with your medical center's official authorization form for requesting release of medical information. The patient takes the responsibility to send the signed release form(s) to the appropriate family member(s), who then send signed release forms to the treating medical facility. The medical records are then sent directly to your office. If the inquiry is via a health professional, there is often no charge to the patient for gathering medical records. Private physician offices and small medical centers may charge fees for this service (this is often true if the patient asks for records to be sent directly to him or her instead of to the inquiring health professional).

Table 6.1 provides a sample letter to accompany the medical release form which provides instructions for the family member on how to fill out the authorization form. I try to be as explicit as possible in requesting information. Each medical center has its own authorization form for obtaining protected health information from another healthcare provider or releasing this information, but here are some general steps for assisting patients in completing such forms. I complete the top of the release form with my address and phone number, and specify the types of medical information I am looking for. I highlight, or mark with a large red X, the sections of the release form the patient must complete.

Depending on the disease, I anticipate the medical records that *might* be available, and I request documentation accordingly. For example:

- Pathology report of a muscle biopsy, creatine kinase levels, electromyogram, and DNA test results for a relative with myopathy.
- Pathology and surgical reports for a relative with cancer, as well as any DNA test results.
- Neurodevelopmental testing, metabolic screening, chromosome analysis, reports of CGH (comparative genome hybridization) arrays, and brain imaging studies for a child with progressive mental delay.
- Birth records, intensive care notes, and autopsy records for a child born with multiple congenital anomalies who died soon after birth.
- Cardiac imaging studies (echocardiogram, CT, MRI) for persons with cardiac disease.
- Autopsy reports when available, particularly from anyone who dies unexpectedly.
- To obtain as much information as possible on deceased family members, I request autopsy information even if my patient is not sure if one was performed.

It is best to provide the Medical Records Department with as much identifying information on the relative as possible. Names should include the first, middle, and last names, all surnames (including maiden names), aliases, and designations such as Junior, Senior, II, or III. Provide complete birth dates (spell out the months so there is no confusion over abbreviations for date or month of birth). In the United States before

TABLE 6.1   Sample Letter to Request a Family Member's Medical Records

Date

Name and Address [Relative of Patient]

Dear _____

Enclosed you will find release forms that will give us permission to obtain your medical records or medical records from a family member. All information obtained will be confidential.

Please send the form directly to the appropriate hospital, physician, or other health professional or agency. They will forward the records directly to us.

The consent form should be signed by the person or his/her legal guardian or next-of-kin whose medical information is being obtained. If the consent form is signed by anyone other than the patient, please note the relationship (for example, daughter—closest surviving next-of-kin; mother—legal guardian).

Please print or type the full name (first, middle, and all last names, including maiden name) and the birth date (write out the name of the month).

If the person is deceased, include the date and year of death.
Include approximate dates of treatment or hospitalization at the medical facility (for example, January 1988, 1960–1967).

Include the person's Social Security number if you know this information (especially if the medical records are being requested from a military medical facility).

If you have any questions about these forms or about your appointment, please call me at
_____.

Thank you for your help in obtaining the information we need.

Sincerely,

[Name of Healthcare Provider or Office Manager]

---

to the enactment of the stringent privacy law HIPAA (Health Information, Portability, Privacy and Accountability Act), Social Security numbers were a traditional way of sorting medical records (particularly in the military).

Obviously, a living family member must sign for the release of his or her own medical records. If an individual is considered mentally incompetent, the legal guardian signs for the records. Some medical records departments require proof of guardianship papers before releasing records. The legal next of kin signs for a deceased individual. The order of legal next of kin is usually, first, the surviving spouse (if married at time of death), followed by the children or parents, and the grandchildren. Siblings can usually obtain records of their deceased brother or sister if the deceased sibling does not have a surviving spouse or offspring. Nieces and nephews of a deceased relative may also be able to obtain medical records if they are the closest surviving next of kin (i.e., John Hancock, grandson, closest surviving next of kin). Release of information authorization forms generally ask that if the authorization is signed by an individual's personal representative or surrogate decision-maker it must include a description of the signatory's authority.

For deceased relatives, it is useful to include a death certificate and any power-of-attorney or estate documentation with the release form. Unfortunately, in the United States it has become harder to obtain records on deceased relatives because of HIPAA because a deceased person cannot consent to release of records. This regulation made it more important to have the legally authorized representative sign the authorization form.

If you are obtaining medical records on several people in a family, it can be crazier than following the plot of a soap opera to keep track of family names. Before I send release of information forms to my patient for distribution to relatives, I always note at the bottom of the form how the relative is related to my patient (e.g., Darwin, Erasmus—grandfather of Darwin, Charles). Such a tracking method is particularly helpful when family members have the same first and last names. I also keep a copy of all release requests and note the date the release was sent to the patient or family members. This serves as a reminder for me to contact the family again in a month or so if I have not received the requested records.

The American Hospital Association (AHA) Guide to the Health Care Field (2009) lists alphabetically all the hospitals in the United States and government hospitals abroad as well as sorting hospitals by city and state. This is a valuable guide for helping patients locate their relative's records. Your patient might know that a deceased relative was seen in a small community hospital in Yakima, Washington, but not know the facility's name and address. With this directory you can easily provide the patient with the names and addresses of all the medical facilities in that community. If your patient does not know the name of the facility, he or she can send medical release forms to each hospital or medical center in that community. The worst that can happen is the receipt of a return letter stating the relative did not receive medical care at that facility. The AHA Guide is produced annually and is available in paperback and CD-ROM.

The information on death certificates can be notoriously inaccurate. (Messite and Stellman, 1996; Magrane et al., 1997). However, it may be that the cause of death listed on a death certificate is the only medical documentation available on a relative. VitalChek Network has a website (www.vitalchek.com) that lists contact information (Fax, e-mail, and telephone number) for obtaining vital records (birth and death certificates and marriage licenses) in each state. There are also links to these services through People Finders (www.peoplefinders.com). There is a small charge for obtaining vital records (the fees are listed on the website). For medical documentation there is no need to incur the added expense of obtaining a certified copy.

6.5 SHIFTS IN MEDICAL TERMINOLOGY

Medical terminology adjusts with time because of factors such as cultural influences, a better understanding of the etiology of a disease, and trends toward names that describe a disease instead of naming a disease after a patient or the physician who described the disease. Some common examples are

- St. Vitus dance or Viper's dance described persons with Huntington disease or children with complications from rheumatic fever.
- Consumption was a descriptor for tuberculosis.
- Apoplexy was a term for stroke.
- Bright's disease was a catch-all label for any person with kidney disease.
- Down syndrome was formerly called Monglism and is now more commonly referred to as trisomy 21.
- Dementia praecox was a term for schizophrenia.

There are several websites that can be searched for historical medical terms and what their contemporary meaning might be, these include

- Nan "Jones" Genealogy (http://users.xplornet.com/~pebbles2/)
- Hall Genealogy (www.rmhh.co.uk/illness.html)
- Genealogy Quest (www.genealogy-quest.com/glossaries/diseases1.html)

6.6 EMPOWERING YOUR PATIENTS WITH TOOLS FOR RECORDING THEIR OWN MEDICAL-FAMILY HISTORIES

Your ability to provide accurate genetic assessment and appropriate genetic diagnostic testing is facilitated if a patient arrives with accurate medical-family history information in hand. There are a growing number of resources to direct people on how to record their own medical-family history. Although they all have similar intent, the resources vary slightly in their methods and approaches for recording family history. Not everyone has ready access to a computer, so many of these resources remain print based, such as Dr. Thomas Shawker's book through the National Genealogical Society: *Unlocking Your Genetic History* (2004). More attention is being given to culturally appropriate ways of helping people ask their relatives about family history. Resources are also being devoted to educating different cultural, religious, and geographic populations about the importance of family health history.

In the United States the Surgeon General's Office in conjunction with the National Human Genome Research Institute, the Centers for Disease Control and prevention (CDC), and the National Cancer Insitute Center for Bioinformatics (NCICB) initiated a family history campaign focusing on the Thanksgiving Holiday as a way to encourage people to begin collecting medical-family history information. They have developed a web-based tool that is available in English and Spanish; the My Family Health Portrait tool (https://familyhistory.hhs.gov/fhh-web/home.action). It has flexibility to record several diseases and to change the orientation of the consuland if that person wants to forward his or her pedigree to a relative to expand and edit.

The CDC project is working to provide health assessment through family history for major diseases such as coronary heart disease, stroke, diabetes, colon, breast, and ovarian cancer (www.cdc.gov/genomics/activities/famhx.htm).

The National Society of Genetic Counselors, the Genetic Alliance and the American Society of Human Genetics also have an initiative encouraging people to record their own family history (www.nsgc.org/consumer/familytree/index.cfm, http://geneticalliance, and www.ashg.org/genetics/ashg/educ/007.shtml). The American Medical Association expanded these printable forms to organize the information that would be collected for a prenatal visit or for a pediatric or adult client (www.ama-assn.org/ama/pub/category/2380.html). The March of Dimes and the Mayo Clinic have used similar approaches (www.marchofdimes.com/pnhec/4439_1109.asp and (www.mayoclinic.com/health/medical-history/HQ01707). Another printable resource is the Utah Department of Health: Family Health History Toolkit (http://health.utah.gov/genomics/familyhistory/toolkit.html).

Through sponsorship from the Genetics Services Branch of the Maternal Child Health Bureau, the Genetic Alliance has worked with several organizations to develop approaches to taking family history as part of collecting family stories and traditions using an educational tool *Does It Run in the Family? A Guide to Family Health History* (www.geneticalliance.org/ws_display.asp?filter=fhh).

There are a growing number of resources for obtaining a directed family history focused on cancer and several other conditions, which include

- James Link: Personalized Cancer Risk Assessment (Ohio State University Comprehensive Cancer Center) (www.jamesline.com/patientsandvisitors/prevention/cancergenetics/jameslink/)
- Evanston Northwestern Healthcare Center for Medical Genetics: MyGenerations, draws a family tree in relation to cancer history and provides interpretation (www.enh.org/clinicalservices/medicalgenetics/mygenerations/default.aspx?id =4411)
- SGgenomics: ItRunsInMyFamily.com is a web-based program for drawing a family history sponsored by SGgenomics, a privately held corporation that funds and develops innovative genetic and health based ideas (www. itrunsinmyfamily.com)

6.7 SOFTWARE PROGRAMS FOR RECORDING FAMILY HISTORIES

Some genealogical software programs incorporate the ability to draw pedigrees (traditionally called a *box chart* in genealogy circles). These programs allow users to create jazzy multimedia "living" pedigrees, with the opportunity to synthesize medical information with family photographs and videotapes, favorite recipes, and even audiotapes of family members reciting the family folklore. A listing of genealogy software programs can be found on the Ancestors.com home page. My current favorites are *Family Tree Maker* (Encore), *Roots Magic Family Tree* (Root Magic), and

Ultimate Family Tree (Palladium Interactive, and its many versions) Many of these software programs coordinate with the online resources discussed in the following section.

6.8 RESOURCES FROM THE GENEALOGICAL GURUS

The Internet has opened wonderful tributaries for genealogical research. A few of the more informative sites include the follwing:

- Ancestry.com: This website has interesting and comprehensive resources, most of which cost money to access. You can design, purchase, and share your own hardcover family history book with pictures, records, etc. (www.ancestry.com).
- Family Search: The Family History Library Catalog of the Church of Jesus Christ Latter-Day Saints. One of the few websites where you can get information at no charge; other information can be purchased. Includes many non-U.S. resources (www.familysearch.org).
- Genealogy.org: Many interesting connections, most of which are available by subscription via (www.genealogy.org).
- My Heritage: This resource is a way to maintain and share family trees, pictures, recipes, and health information, for a subscription fee (http://myheritage.com).
- U.S. Census Bureau: Lots of free and fascinating information. To protect confidentiality, individual records are available only after 72 years (www.census.gov).
- WorldGenWeb Project: A non-profit organization dedicated to providing genealogical and historical records and resources for worldwide access (www.worldgenweb.org).

6.9 SUMMARY

Patients may have incorrect facts about the diseases that have affected their family, and this trend of misinformation intensifies when the information is about more distantly related family members. Obtaining documentation of diagnostic summaries, pathology reports, imaging studies, genetic test results, even autopsy reports provides the most accurate information from which to base health-risk information and guide genetic-testing strategies. Simply obtaining death certificates can provide a wealth of information by confirming the age at death, place and cause of death, and chronic diseases at time of death.

The most time-efficient approach is for a clinician to empower patients to collect and record their own family health information. Because of diverse cultural attitudes regarding family and health as well as varied access to technology, many educational initiatives and family health history tools have been developed. Collection methods are far less important than having the data assembled in the first place. A pedigree can be a short-hand and enjoyable method for a person to collect his or her family health history and share it with other relatives, who in turn can edit and expand on the information. A pedigree is often the easiest way to present a health professional with comprehensive family health history, which can then be interpreted without much difficulty.

Genealogists have been the kin-keepers of families for many generations. Their meticulous tools of research should be applied to collecting family health histories. Families share their environment and health traditions. The melding of family medical history with the collection and storage of family narratives, pictures, occupations, and traditions will be able to provide potentially life-saving health information in a format that can be appreciated by current and future generations.

6.10 REFERENCES

American Hospital Association. (2009). *American Hospital Association (AHA) Guide to the Health Care Field, 2009*. American Hospital Association: Chicago.

Dean, JW, ed. (1863). *New England Historical and Genealogical Register*. Vol XVII. Albany, NY.

Genealogy Quest. (2009). Genealogy Quest. November 2, 2009. Available at www.genealogy-quest.com/glossaries/diseases1.html. Accessed November 22, 2009.

Hall Genealogy Website. (2009). Illnesses encountered in genealogy. October 2, 2009. Available at www.rmhh.co.uk/illness.html. Accessed November 22, 2009.

Hey D. (1993). *The Oxford Guide to Family History*. Oxford University Press: Oxford.

Magrane BP, Gilliland MGF, King DE. (1997). Certificates of death by family physicians. *Am Fam Phy* 56:1433–1438.

Matloff ET. (1997). Generations lost: A cancer genetics case report. *J Genet Couns* 6:169–176.

Messite J, Stellman SD. (1996). Accuracy of death certificate completion: Need for family physician training. *JAMA* 275:794–796.

Nan "Jones" Genealogy Page. (2009). Old diseases and modern definitions. Available at http://users.xplornet.com/~pebbles2/tools.html#top. Accessed November 22, 2009.

National Cancer Institute Center for Bioinformatics (NCICB). (2009). My Family Health Portrait, a tool from the Surgeon General. Available at https://familyhistory.hhs.gov/fhh-web/home.action. Accessed November 22, 2009.

People Finders. (2009). People finders, find anyone, anywhere. Available at www.peoplefinders.com. Accessed November 22, 2009.

SgGenomics. (2008). It Runs In My Family. Available at www.itrunsinmyfamily.com. Accessed February 7, 2009.

Shawker TH. (2004). *Unlocking Your Genetic History*. Nashville, TN: Routledge Hill Press.

Chapter 7

The Challenge of Family History and Adoption

Knowing one's ancestors is not a matter of mild curiosity; it is often part of an attempt to explain life and to understand how we have come to be what we are, not just physically through inherited genes, but how we have come to believe in certain principles or to have acquired the attitudes, prejudices, and characteristics that mould our personality. For very many people, tracing a family tree and discovering the lives of their ancestors is not a task that is undertaken lightly.
—*David Hey (1993)*

7.1 THE PROBLEM DEFINED

A thorough family history is an important part of the adoption process. The lifelong medical care of an individual may be facilitated by access to health and family history information gathered at the time of adoption. Medical information in the adoption records may also be beneficial to an adult making reproductive choices. The availability of sophisticated DNA testing will not obviate the usefulness of a genetic family history, because genetic testing is done in the context of family history. This chapter is for the health professional or professional adoption intermediary involved in gathering medical and family history information for a child being placed for adoption. It also includes resources for searching for information on a birth parent and trying to open sealed adoption records. The information is focused on the system in the United States, although the principles are global, particularly given the increase in international adoptions.

The Practical Guide to the Genetic Family History, Second Edition, by Robin L. Bennett
Copyright © 2010 John Wiley & Sons, Inc.

Any adoption involves a tangled web of interests, including those of the adoptive parents, the birth parents and family, the adopted individual, and the designated intermediaries (e.g., adoption agency, attorney). These parties are often referred to as the *adoption triad* or *adoption constellation*. The legal and emotional needs of these people are complex and are often at odds with each other. Adoptive parents are increasingly interested in genetic testing and family history information about their child. Yet, these same parents may be ambivalent about contact with their child's biological relatives. Biological parents may be interested in information about their child's adjustment in the years following the adoption, and they often want to communicate with their adult child. The trend is toward "open adoptions," in which the birth mother or both parents participate in the selection of the adoptive parents. In parallel, many people who are adopted maintain a healthy curiosity about their biological ancestry, in addition they may seek their biological history for medical reasons. Information about the adopted individual's biological roots may help lessen the impact from the psychological trauma of an identity crisis termed *genealogical bewilderment* (Bender, 1989; Nydam, 1999). All these variables frequently lead to conflicts of interest related to the psychological welfare, medical needs, and legal rights of the parties involved in an adoption.

7.2 EVOLVING ADOPTION LAWS

Adoption is a legal fiction. It assumes that a child's ties to biological parents can be displaced entirely by ties to adoptive parents. Social and psychological evidence suggest, however, that legal rules cannot so easily obliterate the past or prevent adoptees, as they grow older, from desiring to re-establish some lines to their past.

—**Michael Bender (1989) 13.01 §[1][a]**

Before to the early 1900s, adoption in America was a relatively informal matter with few legal adoptions. As an example, recently I learned that in the early 1800s my mother's great-grandparents added a toddler to their brood of six after the boy was orphaned during their westward wagon voyage; in fact, he later married one of the sisters in his adoptive family, a relationship that would be considered illegal (incest) under current statutes.

The first adoption law was codified in Massachusetts in 1851 and contained no requirement that adoption records should be maintained or kept confidential (Bender, 1989). Almost 65 years later, laws were formulated in many jurisdictions to protect the adoption proceedings from public scrutiny. Such laws were enacted to shield birth mothers, as well as their children, from the "shame and stigmatization" of illegitimacy. A 1917 Minnesota statute was the first law to reflect a concern about the privacy of birth parents by requiring that adoption records be kept confidential (Bender, 1989).

As time went on, adoption proceedings became more surreptitious. By the mid-1920s, most states had statutes cloaking the adoption process in secrecy, providing for the sealing of adoption records and the issuance of a new birth certificate. All parties were denied access to these adoption records except under the exceptional judicial finding of "good cause" (Bender, 1989; Lorandos, 1996). Each state in the union and provinces of Canada continue to have varied adoption laws.

Birth parents and adopted persons have challenged the ethos and legality of forced anonymity and secrecy in the adoption process. Many birth mothers and fathers who requested a "closed adoption" often seek a reunion or other connection with their adult child (American Adoption Congress, 2009). The adoption paradigm has shifted from one of magically removing shame to minimizing the pain and loss for each family member in the adoption process (Nydam, 1999). Many state legislatures have responded by enacting laws granting adopted persons and their adoptive families access to appropriate health and family history information. Some laws are even retroactive to opening sealed or closed adoptions. Several states and Canadian provinces have "open adoption records" (including Alabama, Alaska, Delaware, Hawaii, Kansas, New Hampshire, Oregon, Tennessee, Alberta, Newfoundland, and Labrador), by which adult adopted persons and occasionally even their relatives (such as biological siblings or grandparents) can request copies of original birth certificates and sometimes the original adoption documentation (Adoption, 2009; American Adoption Congress, 2009; Child Welfare Information Gateway, 2009). The definitions of an adult range in age from age 18 to 25 years. Most of the laws are nonbinding contracts by which the birth parent or parents can allow direct contact with their adult adopted son or daughter, contact through an intermediary, or no contact at all.

Many states and provinces have implemented adoption registries in which the persons in the adoption constellation can register to seek information about adoptees and birth parents or even their relatives. There are growing resources for children from international adoptions to find information about their birth parents and families.

In Oregon after 10 years of "open" adoption records (1998–2008), the American Adoption Congress website notes that no harm has been done to any party, including birth parents, after the release of 9,267 original birth certificates.

The American Society of Human Genetics (ASHG) has taken the stance that a genetic history should be included in an adopted person's record. They assert that "every person should have the right to gain access to his or her medical record, including genetic data.... When medically appropriate, genetic data may be shared among the adoptive parents, biological parents and adoptees" (ASHG, 2000). At least 25 states actually require compilation of a genetic history (Andrews, 1997). At least 41 states provide, to varying extent, for the collection of medical information from birth parents and the release of this information to adoptive families (Lorandos, 1996). The impetus for change in these laws is partly in response to litigation related to "wrongful adoption." In this type of litigation, adoptive parents attempt to revoke adoptions after discovering genetic, mental, or physical problems in their adopted children (Freundlich and Peterson, 1999; Leshne, 1999; Lorandos, 1996; Zitter, 1987).

Currently no state has an absolute open adoption record policy. Most states now require agencies or private intermediaries to compile comprehensive profiles of children and their biological parents and to share this nonidentifying information with the adoptive parents at the time of adoption (Bender, 1989). Each state has different requirements on the nature of the non-identifying information that is shared with the adoptive parents at the time of adoption (Bender, 1989). The nonidentifying information generally includes

- Date, time, state, and county of the adopted child's birth
- The age of the biological parents at the time of placement and their general physical description (ranging from height and hair color to such subtleties as whether they are right or left handed)
- Race, ethnicity, and religion
- Whether termination of parental rights is voluntary or court ordered
- The facts and circumstances related to the adoptive placement
- The age and gender of the adopted individual's biological siblings
- Medical history of the biological parents and the adopted child
- Information about the parents' educational levels, occupations, skills, and interests (including artistic and athletic abilities)

Some states, such as Alabama, have few provisions for the maintenance and disclosure of the information obtained at the time of adoption. In contrast, Arkansas requires that such information be maintained for 99 years and, upon request, these records are available to the adoptive and biological parents as well as the adult offspring; even the descendants of a deceased adopted individual can have access to the records (Bender, 1989). Michigan's 1998 Adoption Law (Section 710.27) specifically states that the child's health and genetic history information is to be collected and maintained by the adoption agency The law fails to state how this will be done and whether an agency is mandated to monitor the collection, storage, and dissemination of this information.

Although laws may require comprehensive family history and medical profiles to be collected, currently there are no procedures in place to verify that this is followed. Adoption and foster care workers identify many barriers to collecting comprehensive information, including:

- Inability to identify birth father and other extended relatives
- Children in multiple placements because of a history of abuse, neglect, and abandonment
- Lack of continuity of social work staff in agencies
- Time constraints to collecting such data

Biological parents who have their parental rights involuntarily terminated may be unwilling or unavailable to provide family history information. This is a challenging situation that few of the current statutes address.

Adoption is a lifelong process. Ensuing family history data may become relevant after the adoption is finalized. Indeed, some jurisdictions allow for the continued collection of information subsequent to the adoption (Andrews 1997; Bender 1989).

In Delaware, if the family court receives a report stating that a birth parent or the adopted individual has a genetically transmitted disorder or family pattern of disease, a statute requires that the family court instruct the agency that was involved with the adoption to conduct a diligent search for the adult adoptee, the adoptive parents of a minor adoptee, or the birth parents (Andrews, 1997). But who decides what medical and genetic testing information is relevant to share with the parties of the adoption triad in relation to their health monitoring and reproductive decision making? What "burden of disease" is considered great enough to interject this information into the private adoption constellation? How accurate must genetic testing be to warrant disclosure of this information? This is certainly a formidable task that is difficult to regulate through legislation.

There are many websites related to adoption. The following are the web-based resources that I found most reliable and easy to navigate, with summaries of current laws and pending legislation in the United States and Canada as well as many other resources related to books, conferences, and testimonials of persons in the adoption constellation, international adoption, and comprehensive links to other websites:

- American Adoption Congress   • www.americanadoptioncongress.com
- The Child Welfare Information   • www.childwelfare.gov
  Gateway
- Adoption.com   • www.adoption.com
- Adoption Triad Outreach   • www.adoptiontriad.org

7.3   OBTAINING MEDICAL INFORMATION FROM A CLOSED ADOPTION

In the daydreaming and wondering of everyday life, relinquished and adopted people keep their connections with their ancestral history and hold these images "alive," even as they grieve the "death" of the ghost parents whom they never knew as parents.

—Ryan Nydham (1999)

Opening files from a closed adoption can be daunting, even if it is limited to obtaining the nonidentifying information recorded at the time of adoption. Some states do not have a central state registry for adoptive records. The adopted individual must direct inquiries to the court or agency that supervised the placement. The information obtained in the files may be sparse, and the adopted individual may need to search for medical and genetic histories directly from the biological parents. This may be difficult if consents for such disclosures are not on file. Given the mobile nature of our society, it may be difficult to locate biological parents whose surnames and residences have changed over the years.

There are many resources for beginning a search for a birth parent or an adoption record. The availability of social networking web tools and web browsers to search for phone numbers and addresses is a boon to birth parents and adopted persons searching for biological connections. Comprehensive information about such resources is available from several sources as noted in the website listings in the previous section.

7.4 GENETIC TESTING OF CHILDREN BEING PLACED FOR ADOPTION

Few people would argue against medical information, genetic or otherwise, that has an immediate effect on the health of a child being disclosed to the adoptive parents. But what about genetic testing of a healthy child for a medical condition that potentially may affect this person as an adolescent or an adult? Should every child being placed for adoption receive a battery of screening tests for potential genetic diseases, regardless of whether there is a treatment for each condition? Could failure to provide such genetic testing have repercussions for the adoption agency in the form of wrongful birth litigation? For example, should an adoption agency test a healthy infant for the gene mutation for Huntington disease (HD) if the child has a parent affected with this disease? Huntington disease is a progressive neurological condition for which there is no cure. The symptoms of HD are unlikely to develop in this child for another 30 to 40 years. Is this genetic information necessary for the adoptive parents? Or should the adopted person be allowed to make the choice about genetic testing when he or she is an adult?

Among genetic professionals, there is general consensus that a minor should be genetically tested only if there is an obvious medical benefit to the child. Presymptomatic genetic testing for conditions with no available treatment should be postponed until the person is of legal age to make the choice of whether to be tested (American Society of Human Genetics/American College of Medical Genetics Report [ASHG/ACMG], 1995). The fear is that perhaps the healthy child with a known genetic mutation will be treated differently by the parents and other family members, peers, the school system, and society (Bennett et al., 2002). The healthy child may receive increased medical surveillance. There are also concerns that the child may have harmful alterations in self-esteem and self-identity, experience survivor guilt (if tested negative but other relatives have tested positive or are affected by the disease), and feelings of guilt and shame. Specific to adoption, ethicist Dorothy Wertz and co-workers (1994) note, "Testing for untreatable adult-onset disorders prior to adoption make the child into a commodity undergoing quality control."

There are arguments of potential benefit of genetic testing of an asymptomatic minor, even if the test result is positive. Possible testing benefits include "normalization" of health status and that the disease status becomes part of the child's sense of self, anticipatory guidance such as choosing physical activities and steering toward occupation in anticipation of someday being symptomatic, allowing the child and the family time to adjust to future disease status, and resolution of uncertainty (Bennett et al., 2002).

The general approach to genetic testing in the adoption process is to proceed providing it is "(1) consistent with preventive and diagnostic tests performed on all children of a similar age, (2) generally limited to testing for medical conditions that manifest themselves during childhood or for which preventive measures or therapies may be undertaken during childhood, and (3) not used to detect genetic variations within the normal range" (ASHG/ACMG, 2000).

7.5 A MODEL MEDICAL AND GENETIC FAMILY HISTORY FORM FOR ADOPTIONS

To unify the medical and genetic history information collected at the time of adoption, the Education Committee of the Council of Regional Genetics Networks (CORN) developed a model genetic family history form (Appendix A.4). The form consists of a cover page containing identifying information about the birth parents, the child welfare agency, and the agency's file identification code. This identifying information remains with the agency, as specified by the state law, unless the birth parents agree to waive their right to confidentiality. Information is collected about the child's delivery and birth. A comprehensive questionnaire about the medical and genetic history of the birth mother and father is filled out at the time of termination of parental rights with the intent of sharing this information with the foster or adoptive parents.

For optimal use of this form, it is best if a professional adoption intermediary assist each birth parent in completing the questionnaire. Optimally the professional should have some familiarity with the medical and genetic conditions contained in the form. Each user of this model genetic history is encouraged to modify it to comply with local or state regulations. In addition to this form, the Child Welfare Information Gateway (2003a, 2003b) has useful general fact sheets on 'obtaining background information a prospective adopted child' and providing background information to adoptive parents. Both of these resources provide general queries regarding medical and social background for the child, parents, and family and why this information is important.

Genetic counselors and medical geneticists are available to consult with adoption intermediaries about family history interpretation (see Chapter 9).

7.6 SUMMARY

The adoption laws in the United States and Canada are a mishmash of state and provincial regulations that are evolving under the pressures to meet the needs of all persons in the adoption triad or constellation: the birth parents and family, the child placed for adoption, and the adoptive parent or parents. In both the United States and Canada, there is a growing trend toward open adoptions as compared to the forced secrecy and shame associated with adoptions beginning in the early 1900s and extending into the late 1980s and even today.

There is a similar movement for openness in information that is available for children conceived from assisted reproductive technologies (discussed further in Chapter 8). Ideally as much medical information as possible should be obtained at the time of adoption because this information can be important in lifelong health care and decision making for the adopted person and his or her family; Appendix A.4 provides an example of a comprehensive medical history that could be used for adoption. This information also helps with providing an identity for the child.

Not everyone will have success in finding information about the health of their biological parents or their extended family. The routine of asking a person about his or her family health information at a regular medical appointment can make the adopted person acutely aware of how he or she differs from those who were not adopted. Adopted persons can commence the legacy of medical and family history for their descendants.

7.7 REFERENCES

Adoption.com (2009). Adoption.com Home Page. Available at www.adoption.com. 1995–2009. Accessed November 22, 2009.

Adoption Triad Outreach. (2009). Adoption Triad Outreach Home Page. Available at www.adoption.triad.org. Accessed November 23, 2009.

American Adoption Congress. (2009). American Adoption Congress Home Page. Available at www.americanadoptioncongress.org. Accessed November 23, 2009.

American Society of Human Genetics/American College of Medical Genetics. (1995). ASHG/ACMG Report: Points to consider: ethical legal and psychosocial implications of genetic testing in children and adolescents. *Am J Hum Genet* 57:1233–1241.

American Society of Human Genetics/American College of Medical Genetics. (2000). Genetics in adoption—American Society of Human Genetics Social Issues Committee, American College of Medical Genetics Social, Ethical and Legal Issues Committee. *Am J Hum Genet* 66(3):761–767.

Andrews LB. (1997). Gen-etiquette: Genetic information, family relationships and adoption. In: Rothstein MA, ed., *Genetic Secrets: Protecting Privacy and Confidentiality in the Genetic Era*. New Haven, CT: Yale University Press, pp. 255–280.

Bender M. (1989). Legal and social consequences. In: Hollinger JH, ed., *Adoption Law and Practice*. Times Mirror Books, §13.01 [3], [2].

Bennett RL, Hart KA, O'Rourke E, et al. (2002). Fabry disease in genetic counseling practice: Recommendations of the National Society of Genetic Counselors. *J Genet Couns* 11:121–156.

Child Welfare Information Gateway. (2003b). Obtaining Background Information to Adoptive Parents: A Bulletin for Professionals. Available at www.childwelfare.gov/pubs/f_backgroundbulletin.cfm. Accessed February 7, 2009.

Child Welfare Information Gateway. (2003a). Obtaining Background Information on Your Prospective Adopted Child. Available at www.childwelfare.gov/pubs/f_background.cfm. Accessed February 7, 2009.

Child Welfare Information Gateway. (2009). Adoption. Available at www.childwelfare.gov. Accessed November 23, 2009.

Freundlich M, Peterson L. (1999). *Wrongful Adoption: Law, Policy and Practice*. Washington, D.C: CWLA Press.

Hey D. (1993). *The Oxford Guide to Family History*. Oxford: Oxford University Press.

Leshne L. (1999). Wrongful adoptions: Fewer secrets and lies, but agencies still fail at full disclosure. *Trial* 35 (April, 1999).

Lorandos DA. (1996). Secrecy and genetics in adoption law and practice. *Loyola Univ Chicago Law J* 27:277–320.

Nydham RJ. (1999). *Adoptees Come of Age: Living within Two Families*. Louisville, KY: Westminster John Knox Press.

Wertz DC, Fanos JH, Reilly PR. (1994). Genetic testing for children and adolescents, who decides? *JAMA* 272:875–881.

Zitter JM. (1987). Annotation, action for wrongful adoption based on misrepresentation of child's mental or physical condition or parentage. 56 ALR 4th 375:277–319.

Chapter *8*

Family History and Assisted Reproductive Technologies

8.1 GAMETE DONATION ALLOWS COUPLES AT HIGH RISK FOR GENETIC DISORDERS TO HAVE HEALTHY OFFSPRING

For a couple with a high risk to have children with a genetic disorder, certain assisted reproductive technologies (ARTs) can virtually eliminate their chance to pass the condition on to their offspring. Recognizing the inheritance pattern of the condition is essential for providing a couple with appropriate information about reproductive options. Table 8.1 compares how ART using donor sperm or donor ovum can significantly reduce the chance of having an affected child, based on the pattern of disease inheritance and the affected or carrier status of the partner. For example, therapeutic donor insemination (TDI) is an option for a couple in which the healthy male partner is at risk for an autosomal dominant condition, such as Huntington disease, as a way to eradicate his offspring's risk to develop the disease. A healthy woman who carries an X-linked mutation (such as for Duchenne muscular dystrophy) may choose donor ovum as a method to conceive an unaffected pregnancy rather than facing a 50:50 chance to have an affected son. Similarly, a person carrying a balanced reciprocal chromosome translocation may consider donor insemination or donor ovum transfer to avoid his or her increased chance of having a child with an unbalanced chromosome rearrangement. Women who are in their mid-30s and older may choose donor ovum as a way to reduce the risks of chromosomal aneuploidy and to increase the likelihood of harvesting eggs of an adequate number and quality as is needed for in vitro fertilization.

The Practical Guide to the Genetic Family History, Second Edition, by Robin L. Bennett
Copyright © 2010 John Wiley & Sons, Inc.

TABLE 8.1 Comparisons of How Gamete Donation using ART (Assisted Reproductive Technologies) Can Reduce the Risk for a Genetic Disease, Based on Different Inheritance Patterns and the Affected Status of the Partner

Affected Status of Partner	Inheritance Pattern of Condition	Prior Risk of an Affected Child	Risk of an Affected Child after Gamete Donation
Therapeutic Donor Semen Insemination (TDI)			
Male Partner Affected			
Heterozygote	Autosomal dominant	50% son or daughter	Same as background
Hemizygote	X-linked	50% daughter, 0% son	Same as background
Homozygote	Autosomal recessive	75% son or daughter[a]	Carrier test sperm donor for condition (if test available)[b]
Male Partner Asymptomatic Carrier			
Heterozygote	Autosomal recessive	25% son or daughter[a]	Carrier test sperm donor for condition (if test available)[b]
Balanced translocation	Chromosome translocation	Depends on translocation	Same as maternal age-related risk for chromosome anomalies
Donor Ovum			
Female Partner Affected			
Heterozygote	Autosomal dominant	50% son or daughter	Same as background
Homozygote	Autosomal recessive	75% son or daughter[a]	Carrier test ovum donor (if test available)[b]
Heteroplasmic	Mitochondrial	0–100% son or daughter	Same as background
Heterozygote	X-linked	50% son or daughter	Same as background
Female partner asymptomatic carrier			
Heterozygote	Autosomal recessive	TDI is generally favored over donor ovum; although the risk reduction is the same, the pregnancy success rate is higher with TDI, and TDI is not as expensive as donor ovum	
Balanced translocation	Chromosome translocation	Depends on translocation	Based on maternal age risks of egg donor

[a]Assuming that the partner is a carrier for the same autosomal recessive disease.
[b]Risk is usually slightly above background (<1%) but depends on availability and accuracy of carrier testing for donor.

Therapeutic donor insemination is a reasonable option for a healthy couple at 25% risk to have a child with a condition inherited in a classic autosomal recessive pattern. Sperm donors must be screened for carrier status for the same recessive condition. Many gamete donation programs screen a donor for a few genetic disorders based on the donor's ethnic background. For example, a potential sperm donor with ancestors from northern Europe is screened for carrier status for cystic fibrosis, likewise he would be screened for several autosomal recessive disorders common in the Ashkenazi population if he is of that descent (see Table 3.3). For some autosomal recessive disorders carrier testing may not be available or the screening test may not detect 100% of the gene mutations. In this instance, the couple should know that there remains a chance, slightly above the background population risk, to have a child with the genetic disease in question. This is because the sperm donor may by chance also carry the gene mutation for the same recessive gene as the mother. Usually the couple's risk to have a child with the condition will be in the range of 0.5% to 1%, depending on the frequency of heterozygotes for that genetic disorder in the general population.

8.2 SCREENING GAMETE DONORS FOR INHERITED DISORDERS

The American Society of Reproductive Medicine (ASRM) periodically updates guidelines for genetic screening of gamete donors (2006). The recommendations give gamete donation programs leeway to individualize their genetic screening policies, allowing choice about what conditions to screen donors for and flexibility about the extent of family history information that should be collected from donors. A summary of these guidelines follows (adapted from ASRM, 2006):

- A family history should be obtained on the donor, although the extent of the family history to be obtained is not specified. The family history screening form in Appendix A.4 could be used for this purpose (the form was originally designed for a child being placed for adoption).
- A donor should not be used if he or she has a family history of a first-degree relative with a major congenital malformation, a major Mendelian disorder, a common autosomal recessive disorder, or a chromosome abnormality (unless the donor has been adequately screened for the condition in question). Donors who are heterozygous for an autosomal recessive condition are not necessarily excluded if the donor recipient has been adequately screened for the condition.
- Blood type is obtained for issues of maternal-fetal incompatibility (such as Rh factor incompatibility with an Rh^+ fetus and an RH^- mother).
- The donor should not have a major inherited disorder. *Major* is defined as a "malformation that carries serious functional or cosmetic handicap." The interpretation of what constitutes a major problem is a matter of judgment.

- Donors with a history of substance abuse are discouraged. Of interest, donors with two first-degree relatives with a history of substance abuse are also discouraged.
- Donors with a personal or family history of psychiatric dysfunction are discouraged.
- The donor should not be affected with, or have a first-degree relative with, "a significant familial disease with a major genetic component."
- The donor should not carry a chromosomal rearrangement. However, most screening programs do not automatically karyotype the gamete donors because of the expense of a chromosomal study.
- The donor should be screened for any autosomal recessive disorders that are prevalent in the donor's ethnic background and for which heterozygote testing is available—for example, the screening panel for individuals of Ashkenazi ancestry as recommended by the American College of Obstetrics and Gynecologists (ACOG Committee on Genetics, 2004), the American College of Medical Genetics (Gross et al., 2008), the Canadian College of Medical Geneticists and the Society of Obstetricians and Gynaecologists of Canada (Langlois et al., 2006).
- Screening for *FMR1* mutations associated with fragile X mental retardation syndrome is considered optional for women who are oocyte donors. In the United States most women are offered *FMR1* screening in pregnancy. Men who are sperm donors are sometimes screened as well, although this is more controversial (because the risk of the CTG repeat expanding into an abnormal range would be to the male donor's grandchildren).
- Men older than 40 years old probably should not be used as sperm donors (because of the association of new autosomal dominant mutations primarily as a result of single base pair substitutions and advanced paternal age) (Toriello and Meck, 2008). For the offspring of father's over age 40, the absolute risk of birth defects, complex disorders, and chromosome anomalies is low.
- Women 35 years and older should not be used as egg donors because of the increased risk for offspring with chromosomal aneuploidy.

Perceptions of what is a common disorder and what is a burdensome disorder are subject to opinion. As noted, gamete donors heterozygous for an autosomal recessive condition may still be considered suitable donors if the recipient has been appropriately screened.

Most ART programs collect descriptive information on the donor, such as hair color and texture, eye and skin color, body build, and complexion, in an effort to match the donor's characteristics with that of the partner. Some programs even collect "non-genetic" information on donors such as occupation and preferences for music and hobbies to help their clients make a psychological match with the donor.

With increasing availability of genetic testing and new techniques for assisting reproduction, screening protocols for gamete donors continually change. The ASRM online has links to position statements and resources related to this fascinating and controversial field (www.asrm.org).

8.3 INTRACTYOPLASMIC SPERM INJECTION AND GENETIC DISEASE

Infertile men who have azoospermia or oligospermia because of either mechanical means (such as vasectomy) or congenital absence of the vas deferens (absence of the sperm duct) are increasingly turning to removal of the sperm directly from the testes, followed by intrasyctoplasmic sperm injection (ICSI), as a means of conceiving pregnancy. Because there are several inherited conditions associated with male infertility (see Section 4.18.3 and Table 4.32), before using ICSI, men should have a genetic evaluation. At a minimum this assessment should include (ASRM, 2006) the following:

- At least a three-generation pedigree focusing on medical history questions associated with male infertility (see Table 4.33).
- A karyotype (specifically for detection of XXY-Klinefelter syndrome and other sex chromosome anomalies and chromosomal rearrangements).
- Molecular analysis using a panel of Y-probes looking for microscopic Y deletions. Men with proximal deletions, which include the AZFa and AZFb regions, show severe defects in spermatogenesis, whereas deletions of the AZFb and AZFc region can be compatible with residual spermatogenesis and thus success with sperm aspiration and ICSI.
- Men with congenital absence of the vas deferens should have cystic fibrosis gene (*CFTR*) mutation analysis, including the 5T allele. The most comprehensive method is gene sequencing because the spectrum of mutations associated with obstruction is outside of the common *CFTR* screening panels offered (usually 23 mutations) (Danzinger et al., 2004). Partners of men identified with mutations should be offered gene sequencing as well.

8.4 REPRESENTING GAMETE DONATION AND SURROGACY ON A PEDIGREE

When noting on a pedigree that a pregnancy (or child) was conceived through assisted means of reproduction, it is important to trace the biological heritage of the child and birth mother. Although anonymous gamete donation has traditionally been encouraged, a blood relative may be a participant in ART. A gestational carrier (surrogate mother) may carry a pregnancy conceived with her sister's egg and her brother-in-law's sperm (thus the gestational carrier is also a maternal aunt to the fetus). An occasional altruistic mother has been a gestational carrier for a pregnancy conceived with her daughter's egg and her son-in-law's sperm. Rarely, for a lesbian couple, the

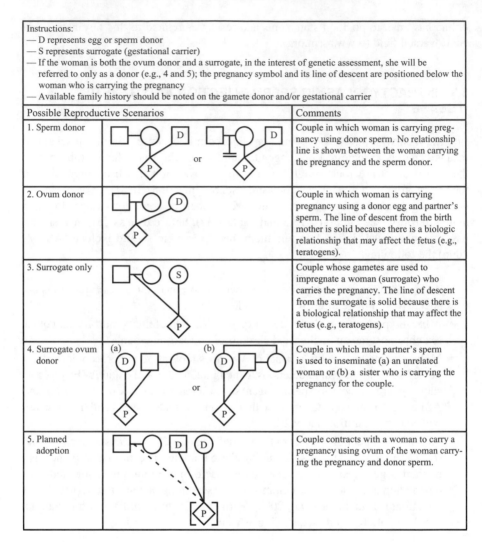

Instructions:
— D represents egg or sperm donor
— S represents surrogate (gestational carrier)
— If the woman is both the ovum donor and a surrogate, in the interest of genetic assessment, she will be referred to only as a donor (e.g., 4 and 5); the pregnancy symbol and its line of descent are positioned below the woman who is carrying the pregnancy
— Available family history should be noted on the gamete donor and/or gestational carrier

Possible Reproductive Scenarios	Comments
1. Sperm donor	Couple in which woman is carrying pregnancy using donor sperm. No relationship line is shown between the woman carrying the pregnancy and the sperm donor.
2. Ovum donor	Couple in which woman is carrying pregnancy using a donor egg and partner's sperm. The line of descent from the birth mother is solid because there is a biologic relationship that may affect the fetus (e.g., teratogens).
3. Surrogate only	Couple whose gametes are used to impregnate a woman (surrogate) who carries the pregnancy. The line of descent from the surrogate is solid because there is a biological relationship that may affect the fetus (e.g., teratogens).
4. Surrogate ovum donor	Couple in which male partner's sperm is used to inseminate (a) an unrelated woman or (b) a sister who is carrying the pregnancy for the couple.
5. Planned adoption	Couple contracts with a woman to carry a pregnancy using ovum of the woman carrying the pregnancy and donor sperm.

Figure 8.1 *Pedigree symbolization of assistive reproductive technologies. Reprinted with permission from Bennett et al. (1995, 2008).*

birth mother may carry a pregnancy conceived with her ovum and sperm from the brother of her female partner.

The pedigree symbols in Figure 8.1 and the pedigree line definitions (see Figure 3.1) can be used to illustrate any combination of parents who use any method of ART. Some simple pedigree drawing rules for symbolizing ART include the following (Bennett et al., 1995, 2008):

- Place a *D* inside the symbol for the game (egg or sperm) donor.
- Place an *S* inside the female circle to represent a gestational carrier (surrogate).

- If a woman is both the ovum donor and the gestational carrier, in the interest of genetic assessment, she is referred to as a donor (thus a *D* is placed within the circle).

- The relationship line is between the couple (heterosexual or same-sex partners). Do not place a relationship line between the pregnant woman and the sperm donor or between the father of the fetus (or child) and the ovum donor.

- The line of descent extends from the woman who is actually carrying the pregnancy.

8.5   THE FORGOTTEN FAMILY HISTORY: THE OFFSPRING OF DONOR-CONCEIVED PREGNANCIES

It is only in the past decade that the story of the "donor adoptee" has begun to be told. Often the person may not be aware until well into adulthood that he or she was conceived with a donor sperm or even less often through a donor egg. Given the legacy of secrecy that was encouraged about the use of donor gametes, often such parenthood disclosures are at a time of crises similar to a death bed confession. The emotional conflicts of having one's heritage described by the method of conception are unique. The barriers faced by a donor adoptee attempting to find health information about his or her biological parent are unquestionably more challenging than those faced by traditional adoptees who at least may find a name on an original birth certificate; sperm donors are often identified only by number. With egg and sperm donors, multiple conceptions may have occurred, compounding the likelihood that the donor adoptee has biological half-siblings. With an estimated 60,000 births a year that originated with a donor egg or sperm, the right of the donor adoptee to his or her genetic origins is likely to become a growing legal and human rights issue (Bauman, 2001; Johnston, 2002; Wallbank, 2004).

8.6   SUMMARY

The methods of ARTs will undoubtedly continue to astonish us, while its application will challenge our legal, ethical and social constructs. By following the rules outlined in Figure 8.1, the genetic and gestational heritage of a fetus or child conceived by any combination of assisted reproductive technologies can be documented on a pedigree. Developing standards for screening gamete donors and gestational carriers for genetic disorders is not so easily accomplished. In putting forth such guidelines, we quickly come to face fundamental issues of what is a "normal" or "abnormal" human and what is a "burdensome" inherited disease. The day that there are simple answers to these questions is the day we must question our humanity.

Bill Cordray (2007), who describes himself as a DI (donor insemination) adoptee, notes his similarities with traditional adoptees by saying, "Our goal as DI adoptees is the same, to be free to connect with our heritage and genealogy." Another DI adoptee notes, "It was not by my choice that my ancestral home is nothing more than a sample jar" (Whipp, 2008). Similar to the transformation that has occurred over the last decade concerning traditional adoption, the trend toward increased openness regarding parentage and family history of persons conceived through gamete donation should continue. The psychological issues faced by persons conceived using donor gametes should be validated and the veil of shame and secrecy lifted (Feast, 2003).

8.7 REFERENCES

ACOG Committee on Genetics (2004). ACOG committee opinion. Number 298, August 2004. Prenatal and preconception carrier screening for genetic diseases in individuals of Eastern European Jewish descent. *Obstet Gynecol* 104(2):425–428.

American Society of Reproductive Medicine. (2006). 2006 Guidelines for gamete and embryo donation. *Fertil Steril* 86(5):S38–S50.

Bauman JH. (2001). Discovering donors' legal rights to access information. *Gold Gate Univ Law Rev* 31:41–45.

Bennett RL, Steinhaus KA, Uhrich SB, et al. (1995). Recommendations for standardized pedigree nomenclature. *Am J Hum Genet* 56:745–752.

Bennett RL, Steinhaus French K, Resta RG, Lochner Doyle D. (2008). Standardized pedigree nomenclature: Update and assessment of the recommendations of the National Society of Genetic Counselors. *J Genet Couns* 17(5):424–433.

Cordray BC. (2008). Reproductive technologies: emotional adoption. Available at www.americanadoptioncongress.org/assisted_cordray_article.php. Accessed June 2, 2008.

Danziger KL, Black LD, Keiles SB, et al. (2004). Improved detection of cystic fibrosis mutations in infertility patients with DNA sequence analysis. *Hum Repro* 19(3):540–546.

Feast J. (2003). Using and not losing the message from the adoption experience for donor assisted adoption. *Hum Fertil* 6:41–45.

Gross SJ, Pletcher BA, Monaghan KG, et al. (2008). Carrier screening individuals of Ashkenazi Jewish descent. *Genet Med* 10(1):54–56.

Johnston J (2002). Mum's the word—Donor anonymity in ART. *Health Law Rev* 11:51–55.

Langlois S, Wilson RD, Genetics Committee of the Society of Obstetricians and Gynaecologists of Canada, Prenatal Diagnosis Committee of the Canadian College of Medical Genetics. (2006). Carrier screening for genetic disorders in individuals of Ashkenazi Jewish decent. *J Obstet Gynaecol Can.* 28(4):324–343.

Toriello H, Meck J (2008). Statement on guidance for genetic counseling in advanced paternal age. *Genet Med* 10(6):457–460.

Wallbank J (2004). Roles of rights and utility in instituting a child's right to know genetic history. *Soc Leg Stud* 13:245–264.

Whipp C. (2008, July 5). Personal correspondence online at www.tangledweb.org.

Chapter 9

Genetic Counseling: Where to Turn, What to Expect, and the Pedigree as a Psychosocial Assessment and Counseling Tool

The family had escaped the persecutions, pogroms, and poverty of Czarist Russia, but for some there would be no escape from a threat hidden within them . . . These were days without hope. Where did it come from? How did it get started? Yet these were modern times. Why did no one know more about the disease? It was hard to believe that in this whole world our family was the only one possessing this trait. Would it ever end?
—*Ben (quoted in Pollen, 1993)*

Nothing is so soothing to our self-esteem as to find our bad traits in our forbears. It seems to absolve us.
—*Van Wyck Brooks (1886–1963)*

9.1 GENETIC CONDITIONS HAVE DISTINGUISHING ASPECTS FROM OTHER MEDICAL CONDITIONS

As more tests are developed that identify a hereditary component to common chronic disorders such as heart disease, cancer, and dementia, genetic disorders are no longer classified in the exclusive realm of rare, mostly pediatric diseases. Competency in genomic medicine is important for all health professionals, and the concept of *genetic exceptionalism* (the idea that genetic information is qualitatively unique from other medical information and therefore raises unique social issues) may no longer be as distinct (Evans and Burke, 2008). But there are still several aspects of genetic information that present important personal, family, and social consequences that often distinguish genetic disorders from other nonhereditary medical conditions.

Schild and Black (1984) first described six features that differentiate genetic disorders from those that do not have a strong hereditary component. Conditions with a genetic etiology are distinctive as follows (Bennett, 2006; Costello, 1988; McConkie-Rosell and DeVellis, 2000; Plumridge et al., 1993; Resta, 2000; Schild and Black, 1984; Weil, 2000):

1. *Familial*. Although genetic information is personal information, it could be considered "family property" because a diagnosis may embrace a whole family, not just an individual. A new genetic diagnosis in a kindred can have profound effects (both positive and negative) on interpersonal relationships among family members. The ramifications of a genetic diagnosis may reverberate beyond the nuclear family, particularly if the condition is inherited in a dominant or X-linked pattern (thus placing many generations at risk). Some areas of family dynamics and functioning in which genetic risk factors can play a role include the following.

   a. *Parental guilt* is a common experience when offspring are affected with a genetic disorder. Children may blame a parent for passing on the "family curse"; offspring may bluntly ask the affected parent, "Will I be like you when I grow up?"

   b. *Familial confidentiality* may be threatened because often it is necessary to obtain medical records and even blood samples from family members affected with the disease or condition as part of a genetic evaluation. In medical genetics the extended family often becomes the client unit, raising unique issues of confidentiality and privacy of health and personal information. This may be felt as an intrusion of privacy, both for the family member being asked to share confidential medical and family information and for the person seeking the medical information: Now other family members will know the person is involved in a genetic evaluation and possibly genetic testing.

   c. *Reproductive plans may be altered* because of knowledge of genetic risk factors, not just for the person seeking this information but also for relatives. Learning genetic carrier status may threaten the individuals' notions of parental roles. There may be challenges to religious and ethical belief systems between couples and their extended families as couples wrestle with core values of biological parenting and views on prenatal diagnosis, assistive reproductive technologies, and potential adoption.

2. *Permanent*. Despite remarkable advances in the general understanding of the mechanisms and management of many genetic disorders, durable cures such

as gene therapy are slow to become reality. The available disease management strategies may be complex, such as lifelong and costly enzyme replacement therapy for a person with Gaucher disease (a lysosomal storage disease); a stringent lifetime diet to prevent the mental impairments associated with phenylketonuria; multiple surgical repairs for the individual with multiple congenital anomalies; or prophyplactic mastectomy for reduction of breast cancer risk for a young woman with a genetic predisposition to breast cancer. There can be a sense of fatalism or hopelessness that the individual cannot alter destiny because the gene alteration is in "every cell of my body."

3. *Chronic*. Genetic diseases often affect individuals in different ways throughout their lifetimes. There can be a continual array of new health challenges throughout a person's lifetime. Many individuals become increasingly impaired by their condition with age. This may create continual strains on the person or family. Depending on the severity of the disease, the family can experience "chronic sorrow" for the person who "will never be" (Olshansky, 1962). For persons with severe disabilities, common life events such as graduations and weddings can remind the person and family of differences from the norm. There can be unresolved grief if a family experiences the death of multiple relatives with the same condition (such as is often the case with families with an inherited cancer syndrome).

4. *Complex*. Genetic conditions often affect multiple organ systems. Persons with a genetic disorder may require the medical expertise of a variety of health professionals. Individuals may need specialized medical tests and procedures that are available only at major metropolitan medical centers. Persons with rare genetic disorders often meet with continual frustration trying to find health professionals who are familiar with their disorder. The rarity of the condition may give the patient and family a sense of isolation. The variable clinical expression of many genetic conditions adds to their complexity; two people with the same gene alteration may have extremely different phenotypes, making prognosis difficult.

5. *Labeling*. As a society we are quick to label. A child with Down syndrome becomes "a Down's," a person with diabetes becomes a "diabetic," or someone with a seizure disorder because an "epileptic." With a genetic label the person may perceive himself or herself as different, flawed, or mutated. The individual (and family) may have trouble with this new identify and grieve for his or her former self. The family may feel their heritage is tainted. Family members and society may stigmatize the individual in blatant or subtle ways. Despite increasing legal protections for people with genetic disorders, fear of genetic discrimination (insurance, employment, and societal) may hinder the willingness of individuals and their families to participate in genetic testing and research. For example, a person with a genetic condition might be considered less desirable as a marriage partner or as a candidate for certain employment opportunities, or a family may steer resources for education toward an unaffected relative.

TABLE 9.1   Common Medical Conditions with Onset in Adulthood for Which Genetic Susceptibility Testing is Potentially Available

Ataxia
Breast cancer
Cardiac arrhythmia
Cardiomyopathy
Colon cancer
Coronary artery disease
Dementia (presenile)
Diabetes
Iron storage disease
Melanoma
Ovarian cancer
Prostate cancer
Thyroid cancer

6. *Threatening*. Genetic disorders threaten at many different levels including the choice of mate, reproductive planning, privacy, self-esteem, and even longevity. The affected or at risk individual (and his or her family) may alter long range plans if facing a degenerative disease or premature death. The life-style of the individual and family unit may be threatened. Parents of a newborn with a severely disabling or life-threatening condition may have trouble bonding with the child.

If Schild and Black were considering this list today, there would be a few other considerations that they would likely add. The ability to test a healthy person for possible future health status provides new challenges to traditional definitions of *healthy* and *diseased*. A well person can choose to be genetically tested for an increasing number of susceptibility mutations for various adult-onset disorders (Table 9.1). These genetic tests cannot predict a precise age of onset of symptoms, nor can they predict the specific manifestations of the disease for any particular patient. Uncertainty will probably always be a pitfall of genetic susceptibility testing. Sometimes a semantic distinction is made between *presymptomatic testing* in which a gene is highly penetrant and thus a person has a strong lifetime probability of developing the disease (approaching 100%), and *susceptibility testing* in which the likelihood of developing manifestations of the disease are lower. In addition a therapeutic gap exists for management of many of these diseases; the technical ability to test for a gene mutation has occurred in advance of the availability of effective therapy. Terms that have been applied to a healthy person who has tested positive for a genetic susceptibility include *unaffected carrier*, *unpatient* (Jonsen et al., 1996), and *pre-vivors* (a description that surfaced in approximately 2000 among the FORCE support network for people who have tested positive for mutations in *BRCA1* or *BRCA2* but who have not developed cancer) (FORCE, 2009). The long-term psychological fallout of making a healthy individual "unwell" is just beginning to be explored.

Survivor guilt is an experience that is common in families with a genetic disorder. The person who is unaffected or who has tested negative for the familial disease susceptibility is conflicted between feelings of relief and joy to have escaped the disease, and sadness and guilt that the condition affects other relatives. Anticipating this reaction is an important genetic counseling message that is given when counseling a healthy person who is considering genetic testing. Clues from the family history may help the clinician further anticipate the likelihood of this occurring (e.g., if the person is the only sibling to test negative for the gene mutation). One of my clients who tested negative for a cancer susceptibility mutation described her experience with survivor guilt as "standing outside a burning house with my family inside."

9.2 THE PEDIGREE AS A TOOL IN PSYCHOSOCIAL ASSESSMENT AND COUNSELING

In Chapter 1 the multipurpose use of a pedigree was discussed in the concrete realms of patient education, assisting with diagnosis and plans for medical management, and identifying at-risk relatives. Beyond these practical uses, the power of a pedigree as a tool for anticipating a client's potential psychosocial needs and issues is immense. The graphic nature of a pedigree can be used by the clinician to anticipate a patient's concerns and fears and as a clue as to how the genetic disorder has been experienced by the patient and his or her family. Sometimes the shade of sorrow that a client must be experiencing from what has happened in the family leaps from the ink of the pedigree portrait and simply cannot be ignored. Family tragedy may have nothing to do with genetics, such as a house fire, a murder, a drowning, or a motor vehicle accident, but it should be acknowledged by the clinician. While taking a family history, even the simple statement "You have been through so much" will be greatly appreciated by the client.

Here are some examples of psychosocial clues from a pedigree:

- *Patient is approaching the age of relatives in the family who have developed a disease or had life-threatening complications.* This may be the reason that the client has chosen now to seek medical interventions or genetic counseling or testing. If many relatives have been severely affected with the condition or have had multiple medical setbacks (such as multiple primary cancer diagnoses) or there have been many deaths in the family, this is a clue that your client may be experiencing a sense of chronic sorrow.
- *Client is the only affected or unaffected relative in the immediate or extended family.* A pedigree can clearly outline relatives who are affected in a family and therefore can guide the clinician as to when to anticipate that a client is likely to have feelings of survivor guilt. The survivor may feel on the outskirts of the family team, despite knowing it is irrational to desire ill health. Alternatively, a client who is the only affected relative in a sibship may have feelings of anger, disbelief, and bewilderment, asking "Why me?"

- *Client is pregnant or experiencing infertility and another close relative is pregnant or has recently given birth.* For a client who is pregnant or experiencing infertility, the pedigree may reveal that another close relative is also pregnant or has a young child or, conversely, has a child or fetus newly diagnosed with the condition. The clinician can anticipate that this simultaneous family experience may be causing some emotional conflicts for the client, and explore her (or his) reactions further.

- *Anticipating a client's reaction to test results based on his or her other relative's experience with genetic testing.* For a healthy person seeking guidance regarding presymptomatic testing, using the pedigree to inquire about who else in the family has been tested and what their experience has been can also help the clinician provide support to the client. For example, your client may feel that his or her risk of disease is higher or lower than the actual risk because of the results of other relatives. The client may feel pressure to be tested because he or she is the only relative yet to be tested in the immediate family. The person may feel ambivalence about genetic testing because of fears about what the next steps in medical management would be based on how other relatives have responded to their results (such as prophylactic surgery for breast cancer risk reduction).

- *How have relatives fared with the disease in the family?* From the pedigree it is often easy to get a sense as to how relatives have lived with their disease. Has there been variability of the disease in the family? Have there been successful medical interventions or screening in other relatives? If relatives have survived their disease then the client is likely to have a different perception from those whose relatives were severely debilitated by the condition. If the course of the disease in other relatives has been grim, it can be important for the clinician to educate the client about how medical care and screening has improved and that the course of the disease that was seen in other relatives can be different in the client and his or her children or siblings.

- *Is there a family history of depression or suicide?* An important risk factor that can be disclosed in family history is a history of suicide in the family. There seems to be a strong correlation with suicide and a family history of suicide (Currier and Mann, 2008; Wasserman et al., 2007).

- *Who in the family is available to turn to for support?* A pedigree can be a graphic display of who may be available as a support person for a client. Does the client have siblings, adult children, parents or a step-parent who can be supportive? Do they live in the area or will they be visiting soon? Are they available to attend a visit where genetic test results and management plans will be discussed? Are there relatives who are not supportive? Will the client be sharing test results with these relatives? The amount of information a client knows about his or her relatives is likely proportional to the support the family will provide for each other and indicates how likely the client's to share information with other relatives (e.g., if the family has not been close for years, a genetic diagnosis probably will not change their communication patterns).

9.3 THE PROCESS OF GENETIC COUNSELING

Genetic disorders can affect so many areas of a person's psychological, medical, financial, and social life. The field of genetic counseling developed from the need to educate, manage, and counsel individuals and families diagnosed with or at risk for genetic disorders. Genetic counseling can help make the difference in the adjustment of a person and family to a genetic diagnosis and help him or her make informed decisions. This is not to imply that every family with a genetic disorder will need long-term support.

Genetic counseling encompasses more than reproductive counseling about inherited disorders or advising about the risks and benefits of genetic tests. Genetic counseling may be of benefit throughout the life cycle, from preconception counseling, prenatal genetic assessment, and assessment of congenital and childhood problems to disorders that affect adults (Ciarleglio et al., 2003). Genetic counseling may involve a one-time crisis intervention dealing with a new genetic diagnosis or may develop into a relationship over many years if the client is treated in a specialty clinic for diseases such as hemophilia, fragile X syndrome, familial cancers, or Huntington disease. Genetic counseling is a multifaceted process, as espoused in the official definition by the National Society of Genetics Counselors (Resta et al., 2006):

> Genetic counseling is the process of helping people understand and adapt to the medical, psychological and familial implications of genetic contributions to disease.
>
> This process integrates:
>
> — Collection and interpretation of family and medical histories to assess the chance of disease occurrence or recurrence;
>
> — Education about inheritance, testing, management, prevention, resources, and research;
>
> — Counseling to promote informed choices and adaptation to the risk or condition.

Genetic counseling is designed to reduce the client's anxiety, enhance the client's control and mastery over life circumstances, increase the client's understanding of the genetic disorder and options for testing and disease management, and provide the client and family with the tools required to adjust to potential outcomes (Bennett, 2006). Genetic counseling can help individuals understand their options and make decisions that are appropriate in view of their perceptions of risk, religion, life beliefs, and family goals.

9.4 WHAT TO EXPECT FROM A GENETICS CONSULTATION

> Genetic consultation offers new, objective, and scientific knowledge from outside the person, but it arouses within the person old, subjective and irrational knowledge of personal griefs, angers, and confusions about the connections between family and illness.
>
> **—Andree Lehmann (1997)**

A first visit for genetic counseling or a clinical genetic evaluation can last between 30 minutes and 2 hours, depending on the complexity of the problem and whether multiple specialists are involved. A written summary of the appointment is often provided to the patient (and family, with the patient's permission). Whether the appointment a one-time visit or ongoing, there are usually three broad areas that are covered in each session: *assessment, education, and counseling*. The areas touched in genetic counseling are briefly summarized as follows (for more detailed information, refer to Bennett, 2006; LeRoy and Walker, 2002; Marymee et al., 1998; McCarthy Veach et al., 2003; National Society of Genetics Counselors, 2007; Uhlmann et al., 2009):

- Contracting—the merging of the counselor's and clients expectations. What are the mutual goals of the session?
- Psychosocial assessment—what are the client's beliefs about about the condition in his or her family, about patterns of inheritance, about his or her risk of developing disease? What emotional, experiential, social, educational, and cultural issues may influence the client's incorporation of information and coping patterns?
- Obtaining and reviewing the client's family pedigree (usually a minimum of three generations). For complicated diagnoses, the pedigree may be obtained over the phone and reviewed during the clinic visit.
- Obtaining and reviewing available medical records on the individual and sometimes extended relatives. Photographs may be helpful for identifying dysmorphic features.
- Obtaining and reviewing a medical history (and developmental history as appropriate).
- Arranging for a physical examination of the patient and other family members (if indicated).
- Establishing a diagnosis or potential diagnosis.
- Reviewing of the inheritance pattern(s) and natural history of the condition, disease monitoring and management, and any preventive measures.
- Discussing options for available genetic testing or diagnostic procedures (including discussion of test sensitivity and specificity) and arranging for tests (as appropriate).
- Assessing personal, social, religious, and ethnocultural issues, including their relationship to the patient's feelings about genetic testing and the possible consequences of such testing.
- Discussion of reproductive options, including prenatal diagnosis and the availability of assistive reproductive technologies (as appropriate).
- Assessing possible ethical concerns such as confidentiality, disparate paternity, insurability, discrimination, employment issues, feelings about prenatal diagnosis, and presymptomatic testing of a minor child.

- Referring to community resources and disease specific advocacy groups, such as the Genetic Alliance, (www.geneticalliance.org) and the National Organization of Rare Disorders, (NORD; www.rarediseases.org).
- Referral to appropriate health specialties/specialists, as needed.
- Supporting a patient's decisions in the context of individual values, beliefs, and goals.
- Providing resources for genetic counseling and/or additional tests/evaluations for other relatives as needed.

Because of the potentially profound influences that a genetic diagnosis may have on the life of the individual being evaluated, test results are often given in person, and a support person is often encouraged to attend such appointments. A follow-up visit or phone call to discuss the patient and family's reaction to the results is often advisable. If the results are the opposite of what the person (or family) anticipated they would be, the client may have trouble adjusting to this new self-identity or state of being. Kessler (1988) describes this phenomenon as "preselection." After presymptomatic testing, individuals may regret past life choices that they might have made differently had they had prior knowledge of their genetic status.

Even good news can have a negative effect on the person receiving this information. The individual may feel an unwelcome burden to care of his or her affected relatives (both physically and financially). A healthy sibling may have a profound sense of survivor guilt as discussed earlier.

9.5   GENETIC COUNSELORS AND OTHER GENETIC SPECIALISTS

The term *genetic counselor* is generally reserved for health professionals who have earned a master's degree and who have extensive training in human genetics and counseling skills. In the United States, the first group of genetic counselors graduated from Sarah Lawrence College in 1971. There are close to 40 programs in the United States and Canada accredited by the American Board of Genetic Counseling (ABGC; www.abgc.net) with similar programs in place around the world (International Genetic Counseling Education; http://igce.med.sc.edu).

Other clinical genetics professionals are typically physicians (medical geneticists) certified by the American Board of Medical Genetics (ABMG; www.abmg.org) or a similar international certification and clinical nurse specialists in genetics who meet genetic competencies through the International Society of Nurses in Genetics (ISONG; www.isong.org) or the Genetic Nursing Credentialing Commission (GNCC; www.geneticnurse.org).

Many other health professionals, such as oncologists, perinatologists, neurologists, and obstetricians, have expertise in genetics and genetic counseling, although they are not specifically certified in this specialty. Many professional societies for specific health professionals have a genetics subcommittee that addresses practice issues and professional guidelines. Often a genetic evaluation involves members from a team of core specialists such as medical geneticists, genetic counselors, nurses and nurse practitioners, nutritionists, social workers, mental health professionals, and clergy.

9.6 LOCATING A GENETICS PROFESSIONAL

The National Society of Genetic Counselors (NSGC) is the leading voice, authority, and advocate for the genetic counseling profession. The NSGC has an online resource directory of genetic counselors in the United States and abroad (www.nsgc.org/resourcelink.cfm). Genetic counselors, medical geneticists, and advanced practice nurse genetics professionals can be located through the NCBI's Gene Tests online (www.geneclinics.org). Many professional societies have listings of members within their specialty with expertise in genetics.

9.7 SUMMARY

Genetic disorders and inherited susceptibility to diseases can occur throughout the lifecycle (Ciarleglio et al., 2003). Although there are many aspects of genetic disease that are issues in noninherited diseases as well (such as fear of discrimination and stigmatization), there are several distinguishing features of genetic disorders that are important to recognize when providing services to clients and their families with an inherited disorder or susceptibility to disease. An important function of a pedigree is to use it as a means of identifying potential psychosocial issues that may be of concern to the client and his or her family (such as survivor or parental guilt, chronic sorrow, perspectives of other relatives, etc.). Genetic counselors, medical geneticists, and clinical genetic nurse specialists are experts in genetic risk assessment, counseling, and care of clients and their families with inherited disorders.

9.8 REFERENCES

American Board of Genetic Counseling. (2009). Welcome to ABGC. Available at www.abgc.net. Accessed September 16, 2009.

American Board of Medical Genetics. (2009). ABMG Home. Available at www.abmg.org. Accessed November 23, 2009.

Bennett RL. (2006). Genetic counseling. In: Runge MS, Patterson C, eds. *Principles of Molecular Medicine*, 2nd ed. Totowa, NJ: Humana Press, pp. 46–52.

Brooks VW, Great–Quotes.com. (2009). Van Wyck Brooks. Available at www.greatquotes.com. Accessed November 23, 2009.

Ciarleglio LJ, Bennett RL, Williamson J, et al. (2003). Genetic counseling throughout the life cycle. *J Clin Invest* 112:1280–1286.

Costello AJ. (1988). The psychosocial impact of genetic disease. In: University of Colorado Health Sciences Center, ed. *Genetics Applications: A Health Perspective*. Lawrence, KS: Learner Managed Designs, pp. 194–165.

Currier D, Mann JJ. (2008). Stress, genes and the biology of suicidal behavior. *Psychiatr Clin North Am.* 31(2):247–269.

Evans JP, Burke W. (2008). Genetic exceptionalism—Too much of a good thing? *Genet Med* 10(7):500–501.

FORCE, Facing Our Risk of Cancer Empowered. (2009). What is a pre-vivor. Available at http://facingourrisk.org/TTInc/viewpage.php?url=.%2Fnewsletter%2F2009winter%2Fraychels_story.html&needle=previvors. Accessed February 7, 2009.

Genetic Counseling Education. Connecting the Global Community. January 30, 2009. Available at http://igce.med.sc.edu. Accessed February 7, 2009.

Genetic Nursing Credentialing Commission. (2009). Available at www.geneticnurse.org. Accessed November 23, 2009.

International Society of Nurses in Genetics. (2009). Genetic Nurse Credentialing Commission Home. Available at www.isong.org. Accessed November 23, 2009.

Jonsen AR, Durfy SJ, Burke W, Motulsky AG. (1996). The advent of the "unpatients." *Nat Med* 2(6):622–624.

Kessler S. (1988). Invited essay on the psychological aspects of genetic counseling. V. Preselection: A family coping strategy in Huntington disease. *Am J Med Genet* 31:617–621.

Lehman A. (1997). Aspects psychologiques du conseil genetique. [Psychological aspects of genetic counseling]. In: J.-Y Bignon, eds. *Oncogenetique: Vers une Medicine de Presumption/Prediction. Cachan*, France: Lavoisier, pp. 383–395.

LeRoy BS, Walker AP. (2002). Genetic counseling: History, risk assessment, strategies, and ethical considerations. In: King RA, Rotter JI, Motulsky AG. *The Genetic Basis of Common Disease*, 2nd ed. New York: Oxford University Press, pp. 87–101.

Marymee K, Dolan CR, Pagon RA, et al. (1998). Development of the critical elements of genetic evaluation and genetic counseling for genetic professionals and perinatologists in Washington State. *J Genet Couns* 6:133–165.

McCarthy Veach P, LeRoy BS, Bartels DM. (2003). *Facilitating the Genetic Counseling Process,* A Practice Manual. New York: Springer.

McConkie-Rosell A, DeVellis BM. (2000). Threat to parental role: A possible mechanism of altered self-concept related to carrier knowledge. *J Genet Couns* 9(4):285–302.

National Organization for Rare Disorders; NORD. (2009). NORD Home. Available at www.rarediseases.org. Accessed November 23, 2009.

National Society of Genetic Counselors. (2007). Scope of Practice. June 2007. Available at www.nsgc.org/client_files/SOP_final_0607.pdf. Accessed February 7, 2009.

Olshansky S. (1962). Chronic sorrow a response to having a mentally retarded child. *Social Casework* 43:190–193.

Plumridge D, Bennett R, Dinno N, Branson C. (1993). *The Student with a Genetic Disorder: Educational Implications for Special Education Teachers and for Physical Therapists, Occupational Therapists and Speech Pathologists*. Springfield, IL: Charles C. Thomas.

Pollen DA. (1993). Hannah's Heirs. New York: Oxford University Press.

Resta RG. (2000). *Psyche and Helix. Psychological Aspects of Genetic Counseling*. New York: Wiley-Liss.

Resta RG, Biesecker BB, Bennett RL, et al. (2006) A new definition of genetic counseling: National Society of Genetic Counselor's Task Force report. *J Genet Couns* 15(2): 77–83.

Schild S, Black RB. (1984). *Social Work and Genetics: A Guide for Practice*. New York: Hawthorth Press.

Simpson JB. (1988). *Simpson's Contemporary Quotations*. Boston: Houghton Mifflin.

Uhlmann WR, Schuette JL, Yashar B. (2009). *A Guide to Genetic Counseling,* 2nd ed. Hoboken: Wiley–Blackwell.

Wasserman D, Geijer T, Sokolowki M, et al. (2007). Nature and nurture in suicidal behavior, the role of genetics: Some novel findings concerning personality traits and neural conduction. *Physiol Behav* 92(1–2):245–249.

Weil J. (2000). *Psychosocial Genetic Counseling*. Oxford: Oxford University Press.

Chapter 10

Pedigree Predicaments

So tangled is the web we weave when once we practice to perceive.
—Michael Bérubé (1996)

10.1 THE TRUTH

A pedigree is unique from other components of a medical record because it contains personal information about extended family members that may not be absolutely factual. Although most pedigrees represent a passable view of the truth, each pedigree will vary, depending on the patient's recall of family data and the type of information solicited from the client by the health professional. For example, if my family physician were to record my medical-family history and compare it to a pedigree taken by my first cousin's primary-care provider, the framework of the two pedigrees would be similar, but the family embellishments would undoubtedly vary. I certainly am more of an authority on my health and the health and ages of my immediate family than I am on the health of my cousin's siblings and parents, and vice versa.

The balance between protecting patient confidentiality and the accuracy of patient information is delicate. A health professional who provides care for multiple members in the same family may encounter a dilemma in how to record a pedigree when the "family facts" are discrepant from one family member to another. Our clinic at the University of Washington Medical Center is a geographic hub for the diagnosis and care of many individuals with rare inherited disorders, thus we often provide services to persons from multiple branches of the same family. Although it is rewarding to follow the generations of an extended family over several years, it also creates some awkward situations. On several occasions, I have discovered during the patient interview that I know more about the family of the patient sitting across from me than

The Practical Guide to the Genetic Family History, Second Edition, by Robin L. Bennett
Copyright © 2010 John Wiley & Sons, Inc.

my patient does. It is a challenge to decide whether to record the pedigree as absolutely reported to me by the patient, or to correct the critical inaccuracies on the pedigree based on the information received from family members I have seen at prior visits.

As health professionals we wear the blinders of our specialty and therefore we naturally seek responses from a patient in relation to our field of expertise. This can dramatically influence the scope of the information recorded on a pedigree. Case in point: Mr. and Mrs. C were referred to our genetics clinic by a respected local pediatric geneticist who, shortly before the death of the Cs first child in the newborn intensive care unit, diagnosed the infant with a lethal unbalanced chromosome rearrangement. We planned to continue the evaluation of the family by obtaining a chromosome study on each parent to determine if one of them carried a balanced chromosome rearrangement then and to proceed with further family studies, if needed. When I greeted the couple in the lobby to escort them to my office, I was puzzled when one of our patients with Huntington disease rose to join them—she was Mr. C's mother! When the initial pedigree had been taken, the fact that Mr. C. had Huntington disease in his family was neither solicited by the geneticist nor volunteered by Mr. or Mrs. C. The chromosome studies found that Mrs. C, two of her siblings, and her father carried a rare balanced reciprocal translocation. We were able to discuss with the Cs the implications of the inheritance of both Huntington disease (with Mr. C's mother's permission) and the chromosome translocation for their future offspring.

A year later, Mrs. C phoned me with the nervous news that she was six weeks along in her pregnancy. She was interested in scheduling an appointment to discuss prenatal testing. After scheduling the appointment, Mrs. C said, "I have one more question, is hemophilia inherited?" When I asked her why she was asking, she replied, "Oh, because two of my brothers and my mother's brother have hemophilia. I'm not really worried about it, I was just curious." How did two genetic professionals miss this classic X-linked genetic disease in the family history? The Cs probably did not think that the information was important at the time of their visit, and the genetic specialists (including me) were guilty of tunnel vision.

The choice of information that is recorded on a pedigree is biased by the cultural and scientific belief systems of the recorder (Resta, 1995). For example, whether I document information on a pedigree about cigarette smoking in family members depends on the family's disease that I am tracking. Given the causal association with tobacco use and disease, I certainly would make pedigree notations regarding family members' usage of tobacco if my client was interested in a hereditary cancer risk assessment (National Cancer Institute [NCI], 2008) or if he or she were inquiring about familial risks associated with cleft lip and palate (Chung et al., 2000, Lorente et al., 2000). I might not record information about the tobacco habits of family members at risk for Huntington disease because my scientific belief system does not register an association with the development of Huntington disease and the use of tobacco products. If a client informs me that a relative has attention deficit disorder, I would record this information on the pedigree if fragile X was a consideration in the family, but I might not if the concern was cystic fibrosis.

My own style of recording pedigrees has evolved over time in synchrony with changes in my scientific knowledge. In the early 1990s, if I were taking a family history from a 25-year-old woman whose mother died of breast cancer at age 42, I probably would have commented to her, "That must have been a difficult time for you." I may have asked, "Do you have other relatives with breast or other cancers?" Even if the consultand had replied yes, I probably would not have explored the family history any further beyond saying, "You should be diligent with your breast self-exams and follow the national guidelines for screening for breast and other cancers." Today, given the availability of genetic testing and options for screening and risk reduction for multiple inherited cancer syndromes, I would ask a whole cascade of medical-family history questions to try to identify patterns of an inherited cancer syndrome (as outlined in Chapter 5). Before the trinucleotide CAG repeat expansion on chromosome 4 was identified as the mutation in Huntington disease in 1993, it was commonplace to record the names and whereabouts of extended relatives because DNA testing required linkage analysis. I recorded the states where they lived because I might need to obtain blood samples from those relatives. Now, with the availability of a direct DNA test, I am more focused on satisfying myself that the family pedigree appears autosomal dominant and that an affected family member has had a positive DNA test. Just as family dynamics change, so does our focus in genetics.

10.2 LESSONS FROM HISTORY

At the turn of the 20th century, the Eugenic Record Office (ERO) at Cold Spring Harbor was filled with serious and responsible scientists concerned about the civic duties of science and its application to human problems. Pedigrees were a part of this movement because they could demonstrate, as eugenicist Karl Pearson put it, "the facts of heredity, free of all more or less contentious interpretations" (quoted in Mazumdar, 1992). The early pioneers of pedigrees distributed standardized forms for making a eugenical family history to the general public to encourage people to "register their family network" (Figure 10.1) (Davenport and Laughlin, 1915). Families and their physicians were charged to describe both the good qualities and defects of family members with "care, accuracy, and frankness." Some of the objective traits to be marked were "meane, feebleminded, pauper, epileptic, wanderlust, musical ability, and alcoholic" (Laughlin, 1914; Mazumdar, 1992). It is easy to see why the *Oxford English Dictionary* defines the term *pedigree* as a colloquial term for an individual's criminal record (Resta, 1993). I presume a quantitative or objective measure of "meane" or "wanderlust" is a challenge even in modern times.

In the United States, data from collections of pedigrees were used to champion state laws allowing involuntary sterilization of persons considered unfit for reproduction. Similar sterilization programs were implemented in the UK, Norway, Sweden, Denmark, Finland, and Germany (Cowan, 2008). In hindsight we look at these historical pedigrees, taken by well-meaning geneticists intending to better the world with science and we shudder at the realization that herein lie the tarnished roots of the Nazi eugenic pogroms of the 1930s and 1940s.

About 100 years after the Eugenics Records Office national campaign, several other campaigns in the United States have been initiated promote to the gathering

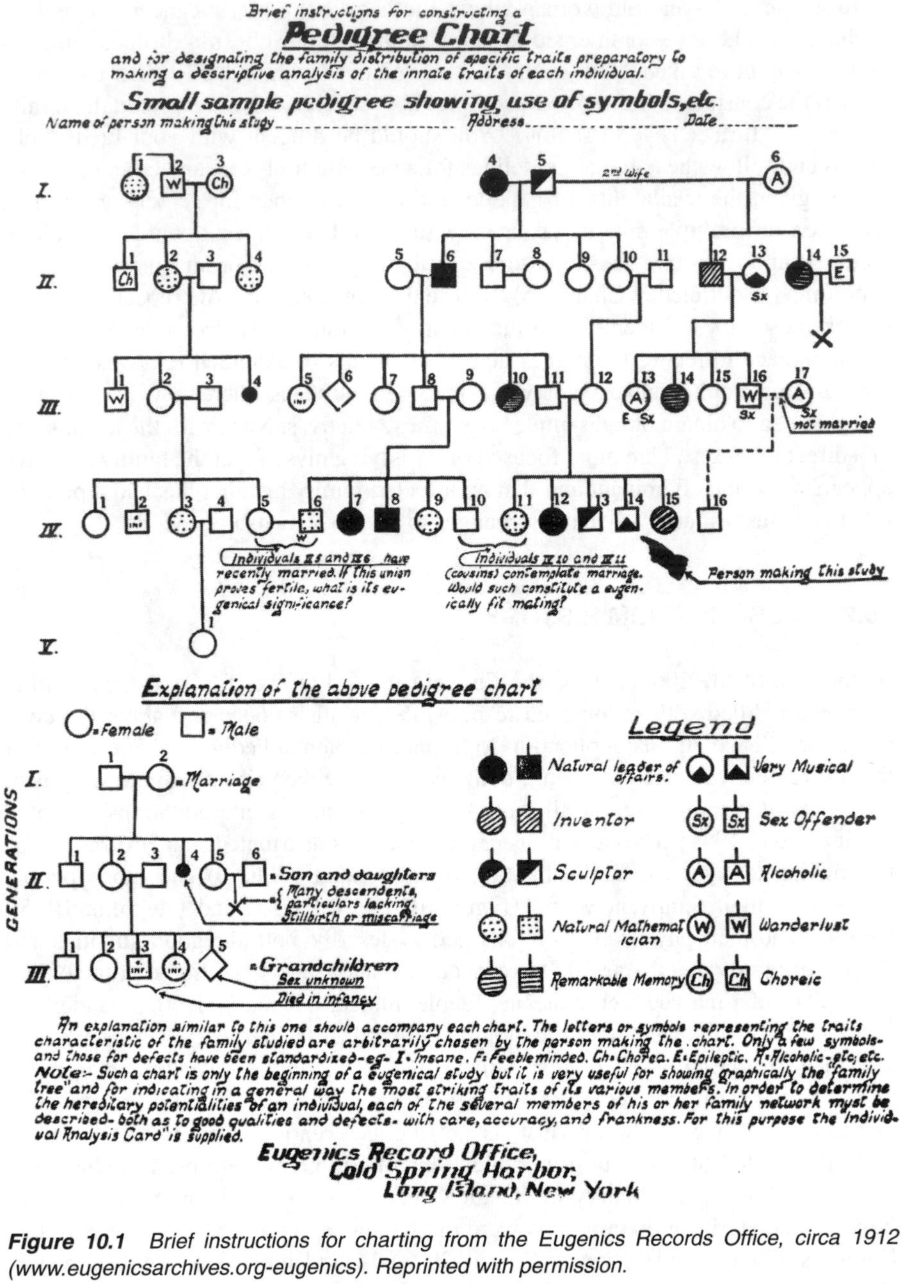

Figure 10.1 Brief instructions for charting from the Eugenics Records Office, circa 1912 (www.eugenicsarchives.org-eugenics). Reprinted with permission.

of family health history such as the U.S. Surgeon General's "My Family Health Portrait," (http://familyhistory.hhs.gov/fhh-web/home.action) with similar initiatives in other parts of the world including the UK (www.clingensoc.org/Docs/Standards/CGSPedigree.pdf) and Mexico (www.inmedgen.gob.mx). Such initiatives highlight that gathering medical family history and sharing this information with various health professionals can potentially save a life. We hope that the past abuses of the application of family history serve as a lesson and a guide to prevent future misuse.

10.3 THE RESEARCHER AND FAMILY STUDIES

Because specialists in all medical disciplines care for individuals with genetic disorders, any health professional may someday be involved with a person participating in a genetic research study. Research studies in which a subject has a genetic disorder (or potentially inherited condition) are different from the study of an individual for a nongenetic indication. Table 10.1 compares the traditional model of individual subject research to that of a family studies model (Frankel and Teich, 1993). Areas of subject recruitment, voluntary consent, and subject withdrawl must be carefully considered when research involves individuals and families with inherited disorders. Genetic research of minors should be approached with particular caution. Because the study

TABLE 10.1 Unique Issues in Family Studies

Traditional Research Model	Family Studies Model
1. Subject consents to be studied as an individual	1. Subject has ties to other research participants because of shared genetic heritage
2. Subject has no ties to other research participants	2. Information learned from research affects the family, and what researchers learn about the family affects what the subject knows about self
3. Information learned from the research affects only the subject	3. Other family members become part of study without their consent because they are members of a family under study
4. Subject recruitment is entirely voluntary and is usually based on specific medical features under study (or demographics such as in a population-based association study)	4. Subject recruitment may not be entirely voluntary because other family member(s) may benefit if family members participate; therefore, subject may feel coerced to participate by the other family member(s) already participating in the study
5. Subject can withdraw from study at any time for any reason	5. Although subject can withdraw from study (i.e., by requesting destruction of subject's blood or tissue sample), there typically are not mechanisms for the withdrawal or destruction of family history information (If such mechanisms did exist, would that mean if one relative withdraws from the study, the entire family history must be withdrawn or only that individual's information?)

Source: Adapted from Frankel and Teich, 1993.

results may affect multiple family members, a discussion of if, how, and to whom results will be given must be a critical component of the informed consent process.

10.4 PEDIGREES AND PUBLICATIONS

The pedigree can be a powerful and succinct presentation of scientific data, and it is common to publish a pedigree as part of a case study or genetic research. Caution must be used to protect privacy and confidentiality of family members in the decision to publish a pedigree.

Two groups have addressed the complex issues of privacy and confidentiality in the publication of pedigrees. In a 1993 guidebook, *The National Institutes of Health's Office of Protection from Research Risks* (OPRR) addresses the issues of publication of pedigrees by stating "Where a risk of identification exists, participants must consent, in writing, to the release of personal information." Furthermore, Institutional Review Boards (IRBs) should address the following questions:

- Is the pedigree essential to the publication?
- Can identifying data be omitted?
- If an identifying pedigree is to be published, have subjects given consent for publication?

Guidelines by the International Committee of Medical Journal Editors (ICMJE) released in 1995 state:

Patients have rights to privacy that should not be infringed without informed consent. Identifying information should not be published in written descriptions, photographs, or pedigrees unless the information is essential for scientific purposes and the patient (or parents or guardian) gives written informed consent for publication. Informed consent for this purpose requires that the patient be shown the manuscript to be published. Identifying details should be omitted if they are not essential, but patient data should never be altered or falsified in an attempt to attain anonymity. Complete anonymity is difficult to achieve, and informed consent should be obtained if there is any doubt. For example, masking of the eye region in photographs of patients is inadequate protection of anonymity. The requirement of informed consent should be included in the journal's instructions for authors. When informed consent has been obtained it should be indicated in the published article.

The practice of masking or altering pedigrees to protect privacy and confidentiality is controversial. Botkin and his colleagues (1998) define *masking* as using symbols in a way that is obvious to the reader that information is being withheld; such as choosing diamonds to mask the gender of individuals, or giving approximate instead of absolute ages. The purpose of masking could be compared to using black bands across the eyes to disguise a patient in a published photograph. In contrast, *alteration* is used in reference to changing symbols or the framework of the pedigree in ways that may not be evident to the reader—for example, altering the birth order, changing gender, or not including all members of a sibship.

CHART SHOWING THE

INHERITANCE OF ABILITY

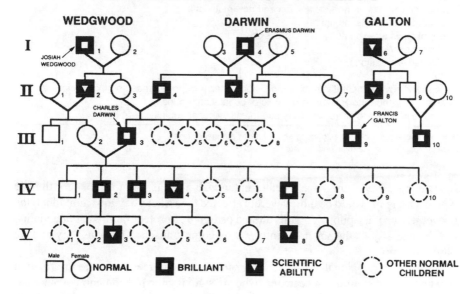

Figure 10.2 *A pedigree of the Wedgwood-Darwin-Galton family. Generation and individual numbers and names have been added to the original pedigree for ease in identification. Courtesy of Robert Resta, reprinted from Mazumdar (1992) with permission from Routledge, Chapman and Hall, Inc.*

One of the earliest examples of an altered pedigree is a pedigree published by the Eugenics Education Society (Mazumdar, 1992) showing the inheritance of brilliance and scientific ability in Darwin's own family (Figure 10.2). The pedigree is striking for its holandric (Y-linked) inheritance of ability in that only the male relatives are gifted. If one compares this pedigree to Figure 3.11 you will note the pedigree is biased by the absence of some contributory family facts, including intellectual disability in Darwin's multiple family members and hereditary deafness in the Wedgwood family (Bowlby, 1992; Resta 1995). The pedigree data may have been modified by Darwin's son Leonard (who was president of the Eugenic Education Society) to bolster the theory of the hereditary nature of his own family's genius (Robert Resta, personal communication, 1998).

A well-known example of a pedigree that was masked and altered in a nationally recognized journal was a pedigree diagram published in 1987 by Nancy Wexler and colleagues (1987) of a couple that each had Huntington disease. Their 14 children were represented as diamonds on the pedigree as a way of showing that four of the 14 siblings were homozygous for the HD mutated allele. The pedigree was published in this manner to protect the privacy of these homozygous individuals because 100% of their children are at risk to develop Huntington disease. Until the publication of

TABLE 10.2   Examples of Major Human Genetic Paradigms That May Be Missed If Critical Data[a] in a Pedigree Are Omitted, Masked, or Altered.

Anticipation
Parental age effects on non-disjunction and new mutations
Parent of origin effects in imprinting
Parent of origin effects in disease expression
Sex-linked expression
Sex-limited expression
In utero lethality
Genetic and environmental variables modifying patterns of penetrance and expression
Skewed gene frequencies in certain ethnic or population groups
Recessive inheritance or autozygosity suggested by consanguinity

[a]For example, ages, birth order, gender, sex, ethnicity, pregnancy loss.
Source: Adapted with permission from Bennett, 2002.

this pedigree, it was unknown whether individuals who are homozygous for the HD expansion alleles would be more severely affected than a heterozygous individual (the answer was no). By publishing this altered pedigree to protect family confidentiality, was the integrity of the scientific information compromised? Opinions vary and we may never know.

But the fact remains that by altering or masking pedigrees, valuable information may be lost. For example, researchers who are studying the phenomenon of anticipation in a specific disease often review published pedigrees to determine whether there is a trend for earlier ages of disease onset and more severe disease manifestations in successive generations. To recognize diseases with imprinting or mitochondrial inheritance, it is critical to record the sex of the transmitting parent. If the ages and sexes of individuals on the pedigree are altered, important patterns in disease expression may be missed or incorrectly interpreted. Examples of major human genetic paradigms that may be missed if critical data (e.g., ages, birth order, sex, ethnicity, miscarriages) in a pedigree are omitted, masked, or altered are shown in Table 10.2.

In reference to the pedigree published by Wexler et al., we now know that the age of onset of Huntington disease symptoms is influenced by the size of the triplet repeat; larger CAG repeat sizes are associated with earlier onset of disease, and the CAG repeat is more likely to be larger in an offspring if the parents have a large repeat size (greater than 50), particularly if the parent is a male (Brinkman et al., 1997). Would the information gained from this published pedigree be different if we had more complete information for the benefit of our interpretation?

One could argue that the practice of masking and altering pedigrees is fudging the data and is no more acceptable than if an investigator modifies aberrant research data to fit a hypothesis. A survey of investigators who published pedigrees in well-respected scientific journals reports that 19% of 177 respondents have published an altered pedigree, and 45% of these individuals did not disclose their alterations to the journal editor (Botkin et al., 1998).

All published pedigrees are truncated because an investigator must use discretion in how many generations in a pedigree are necessary to prove or illustrate the hypothesis. For example, a pedigree demonstrating familial Alzheimer disease might not include the grandchildren of affected individuals since they are not of an age to show symptoms. Likewise, a published pedigree will probably extend back only to the parents in the first affected generation, even if more information is known about prior generations. If full genealogical charts were published, the pedigrees would be cluttered and fill costly journal space.

Who decides which information is trivial or what information is significant enough to record on a pedigree? For example, information such as miscarriages or stillbirths may seem irrelevant with respect to a disease under study, yet a certain genotype may be lethal at the embryonic stage (such as carrying two *BRCA1* mutations: homoyzgosity or autozygosity) (Gowen et al., 1996). Current practices demonstrate that the line between the protection of identifying information and the reporting of pure data is fuzzy.

We must assume that any pedigree is potentially identifiable. With the increasing public access to medical literature through the Internet and through communication with disease-specific patient advocacy groups, any patient or research subject and his or her relatives may see the published pedigree. Here are some points to consider if you are in the position to publish a pedigree, if you are reviewing an article for publication in a journal or even if you are a participant on a human subjects' review board (Bennett, 2000):

- Did family members give consent for the publication of a pedigree? If yes, were they shown a copy of the pedigree that will be published?
- Does the pedigree contain sensitive information that is unknown to the subject (e.g., mental illness, presymptomatic testing information, or information on minor children)? Examples of sensitive information that may be published on a pedigree are included in Table 10.3. Might family members find out information about a risk to themselves that they were not aware of?
- Does the pedigree add to the understanding of the publication? Does it contain the necessary information needed to support or refute the hypothesis?
- If the pedigree is masked, is it still the best vehicle for relaying the data? Is a neutered pedigree, which uses diamonds to mask gender, still an effective visual communication tool?
- In reference to publication, have alterations to the pedigree been disclosed to the reader (such as a footnote stating that birth order is changed to preserve confidentiality)?
- And, perhaps the most telling question—If this was your family pedigree, would you be upset by disclosure of the information?

10.5 PEDIGREES AND THE ELECTRONIC MEDICAL RECORD

Brief family history information has been a part of the electronic medical record in text format, usually in reference to a particular clinical encounter. Complete pedigrees, however, are just beginning to be incorporated into electronic medical records. Family

TABLE 10.3 Examples of Potentially Identifying Information That May Be Sensitive or Concerning to the Patient or Family That Might Be Omitted from a Pedigree, and Why It Can Be Useful to Retain This Information on the Pedigree

Information Recorded on Relatives	Examples of Why Information of Potential Concern to Patient/Family	Why Information Useful
Age	Stigma if unmasks conception outside of marriage	Document age of disease onset Evaluate penetrance
Cause of death	Stigma related to some causes of death (e.g., suicide, substance abuse)	Document natural history of disease and penetrance Provide counseling related to disease management and prevention (e.g., anticipatory guidance)[a]
Physical characteristics (e.g., height, weight)	Stigma related to some physical features (e.g., obesity, unusually tall or short stature) Feelings of guilt related to control of disease (e.g., obesity and relation to risk of disease)	Obesity alters risk for disease (e.g., type 2 diabetes, uterine cancer) Obesity manifestation of disease (e.g., Beckwith Wiedemann syndrome.) Stature may be manifestation of disease (e.g., Marfanoid phenotype)
Genotype/carrier status (obligate or presymptomatic)	Parental guilt Survivor guilt Fear of discrimination	Genetic risk assessment Opportunity for genetic counseling Genetic testing strategy Counseling related to disease management and prevention (e.g., anticipatory guidance)
Mental illness, psychiatric history	Fear of stigma and discrimination Guilt	May be manifestation of disease (e.g., 22q11.2 deleton syndrome, Huntington disease) Counseling for psychological or medical intervention (e.g., anticipatory guidance)
Substance abuse	Fear of stigma and discrimination Guilt Shame	Teratogen exposure May influence manifestation of disease (e.g., tobacco) Referral to cessation program
Termination of pregnancy	Fear of stigma Guilt Shame Adverse effect on family relationships	Document ability to conceive

(Continued)

TABLE 10.3 (*Continued*)

Information Recorded on Relatives	Examples of Why Information of Potential Concern to Patient/Family	Why Information Useful
Misattributed paternity	Fear of stigma Guilt Shame Adverse effect on family relationships	May alter genetic risk assessment
Infertility	Adverse effect on family relationships Wrongly associated with reduced or impaired sexuality/virility	Documentation of disease process Possible embryonic/fetal lethality
Pregnancies or persons conceived using donor gametes	Fear of stigma Guilt Effect on family relationships Wrongly associated with reduced or impaired sexuality/virility	May be associated with disease May alter genetic risk assessment Potential to understand family dynamics
In vitro fertilization	Wrongly associated with sexuality/virility	Possible teratogenic effect
Adoption	Fear of stigma if unmasks conception outside of marriage Guilt Adverse effect on family relationships	May alter genetic risk assessment Potential to understand family dynamics
Ethnicity	Fear of stigma and discrimination Fear of racism	May alter genetic testing strategies and effect interpretation of test results
Consanguinity (relationships of first cousin and more distant)	May be confused with incestual relationship Fear of stigma and discrimination Effect on family relationships	May alter genetic risk assessment Opportunity for genetic counseling Potential to understand family dynamics
Incest (relationship between first degree relatives)[b]	Fear of stigma and discrimination Guilt Shame Criminal consequences Adverse effect on family relationships	May alter genetic risk assessment Opportunity for genetic counseling Potential to understand family dynamics

[a] *Anticipatory guidance* is a term that is used to describe a proactive approach to providing information that is given to a person or family in anticipation of physical or behavioral changes, and/or to promote health and well-being (Pridham, 1993).

[b] In some countries a marriage between an uncle and a niece (second-degree relatives) is a preferential union, but this is considered an incestual relationship in many countries (including the United States).

history data in a genealogical tree or as a pedigree may be brought to a clinic visit by the patient or provided by another relative. Pedigrees drawn by the health professional may be scanned into the medical record or even directly entered as a pedigree into the electronic medical record; downloading and updating pedigrees entered by the patient into the formal medical record is also an option. With all these possibilities there are a cacophony of challenges involving issues of ethics, security, privacy, confidentiality, and the validity or accuracy of the information provided (Bennett et al., 2008).

A utopian look might be to create a pedigree that travels from birth to grave through a person's electronic health record. The pedigree would need to have a way of being updated but also referenced to time, as medical recommendations would be made in reference to the family history data available at a set time point. Ideally electronic risk assessment and automatic updates would be done. A record would soon be cluttered with information relevant to one health professional but not another (imagine information relevant to a pediatric visit as compared to a geriatric visit). Is there information that might be too sensitive to include in a pedigree? By not including potentially sensitive information, as outlined in Table 10.3, there may be a risk of missing important medical paradigms (similar to those reviewed in Table 10.2) that could shift essential medical and screening recommendations for the patient and his or her family. A litmus test might be similar to the one noted for showing a research pedigree to the participant and relatives: Would you be willing to have your patient walk away with the pedigree you have recorded (Bennett et al., 2008)?

One approach to determining the information to include in the electronic health record is to consider the core data elements of a pedigree and the purpose of their inclusion on a pedigree. In a series of meetings sponsored by the Division of Medical Genetics of the University of Washington, and the Genetic Services Section of the Washington State Department of Health (Bennett et al., 2007, 2008), the participants determined the main reasons to include data on a medical pedigree are for:

1. *Orientation* (e.g., an arrow to identify the proband or consultand; the family relationship lines to understand biological relationships to the proband/consultand; a key to understanding shading of symbols; information on who took the pedigree, when and why)
2. *Diagnosis and risk assessment* (such as who is affected and relatives' ages and ages of disease onset; relationship lines documenting biological relationships and degrees of relatedness; other pertinent healthcare information such as screening and habits; ancestry and consanguinity)
3. *Ease of reading by multiple users* (such as using standardized pedigree symbols and including a key)
4. *Validation* (such as documenting that records were reviewed)
5. *Accountability, to the patient and for legal purpose* (reflecting accurate information on a pedigree is as important as the accuracy of a clinic note)
6. *Education of the patient and to develop plans for /health promotion and intervention* (discussed in detail in Chapter 1)
7. *Communication, to the patient and between health professionals*

The Personalized Health Care Work Group of the American Health Information Community has also worked to develop similar core data elements for inclusion in the electronic medical record, particularly for use by primary care professionals (Bigley and Feero, 2008). Careful consideration is necessary as these programs are developed; implementing changes will be difficult at best once these large hospital-based systems are in place. Representatives from all stakeholders in the system should be included beyond just the hospital administrators and software developers, to include the health professionals that will be inputting and interpreting the data and the patients and families the systems effect.

10.6 SUMMARY

Medical-family histories are a critical component of clinical medicine and research. Recording this information in the form of a pedigree is a shorthand method of tracking key elements (such as age, health status, age at disease onset, and environmental exposures in multiple family members over several generations) (Bennett et al., 2008). Because the identification of a genetic disorder in a family can be perceived as a stigma by the family and society, there are unique ethical issues to consider in the delivery of clinical services, the provision of informed consent for participation in research studies, and the publication of pedigrees.

The medical-family history information that is elicited from a patient and then recorded on a pedigree is prejudiced by the cultural and scientific belief systems of both the patient and the healthcare provider. Is documenting information on a pedigree such as misattributed paternity, depression, sexual orientation, abortions, drug and alcohol abuse, behavioral problems, or criminal behavior a record of medical facts or social information? Our biases may not be easily recognized, as Resta (1995) notes:

> In genetics, as in all scientific pursuits, the construction and interpretation of a pedigree can be influenced by the political and social beliefs of all-too-human geneticists. Those beliefs may be so ingrained that we mistake them for biological laws. It is, I suspect, beyond our ability to know which of our personal biases we are disguising as scientific truths. The whisper and hints of our biases may be heard only by future generations.

The use of pedigrees in clinical medicine has been evidenced for more than a century (Resta, 1993). Even with the advent of molecular and genomic medicine, pedigrees are not a tool of the past but remain an art of the future. The ability to data mine pedigrees in an electronic medical record may be of clinical utility in patient care and may also advance the understanding of disease mechanisms, particularly for common disease.

We should proceed with caution as campaigns such as the U.S. Surgeon General's Family Health Portrait initiative are advocated. The seemingly benign study of pedigree icons as an exercise in understanding human variation and disease can become a potential vehicle for the labeling of normality and abnormality and of distinguishing desirable from undesirable traits (Bennett, 2000). A similar program was instigated in the United States in the early 1920s by the Eugenic Record's Office (www.eugenicsarchive.org). Individuals were encouraged to use a standard pedigree format for collecting family history information (Figure 10.1). Scientific data were collected for conditions such as "meane, wanderlust, criminal activity, musical ability, and chorea" and given scientific status. By collecting this information, it was expected that persons would be able to make "fit marriages." The eugenics movement was born. What began with good intentions, at its hey day resulted in mass sterilization programs of those determined to be unfit and the ethnic cleansing horrors of Nazi Germany. Today, crimes against humanity continue under the guise of ethnic cleansing; we must continually monitor that our scientific truths are implemented with ethical clarity.

10.7 REFERENCES

Bennett RL. (2000). Pedigree parables. *Clin Genet* 58:241–249.

Bennett R, Lochner Doyle D, Harrison T, Byers P. (2007). Core elements of the pedigree in the era of electronic medical records. In Cooper S, Austin J, eds., Abstracts from the Twenty-Sixth Annual Education Conference of the National Society of Genetic Counselors, Kansas City, Missouri, October 2007. J Genet Couns 16:687.

Bennett RL, Steinhaus French K, Resta RG, Lochner Doyle D. (2008). Standardized pedigree nomenclature: Update and assessment of the recommendations of the National Society of Genetic Counselors. *J Genet Couns* 17(5):424–433.

Bérubé M. (1996). *Life as We Know It: A Father, a Family and an Exceptional Child*. New York: Pantheon Books.

Bigley MB, Feero WG. (2008). United States Department of Health and Human Services A report of the Family Health History Multi-Stakeholder Workgroup, October 25, 2007. Available at www.hhs.gov/healthit/ahic/materials/10_07/phc/report.html. Accessed August 5, 2008.

Brinkman RR, Mezei MM, Theilmann J, et al. (1997). The likelihood of being affected with Huntington disease by a particular age, for specific CAG repeat size. *Am J Hum Genet* 60:1202–1210.

Botkin JR, McMahon WM, Smith KR, Nash JE. (1998). Privacy and confidentiality in the publication of pedigrees: A survey of investigators and biomedical journals. *JAMA* 259:1808–1812.

Bowlby J. (1992). *Charles Darwin: A New Life*. New York: Norton.

Chung KC, Kowalski CP, Kim HM, Buchman SR. (2000). Maternal cigarette smoking during pregnancy and the risk of having a child with cleft lip/palate. *Plast Reconstr Surg* 105 (2):485–491.

Clinical Genetics Society, Clinical Governance Subcommittee. (2001). Guidelines for pedigree drawing, Paper 2 (Version A, 5/7/2001). Available at www.clingensoc.org/Docs/Standards/CGSPedigree.pdf). Accessed February 7, 2009.

Cold Springs Harbor Laboratory. (2009). Eugenics Archives. Brief instructions for charting, circa 1921. Available at www.eugenicsarchive.org/html/eugenics/index2.html?tag=922. Accessed February 15, 2009.

Cowan RS. (2008). *Heredity and Hope: The Case for Genetic Screening*. Cambridge: Harvard University Press.

Davenport CB, Laughlin HH. (1915). *How to make a eugenical family study. Bulletin 13*. Cold Spring Harbor, NY: Eugenics Records Office.

Frankel MS, Teich A. (1993). *Ethical and Legal Issues in Pedigree Research*. Washington, DC: American Association for the Advancement of Science.

Gowen LC, Johnson BL, Latour AM, et al. (1996). Brca1 deficiency results in early embryonic lethality characterized by neuroepithelial abnormalities. *Nat Genet* 12 (2):191–194.

International Committee of Medical Journal Editors. (1995). Protection of patient's rights to privacy. *BMJ* 311:1272.

Laughlin HH. (1914). Report of the committee to study and to report on the best practical means of cutting off the defective germ-plasm in the American Population. Bulletins 10A and 10B. Cold Springs Harbor, NY: Eugenics Record Office.

Lorente C, Cordier S, Goujard J, et al. (2000). Tobacco and alcohol use during pregnancy and risk of oral clefts. Occupational exposure and Congenital Malformation Working Group. *Am J Pub Health* 90 (3):415–419.

Mazumdar PMH. (1992). *Eugenics, Human Genetics and Human Failings*. London: Routledge.

NCICB, National Cancer Institute Center for Bioinformatics. (2009). My Family Health Portrait, a Tool from the Surgeon General. January 13, 2009. Available at https://familyhistory.hhs.gov/fhh-web/home.action. Accessed February 7, 2009.

National Cancer Institute. (2008). Prevention and cessation of cigarette smoking: control of tobacco use. February 22, 2008. Available at www.cancer.gov/cancertopics/pdq/prevention/control-of-tobacco-use/Patient/page2. Accessed February 7, 2009.

Office for Protection from Research Risks. (1993). *Protecting Human Research Subjects: Institutional Review Board Guidebook*. U.S. Government Printing Office, Washington, DC. 5–42—5–56.

Pridham K. (1993). Anticipatory guidance of parents of new infants: Potential contributions of the internal working model construct. *J Nurs Scholarsh* 25(1):49–56.

Resta RG. (1993). The crane's foot: The rise of the pedigree in human genetics. *J Genet Couns* 2:235–260.

Resta RG. (1995). Whispered hints. *Am J Med Genet* 59:131–133.

Wexler NS, Young AB, Tanz RE, et al. (1987). Homozygotes for Huntington's disease. *Nature* 326:194–197.

Glossary

acanthocytosis The presence in the blood of distorted red cells with a "thorny" appearance.

age of onset Age at which the effects of a genetic disorder become evident.

allele Alternative forms of the gene occupying a specific site on a chromosome.

allelic heterogeneity Multiple gene mutation in the same locus that are each capable of producing an aberrant phenotype.

amino acids The major building blocks of polypeptides: Each of the 20 amino acids is encoded by one or more mRNA codons.

amniocentesis Removal, through a needle inserted through the abdomen and uterus, of a small amount of the amniotic fluid, which is analyzed for fetal testing.

amniotic bands Strands of tissue, thought to be from the rupture of the amnion (the sac around the fetus), leading to disruption of fetal development resulting in asymmetric congenital abnormalities (such as amputated digits, facial clefting).

anal atresia (imperforate anus) Congenital absence of an anal opening.

anencephaly Failure of the anterior neural tube to close, leading to complete or partial absence of the cranial vault (forebrain, overlying meninges, skull, and skin); a neural tube defect.

aneuploidy Cells that contain a variant number of the normal diploid number of 46 chromosomes (either extra or missing chromosomes). Tripoloidy with 69 chromosomes is polyploidy.

aniridia Absence of the iris of the eye.

The Practical Guide to the Genetic Family History, Second Edition, by Robin L. Bennett
Copyright © 2010 John Wiley & Sons, Inc.

anophthalmos   Congenital absence of the iris of the eye.

anosmia   Absence of smell.

anotia   Congenital absence of the pinna (external ears).

anticipation   The observation in a pedigree of a disease occurring at earlier ages or with increased severity in successive generations. In many instances, this is attributed to unstable trinucleotide repeats.

arachnodactyly   Long thin fingers and toes.

artificial insemination   See THERAPEUTIC INSEMINATION.

arthrogryposis   Congenital joint contractures.

Ashkenazi   A Jew whose ancestors were from central and eastern Europe.

assortative mating   A term used by geneticists to explain that humans do not choose their mating partners randomly.

asymptomatic carrier   A person who carries a gene alteration but will not develop the disease.

ataxia   Poor coordination of movement with a wide-based unsteady gait; often associated with poor coordination of the limbs and slurred speech.

atresia   Congenital absence or closure of a normal body orifice or tubular organ (e.g., anal atresia, esophageal atresia).

autosome   Describes the 22 pairs of chromosomes excluding the sex chromosomes (X and Y).

autoimmune disease   A disease characterized by the action of the body's own immune system against itself.

autozygous   Not only homozygous but both gene copies are identical by descent (i.e., can be traced to the same ancestral gene copy).

azoospermia   The absence of sperm in the seminal fluid; may be due to a blockage or an impairment of sperm production.

benign   A condition tumor or growth that is not cancerous; it does not spread (metastasize) to other parts of the body or invade surrounding tissue.

bialellic   Pertaining to both alleles (both alternative forms of a gene).

bifid uvula   A cleft in the uvular; a minor manifestation of cleft palate. The *uvula* is the small, conical, fleshy mass of tissue suspended from the center of the soft palate above the back of the tongue.

blepharphimosis   Narrowing of the horizontal apertures of the eyelids.

brachydactyly   Abnormal shortness of the fingers and/or toes.

brachial cysts or fistulas   Vestiges of the embryonic branchial grooves. Found in the lower third of the neck and may be bilateral. They are associated with hearing loss, specifically with the branchio-oto-renal (BOR) syndrome.

brushfield spots   Speckled, mottled, or marbled rings about two thirds of the distance to the periphery of the iris.

café au lait spots   Area of brown skin pigmentation with irregular borders.

canthus   Inner or outer edge of the eye (as in inner canthus or outer canthus).

carrier An individual who has one copy of a disease causing gene but who does not express the disease. An *asymptomatic carrier* is some one is not expected to develop the disease (e.g., the parents of a child with Tay-Sachs; an autosomal recessive condition). A *presympomtatic carrier* is someone who is expected to develop the disease sometime in his or her lifetime (e.g., Huntington disease).

centromere A constriction seen in each chromosome.

chorionic villus sampling (CVS) A technique for obtaining tissue from the developing placenta (the chorionic villi) for the purpose of prenatal testing; usually performed at 10 to12 weeks of pregnancy.

choroid The dark brown vascular coat of the eye between the sclera (white of the eye) and the retina (the light-sensitive membrane of the inner eyeball).

chromosomes Thread-like structures in the nucleus of the cell that are composed of DNA. Human have 23 pairs of chromosomes, with one of each pair inherited from the mother and one from the father. The egg and sperm have one of each chromosome.

clinical heterogeneity The existence of clinically different phenotypes from mutations of the same gene.

clinodactyly An incurving finger.

compound heterozygote The presence of two different mutant alleles at a particular gene locus, one on each chromosome.

coarctation of the aorta Narrowing of either a short or long segments of the aorta.

codominance The expression of both alleles in a heterozygous individual.

codon A group of three mRNA bases, each of which specifies an amino acid when translated.

coloboma A fissure (cleft or groove), especially of the eye (may involve the iris, retina, lid, etc.), which can be congenital or traumatic in origin. An *iris coloboma* has a keyhole appearance.

comparative genomic hybridization (CGH) A molecular–cytogenetic method for analysis of copy number changes (gains and losses) in the DNA.

conductive hearing loss Hearing loss caused by a physical problem of the external and/or middle ear.

congenital A characteristic that is present at birth (not necessarily inherited).

consanguinity In medical genetics, used to refer to any union between biological relatives (e.g., first cousins). The term *incest* is usually reserved for sexual unions between couples who are related as first-degree relatives (e.g., father–daughter, brother–sister).

consultand The individual seeking genetic services. The consultand may or may not be affected.

contiguous gene syndrome A disease associated with a microscopic deletion or duplication involving several consecutive genes located on a chromosome arm. See MICRODELETION SYNDROME.

craniosynostosis A mis-shaped head due to premature fusion of the cranial bones.

cubitis valgus   Increased carrying angle at the elbow.

cystic hygroma(s)   Congenital cyst(s) of the lymphatic system most commonly found within the soft tissues of the neck.

deformation   An abnormal shape or position of a part of the body caused by in utero mechanical forces.

deletion   A missing sequence of DNA or part of a chromosome.

dementia   A general description for mental deterioration, loss of mental capacity.

diaphragmatic hernia   Some portion of the abdominal contents protrude through the diaphragm into the chest cavity.

digenic   Inheritance of genes at two different chromosome locations.

diploid   Cells possessing pairs of chromosomes (two of each type).

dizygotic twins   Nonidentical (fraternal) twins; twins produced by two fertilized eggs (fertilized separately).

disruption   The result of interference with an originally normal development process, resulting in a birth defect.

double-outlet right ventricle   Classification of a group of congenital heart defects in which both great arteries arise from the morphological right ventricle.

DSM-IV   Abbreviation for *Diagnostic and Statistical Manual of Mental Disorders*, 4th edition, a book containing diagnostic criteria for mental disorders.

duplication   A repeat of a gene or DNA sequence; presence of an extra piece piece of a chromosome.

duodenal atresia   The absence, blocking, or narrowing of a portion of the duodenum (small bowel).

dynamic mutation   A gene mutation that is unstable when transmitted from parent to child. The term is usually used in reference to trinucleotide repeat disorders.

dysarthria   Slurred speech.

dysostosis multiplex   Defective ossification leading to a pattern of skeletal abnormalities, including a large skull with deep, elongated, J-shaped sella, oar-like ribs, deformed hook-shaped lower thoracic and upper lumbar vertebrae, pelvic dysplasia, shortened tubular bones with expanded diaphyses, and dysplastic epiphyses. A common characteristic of the mucopolysaccharide storage diseases.

dysplastic   Abnormal development or growth of tissues, organs, or cells.

dystonia   Disordered muscle tone or tension; a neurological movement disorder in which sustained muscle contractions cause twisting and repetitive movements or abnormal postures.

dystopia canthorum   Short palpebral fissures with displacement of inner canthi, giving the impression of hypertelorism.

Ebstein anomaly   Displacement of the septal and posterior leaflets of the tricuspid valve toward the apex of the right ventricle.

ectopia cordis   The heart is totally (or partially) outside of the chest.

ectopia lentis   Dislocate lens(es) of the eye(s).

ectopic pregnancy   An embryo that grows outside of the uterus, usually in a fallopian tube.

empirical risk   The probability that a trait will recur based on its observed incidence in a particular population.

encephalocele   A type of neural tube defect in which the brain tissue protrudes through a defect in the skull.

encephalopathy   A degenerative disease of the brain.

endocardial cushion defect   Term used to describe a spectrum of heart defects involving an atrial-septal defect (ASD) associated with ventricular septal defects (VSD) and abnormalties of the atrioventricular (AV) valves.

epicanthal folds   Congenital vertical fold of skin medial to the eye and lateral to the nose, sometimes covering the inner canthus.

epicanthus inversus   Skinfold arising from the lower eyelid and running inward and downward.

esophageal atresia   A blind-ending esophageal pouch often associated with a tracheoesophageal fistula (TEF).

ethnicity   A group whose member's identify with each other on the basis of presumed common geneaology or ancestry.

ethnic identity   A group's distinctive common cultural, linguistic, religious, and biological traits.

etiology   Cause of a disease.

expressivity   The degree to which a heritable trait is expressed in an individual; the clinical severity of the trait(s).

exencephaly   A problem with closure of the neural tube, leading to the brain lying outside of the skull.

exon   Portion of genes that encode amino acids that are retained after the primary mRNA transcript is spliced.

F1   The first generation of a pedigree (a pedigree is numbered by each subsequent generation forward: F1 (great-grandparents), F2 (grandparents), F3 (parents), F4 (children).

familial   The occurrence of a trait in more than one family member at a greater frequency than expected by chance alone; not synonymous with *hereditary*.

fibroid   Noncancerous tumor composed mainly of fibrous or fully developed connective tissue.

first-degree relatives   An individual's children, full brothers, full sisters, and parents.

founder effect   An inherited disorder that spreads when a small group of people found a new population. The genetic background of the small group of persons in the founding group may contain common gene mutations. The disease may occur at high frequency in this population.

gamete An egg or sperm.

gastroschisis The intestine is entirely ouside of the body through a defect in the umbilical wall.

gene The basic unit of hereditry; a specific portion of the DNA sequence.

genome The entire sequence of an organism's DNA; includes all the DNA found within the chromosomes and the mitochondria.

genomic medicine The functions and interactions of all the genes in the genome.

genotype The genetic constitution of an individual as applied to a single locus or all the loci collectively.

germline The line of germ cells that have genetic material that may be passed to offspring.

gestational carrier (surrogate) A woman who carries a fetus for a couple in her uterus with the intention of legally giving up the child to the couple at birth. She may also provide the oocytes.

gonadal agenesis Absent or rudimentary testis/testes, or ovary/ovaries.

gonads Sites of sperm and egg production (testes and ovaries, respectively).

gynecomastia Excessive development of breast tissue in a male.

hamartoma A benign tumor-like nodule composed of an overgrowth of mature cells and tissues that normally occur in the affected body part or organ.

hematuria Blood in the urine.

hemizygous Possessing only one of a pair of genes that influence the determination of a particular trait. A *hemizygote* is a person who is hemizygous for a particular gene.

hereditary Traits under genetic control that may be transmitted to the next generation.

hepatosplenomegaly Enlarged liver and spleen.

heterochromia Different colored irises (i.e., one brown eye and one blue eye).

heterogeneity The occurrence of the same or similar phenotypes from different genetic mechanisms.

heterozygote (heterozygous) An individual (or genotype) with two different alleles at a given locus.

hirsute Excessive body hair.

historian The person providing medical-family history information to the clinician.

holoprosencephaly A term used to describe the spectrum of anomlies resulting in abnormal cleavage of the embryonic forebrain and midline facial anomalies. Three subtypes are seen: alobar, lobar, and semilobar.

homozygote (homozygous) An individual (or genotype) with identical alleles at a given locus.

Hutterites Isolated German-speaking people originating from a European Anabaptist group in the 1530s.

hydrocephalus Abnormal accumulation of cerebrospinal fluid with the cranial vault, resulting in an englarged head, prominent forehead, and usually mental deterioriation and seizure.

hypertelorism An increased distance between two organ or parts, commonly used to refer to ocular hypertelorism (increased interpupillary distance).

hypotonia/hypotonic Low muscle tone (floppy).

idiopathic Of spontaneous origin.

imprinting The process by which genetic material is expressed differently when inherited from the father than when inherited from the mother.

inborn error of metabolism An inherited biochemical disorder resulting from a malfunctioning or absent enzyme in a metabolic pathway.

incidence An expression of the rate or frequency at which a certain event (or disease) occurs such as the number of persons diagnosed with a disease per year.

index case The first affected person to be studied in the family.

individual's line The vertical line in a pedigree extending up from an individual's symbol to connect to a sibship line. If an individual has no siblings, the individual's line connects directly to the horizontal relationship line. In this case the vertical line of descent and the individual's line are the same. Multiple births have a single individual's line that forks for each individual.

iniencephaly Extremely short cervical spine with missing vertebrae and extension of the fetal head in association with neural tube defects (e.g., anencephaly).

intracytoplasmic sperm injection (ICSI) A procedure of therapeutic insemination by which a single sperm is directly inserted into an individual egg.

intron The noncoding DNA sequence found between two exons. Introns are transcribed into primary mRNA but spliced out in the formation of the mature mRNA transcript.

Inuit (pl. Inuits) A member of a group of indigenous people of Northern North America inhabiting areas of Greenland, Eastern Canada, and Alaska (formerly called Eskimo).

in utero Within the uterus.

inversion A chromosome alteration in which a segment has been reversed because of breakage, 180° rotation, and reunion. A *DNA inversion* is when a section of DNA is reversed (this may involve only a few base pairs).

ischemia Deficiency of blood supply to a part of the body due to obstruction or constriction of a blood vessel.

karyotype The standardized arrangement (chart) of chromosome pairs in a single cell by number.

key Used in medical pedigrees to define unusual symbols and shading to assist interpretation. Sometimes referred to as a *legend*.

kindred A family grouping.

leiomyoma   A benign tumor of smooth muscle usually found in the uterus (fibroid), skin, or digestive tract.

legend   See KEY.

line of descent   The vertical line on a pedigree connecting the horizontal relationship line to the horizontal sibship line. If an individual does not have siblings the line of descent and the individual's line is the same.

lipoma   Fatty, benign tumor.

locus   (plural, loci) The chromosomal location of a specific gene.

Lyonization   See X-INACTIVATION.

macrocephaly   Unusually large head circumference (greater than the 98th percentile).

macule   A flat, disclored spot on the skin.

malformation   Defects in an organ, or part of an organ, resulting from an intrinsically abnormal development process.

meconium   The dark green intestinal waste in a full-term fetus. Presence of meconium in the amniotic fluid is a sign of fetal distress.

Mendelian inheritance   The transmission of single-gene traits or disorders following the rules described by Gregor Mendel.

meningomyelocele   A common neural tube defect involving protrusion of the cord and its meninges through a defect in the vertebral canal.

metachronous   Occurring at different times. Used in reference to primary cancers that are diagnosed at separate intervals.

metastasis   The spread of malignant cells from one site in the body to another (the verb is *metastasize*).

methylation   The attachment of methyl group ($-CH_3$) to cytosine in DNA. Hypermethylation of cytosine within or near a coding sequence is associated with reduction in gene a activity. Genes that are permanently active in all cells lack methyl groups.

microcephaly   Unusually small head circumference (less than 2 standard deviations below the mean).

microdeletion syndrome   A chromosome deletion that is too small to be visible under a microscope.

micrognathia   Small, recessed jaw or chin.

microphthalmos   Abnormally small eyes.

microtia   Small, underdeveloped ear with a blind or absent external auditory canal.

misattributed paternity   The presumed father is not the biological father.

mitochondria   Small, spherical to rod-shaped organelles found in the cytoplasm (outside the nucleus) of cells. They are a major source of energy for the cell.

monoalellic   Involving a single allele.

monosomy   Missing one of a chromosome pair or partial chromosome pair in a normally diploid cell.

monozygotic twins   Identical twins who originated from a single fertilized egg.

mosaic   The existence of two or more genetically distinct cell lines in an individual.

multifactorial   The interaction of many genes and the environment.

mutation   A change in DNA sequence.

myoclonus   Shock-like contractions of a muscle or muscle group; abrupt jerking movements of muscle groups and/or entire limbs.

myopathy   Any disease of a muscle (e.g., cardiac myopathy).

myopia   Commonly referred to as nearsightedness.

neonate   A newborn infant.

neural tube   An embryonic structure that develops into the brain and spinal cord.

neuropathy   A general term referring to functional or pathological changes in the peripheral nervous system.

nevi   Moles.

nitrogenous bases   Components of nucleic acids consisting of purines (adenine and guanine) and pyrimidines (cytosine, thymine, and uracil).

nondisjunction   Failure of chromosomes to separate properly in the process of mitosis or meiosis, resulting in cells or gametes with too few, or too many chromosomes.

nonpaternity   The biological father is not as stated.

nucleus   The structure within the cell that contains the chromosomes.

nystagmus   Involuntary rapid movement of the eyeball (may be horizontal, vertical, mixed, or rotary).

obligate carrier   A person who carries a gene or chromosome alteration (known by pedigree analysis or genetic testing) who will not clinically manifest the disease.

oligohydramnios   Decreased amniotic fluid. *Anhydramnios* is absence of amniotic fluid.

oligozoospermia (oligospermia)   An abnormally low number of sperm in a specimen.

omphalocele   Protrusion of the intestines and/or other abdominal organs through a defect in the abdominal wall into a transparent sac.

p arm   In cytogenetics, refers to the short arm of the chromosome (from the French *petit*).

palpebral fissure   Eye opening.

paracentric inversion   A segment of a chromosome that is inverted but does not include the centromere (the site where the chromosome constricts).

parganglioma   Tumors that arise within the sympathetic nervous system, originating anywhere from the neck to the pelvis in locations paralleling the sympathetic ganglion chain. Tumors of both adrenal and extra-adrenal origin are often active secretors of catecholamines and can cause symptoms such as labile hypertension, palpitations, headache, and sweating. Most are benign, approximately 10% of paragangliomas metastasize.

pectus excavatum Depression of the breastbone (sternum). Sometimes referred to as a "funnel chest."

pedigree A diagram representing family relationships, medical histories, and health status.

penetrance The likelihood that a genetic condition is actually expressed in a population; usually phrased as a percentage of expression at a certain age or time (e.g., 60% penetrant at birth, 100% penetrant by age 40 years). A trait can be fully penetrant but vary its level of expression or degree of severity.

pericentric inversion A segment of the chromosome that is inverted and includes the centromere (the site where the chromosome constricts).

periungual fibromas Small wart-like tumors that develop around and under the finger and toenails; diagnostic of tuberous sclerosis.

phakomatoses A collection of disorders predisposing to hamartomas and other tumors involving the skin and/or eyes, nervous system, and one or more body tystems. Derived from the Greek work *phakos* for "mother spot" or "birthmark."

pheochromocytoma Endocrine secreting tumor (produces norepinephrine and epinephrine).

philtrum Vertical groove in the midline of the upper lip, extending from beneath the nose to the top of the upper lip.

phyllodes tumor (cystosarcoma phyllodes) A nonepithelial breast tumor that may be benign or malignant.

pokiloderma The constellation of hyperpigmentation and hypopigmentation, atrophy, and telangiectasia

polydactyly Extra fingers or toes. *Postaxial polydactyly* means the extra finger is lateral to the fifth finger. *Preaxial polydactyly* means the extra digit is medial to the thumb.

polygenic A trait caused by the combined effects of multiple genes.

polyhydramnios Increased amount of amniotic fluid.

premutation An unstable allele that can expand in size to a full mutation in the next generation.

prenatal diagnosis Testing to identify a disease or anomaly in a fetus or embryo.

prevalence The total number of cases of a disease in existence at a certain time in a designated area (e.g., the prevalence of *x* disease at birth among Caucasians in North America is 1/10,000).

proband The first affected family member coming to medical attention independent of other family members.

prognathia A protruding jaw.

ptosis Drooping of the upper eyelid.

q arm In cytogenetics, refers to the long arm of the chromosome.

relationship line The horizontal line on a pedigree joining mating partners. A break in this lines indicates a divorce or separation in the union.

renal agenesis Absence of the kidney(s).

retina A multilayer light-sensitive membrane lining the inner eyeball that sends visual signals to the brain through the optic nerve.

ribosomes Small particles in the cell cytoplasm serving as the sites of protein synthesis; they attach to the messenger RNA.

sarcoma From the Greek word for "fleshy growth," malignant tumors that originate in the soft tissues of the body (muscle, fat, blood vessels, nerves, tendons, and synovial tissues (lining of the joints).

sclerae Whites of the eyes.

scoliosis Curvature of the spine; a lateral (sideways) deviation of the normally straight line of the spine.

SCTAT (sex cord tumor of the ovaries with annular tubules) Benign neoplasms associated with Peutz-Jeghers syndrome.

second-degree relative An individual's aunts, uncles, grandparents, nieces, and nephews, grandchildren, and half-siblings.

sex chromosomes The X and Y chromosomes.

sex-influenced gene expression A gene whose expression is modified by the gender of the individual possessing the gene alteration (e.g., breast cancer).

sex-limited gene expression A trait that is expressed only in one sex or the other (e.g., ovarian cancer, prostate cancer).

sex-linked A gene that is located on the X or Y chromosome.

sib A brother or sister.

sibling A person's brother or sister. Full siblings share the same mother and father.

sibship line The horizontal line used in a medical pedigree to connect individuals related as brothers and sisters (both full and half-siblings). Each sibling is connected to the sibship line by a vertical *individual's line*. A vertical *line of descent* connects directly from the symbol for a parent (or from the horizontal *relationship line* between parents) to the sibship line.

simian crease A single palmar crease. (Typically individuals have a transverse double horizontal crease across each palm.)

spasticity Increased muscle tone.

spina bifida An early embryonic defect resulting in an opening anywhere along the spinal column.

spontaneous pneumothorax An accumulation of gas or air in the chest cavity that may lead to a collapsed lung.

sporadic The occurrence of a disease in a family with no apparent genetic transmission pattern.

surrogate See GESTATIONAL CARRIER.

synchronous   Occurring at the same time. Used in reference to cancers that are diagnosed at the same time (such as two areas of colon cancer or breast cancer).

syndactyly   Webbing or fusion of the fingers and/or toes.

syndrome   A collection of characteristics that are recognized as a distinct clinical diagnosis.

synophrys   Eyebrows (often bushy) that meets at the midline.

telangiectasia   "Spiderweb" blood vesssels usually found on the skin and whites of the eyes.

teratogen   An environmental agent capable of causing malformations of the embryo.

tetralogy of Fallot (TOF)   The combination of a ventricular septal defect (VSD) with pulmonary stenosis at the infundibular level (with or without associated valve stenosis) and right ventricular hypertrophy, with an aorta that overrides the ventricular septal defect.

therapeutic insemination (TI)   A means of conceiving a pregnancy whereby that semen is obtained from the male and placed into a woman's reproductive tract. The term is preferred over the commonly used *artificial insemination*.

third-degree relative   An individual's first cousins, great-grandparents, half-aunts, and half-uncles, great-grandchildren, and great-aunts and great-uncles.

tracheoesophageal fistula (TEF)   An abnormal passageway between the trachea and the esophagus.

translocation   A chromosome rearrangement between two chromosomes.

transposition of the great vessels.   The aorta arises entirely from the right ventricle and the pulmonary artery from the left ventricle, resulting in complete separation of the circulation.

trinucleotide repeat   A repeated sequence of three bases (e.g., CAG, CCG) that is expanded and unstable in some genetic disorders (triplet repeat disorders).

trisomy   An extra copy of all or part of a chromosome normally present in a diploid state.

uniparental disomy   Both copies of a chromosome pair are inherited from the same parent instead of inheriting one copy of each chromosome pair from the mother and the father.

URL   The address of a site on the Internet.

variable expression   A trait in which the same genotype may produce phenotypes with different manifestations and severity.

velopharyngeal insufficiency   Referring to the incompetence of the soft palate indicative of a submucosal cleft. Often evidenced by nasal speech tone.

ventricular septal defect   Absence of part or all of the wall (septum) between the ventricles (lower chambers of the heart).

xanthoma   A yellow colored nodule, papule, or plaque in the skin due to lipid deposits.

X-inactivation   A random process occurring soon after fertilization in which one of the X-chromosomes becomes inactivated so that a single X-chromosome remains active in each cell.

X-linked   Genes that are located on the X chromosome.

Y-linked   Genes that are located on the Y chromosome.

Yup'ik (pl. Yupiit)   People with ancestry of Western and Southwestern Alaska, believed to have their origin in Eastern Siberia.

Appendix A.1

Handy Reference Tables of Pedigree Nomenclature

Some of the figures were previously published in RL/Steinhaus KA, Uhrich SB, Bennett et al. (1995). Recommendations for human standardized pedigree nomenclature. Am J Hum Gen 56:745–752. Republished with permission of the University of Chicago Press.

STANDARDIZED SYMBOLS AND NOMENCLATURE FOR HUMAN PEDIGREES
(Adapted from Bennett RL et. al., Am J Hum Genet, 56:7445, 1995)

Information to include in a pedigree

- Age/birth date, or year of birth
- Age at death (year if known)
- Cause of death
- Full sibs versus half sibs
- Relevant health information (e.g., height, weight)
- Age at diagnosis
- Affected/unaffected status (define shading of symbol in key/legend)
- Personally evaluated or medically documented (*)
- Testing status ("E" is used for evaluation on pedigree and defined in key/legend)
- Pregnancies with gestational age noted LMP or EDD - estimated date of delivery
- Pregnancy complications with gestational age noted (e.g., 6 wk, 34 wk), miscarriage (SAB), stillbirth (SB), pregnancy termination (TOP), ectopic (ECT)
- Infertility vs. no children by choice
- Ethnic background of each grandparent
- Use a "?" if family history is unknown
- Consanguinity (note degree of relationship if not implicit in pedigree
- Family names (if appropriate)
- Date pedigree taken
- Name of person who took pedigree and credentials (MD, RN, MSW, CGC)
- Key/legend

Pedigree Symbols

	Male	Female	Sex Unkown
Individual (assign gender by phenotype)	□ b. 1925	○ 30	◇ 4 mo
Clinically affected individual (define shading in key/legend)	■	●	◆
Affected individual (> one condition)	■	●	◆
Multiple individuals, number known	5	5	5
Multiple individuals, number unknown	n	n	n
Deceased individual	⊘ d. 35 y	⊘ d. 4 mo	⊘
Stillbirth (SB)	⊘ SB 28 wk	⊘ SB 30 wk	⊘ SB 34 wk
Pregnancy (P)	P LMP: 7/1/94	P 20 wk	P 16 wk
Spontaneous abortion (SAB), ectopic (ECT)	△ male	△ female	△ ECT
Affected SAB	▲ male	▲ female	▲ 16 wk
Termination of pregnancy (TOP)	△ male	△ female	△ 12 wk
Affected TOP	▲ male	▲ female	▲ 12 wk
Consultand	□ b. 4/24/59	○ 35y	
Proband	P■	P●	

STANDARDIZED SYMBOLS AND NOMENCLATURE FOR HUMAN PEDIGREES
(Adapted from Bennett RL et al., Am J Hum Genet, 56:7445, 1995)

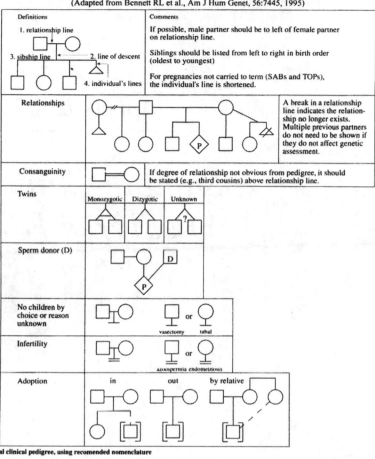

Hypothetical clinical pedigree, using recomended nomenclature

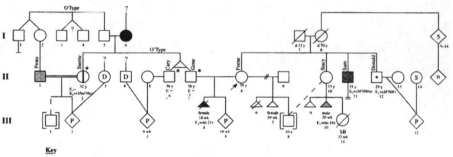

Key

- ▲ = Down Syndrome
- △ = Neural tube defect
- ▨ = Cystic fibrosis
- ▨ = Red/green color blindness
- ● = Huntington disease (affected)
- ▯ = Huntington disease (presymptomatic)
- ⊡ = Cystic fibrosis asymptomatic carrier

E_1 = Karyotype
E_2 = Cystic fibrosis mutation study
E_3 = Neurologicalexam
E_4 = Huntington disease mutation study
* = Examined personally
S = Surrogate mother
D = Gamete donor

Consultand: Feene O'Type
Taken by: Gregor Mendel
Historians: Gene and Feene O'Type
Date of intake: April 1, 1998

Appendix A.2

Sample Clinical Pedigree Form

The Practical Guide to the Genetic Family History, Second Edition, by Robin L. Bennett
Copyright © 2010 John Wiley & Sons, Inc.

FAMILY PEDIGREE

Record #: _____   Medical Center Location: _____

Consultand: _____   Historian: _____   Recorder: _____   Date: _____

Diagnosis: _____

Ancestry: _____   Consanguinity? _____   KEY: ☐ -

☐ -

Sample Genetic Screening Form for Familial Cancer Risk Assessment

This form can be completed by healthy individuals or persons with cancer to assist the healthcare provider in identifying individuals who might be at an increased risk of developing cancer or another primary tumor. For those individuals with a possible contributory history (see Tables 5.1 and 5.2), a personal interview and the recording of a pedigree can be used to explore the family history further.

The Practical Guide to the Genetic Family History, Second Edition, by Robin L. Bennett
Copyright © 2010 John Wiley & Sons, Inc.

Familial Cancer Risk Assessment Form

Date _____

Patient # _____

Name _____ Birthdate _____ Phone _____

Street Address _____ City _____ State _____ ZIP _____

Your answers to the following questions will help us evaluate your chances of developing cancer. We are interested in any cancer in a blood relative (for example, breast, colon, lung, uterine, pancreatic, prostate, ovarian, kidney, skin, leukemia, lymphoma, etc). Be as specific as possible.

A **maternal relative** is on your mother's side of the family. A **paternal relative** is on your father's side of the family.

Have your or any of the following blood relatives ever had cancer?

Relative	*Living?*	*Type(s) of cancer*	*Age when cancer(s) found*
Yourself		_____	_____
Mother	yes no	_____	_____
Maternal grandmother	yes no	_____	_____
Maternal grandfather	yes no	_____	_____
Father	yes no	_____	_____
Paternal grandmother	yes no	_____	_____
Paternal grandfather	yes no	_____	_____

How many blood-related **sisters** do you have? _____
How many of them have ever had cancer? _____
For each blood-related sister who had cancer, list the type(s), and her age when the Cancer was found. For a half sister, write *M* for maternal or *P* for paternal.

Sister	*Half?*	*Living?*	*Type(s) of cancer*	*Age when cancer(s) found*
1	_____	yes no	_____	_____
2	_____	yes no	_____	_____
3	_____	yes no	_____	_____
4	_____	yes no	_____	_____

How many blood-related **brothers** do you have? _____
How many of them have ever had cancer? _____
For each blood-related brother who had cancer, list the type(s), and his age when the cancer was found. For a half brother, write *M* for maternal or *P* for paternal.

Brother	*Half?*	*Living?*	*Type(s) of cancer*	*Age when cancer found*
1	_____	yes no	_____	_____
2	_____	yes no	_____	_____
3	_____	yes no	_____	_____
4	_____	yes no	_____	_____

Turn Page Over and Continue

Name _____ ID#_____ Page 2

How many blood-related **children** do you have? _____

How many of them ever had cancer? _____

For each of your blood-related children who had cancer, list the type(s), and how old he or she was when the cancer was found.

Child	Living?	Type(s) of cancer	Age when cancer found
1	yes no	_____	_____
2	yes no	_____	_____
3	yes no	_____	_____

Do you have any **other blood relatives** who have had cancer?   Yes   No

For each of your blood relatives who have had cancer, list how he or she is related to you (your maternal aunt, paternal uncle, maternal first cousin, etc.), the type(s) of cancer, and how old he or she was when the cancer was found.

Relation	Living?	Type(s) of cancer	Age when cancer found
_____	yes no	_____	_____
_____	yes no	_____	_____
_____	yes no	_____	_____

Have ANY of your relatives had breast cancer in both breasts?   Yes   No

If yes, which relative(s)? _____

Have **you** had a colonoscopy?   Yes   No   If yes, at what age(s) _____

Have you ever had colon polyps?   Yes   No   If yes, how many _____

Have any of your relatives had polyps in the colon or rectum?   Yes   No

If yes, which relative(s)? _____

To what country or countries do you trace your ancestors (for example, France, Germany, China, Japan, Mexico, Africa, Philippines.)?

Your Mother's Father _____Your Mother's Mother _____

Your Father's Father _____ Your Father's Mother _____

If you family of eastern European/Jewish ancestry?   Yes   No   Don't know

Would you be interested in meeting with a genetic counselor regarding your family history of cancer?   Yes   No   Maybe

Have you, or anyone else in your family had genetic testing? If yes, explain _____

_____

Do you have any other concerns? _____

Appendix A.4

Sample Adoption Medical-Family History Form

MODEL MEDICAL GENETIC HISTORY FORM FOR ADOPTIONS

This model medical genetic family history form is intended for use in adoptions. It is assumed that each user of this model form will modify it to comply with local or state regulations.

In documenting medical genetic histories, it is optimal if *each* birth parents is assisted in completing the questionnaire by a trained adoption professional who appreciates the importance of collecting this information and has an awareness of the medical and genetic conditions included in the form.

The form consists of the following segments:

- A **cover page** containing identifying information about the birth parents, child welfare agency, and an agency file identification code. This page is filed with the agency designated in each state to retain such identifying information. The cover page is not intended to be shared with the birth parents, unless they agree to waive their rights to confidentiality.

- A one-page **pregnancy care information sheet** to be completed by the birth mother.

- A one-page **delivery, birth and medical information sheet** to be completed by the birth mother or the adoption professional.

- An eight page **medical genetic family history questionnaire**. One copy of this form should be completed by *each* birth parent.

The Practical Guide to the Genetic Family History, Second Edition, by Robin L. Bennett
Copyright © 2010 John Wiley & Sons, Inc.

Todays date: _____

COVER PAGE: Medical-Genetic Family History Questionnaire

You are being asked to provide family history information at a time that we know is difficult for you; however, this information may be important at some point in providing medical care for your child. There are many medical conditions that can run in families. We are trying to obtain a complete medical history because your child may need this information in the future. Please answer the questions as best as you can. If you have any questions about how to answer anything, please ask your adoption worker for help. Each birth parent should complete a Medical-Genetic Family History Form.

This page contains information that is needed for the child's records. It will be shared with the child or the adoptive parents *only* if you sign a special sheet giving your permission to release this information for their use.

Child's Name: _____
                   Last   First   Middle

Date of Birth: _____

Birthplace: Please Circle: Hospital   Home   Other _____

Provide name and address of birth location as well as the name of the doctor or health provider who delivered the baby:

_____

_____

Birth Mother's Name: _____
                          Last   First   Middle

Date of Birth: _____

Current Permanent Mailing Address:

_____

Birth Father's Name: _____
                         Last   First   Middle

Date of Birth: _____

Current Permanent Mailing Address:

_____

Case Identification Number: _____

Name and Address of Agency involved in the Adoption: _____

_____

PREGNANCY CARE WITH THIS CHILD   Agency #_____   Today's date _____   **p. 1 of 1**

In what month of your pregnancy did you first see a health care worker? ___ 1 mo ___ 2 mos
___ 3 mos ___ 4 mos ___ 5 mos ___6 mos ___ 7 mos ___ 8 mos ___ 9 mos ___ no prenatal care

Did you have, or were you exposed to, any of the following in pregnancy?

	Yes	No	Don't Know	What Months In Pregnancy?	If Yes, Please Explain
Fever (101 degrees or over)	—	—	—	_____	_____
Rashes	—	—	—	_____	_____
Infection	—	—	—	_____	_____
X-rays/radiation	—	—	—	_____	_____
Chemicals	—	—	—	_____	_____
Toxic/hazardous wastes	—	—	—	_____	_____
Sexually transmitted diseases	—	—	—	_____	_____
HIV/AIDS	—	—	—	_____	_____
Diabetes	—	—	—	_____	_____
Measles (or rubella)	—	—	—	_____	_____
Mumps or chicken pox	—	—	—	_____	_____
High blood pressure	—	—	—	_____	_____
Toxemia	—	—	—	_____	_____

Did you take any of the following? If yes, when in pregnancy, and how much per week did you take?

	Yes	No	Don't Know	What Months In Pregnancy?	How Much Per Week?
Alcohol (include beer and wine)	—	—	—	_____	_____
Cigarettes	—	—	—	_____	_____
Cocaine/crack (circle)	—	—	—	_____	_____
Heroin/Methadone (circle)	—	—	—	_____	_____
LSD/acid	—	—	—	_____	_____
Marijuana/pot	—	—	—	_____	_____
Amphetamines (uppers)	—	—	—	_____	_____
Barbiturates (downers)	—	—	—	_____	_____
Others (specify)___	—	—	—	_____	_____

Did you take any of the following medications? If yes, name the medication, and explain when and how much was taken during the pregnancy.

	Yes	No	Don't Know	What Months In Pregnancy?	Name of Medication/ How Much Per Week?
Prescription medicines	—	—	—	_____	_____
	—	—	—	_____	_____
	—	—	—	_____	_____
Over the counter medications	—	—	—	_____	_____
	—	—	—	_____	_____
	—	—	—	_____	_____
Seizure medications	—	—	—	_____	_____
	—	—	—	_____	_____
	—	—	—	_____	_____
Other _____	—	—	—	_____	_____

Did you have any genetic tests in pregnancy? ___ Yes ___ No ___ Don't Know If Yes, please explain_____

DELIVERY AND BIRTH INFORMATION OF THE CHILD Agency #____ Date _____ p. 1 of 2

How many hours were you in labor? _____ *The delivery was:* _____ Vaginal _____ Cesarean

If cesarean, why? _____

Were there any problems during this delivery? ____ Yes ____ No ____ Don't Know
If Yes, please explain _____

The baby was born ____ Breech ____ Head first ____ Don't Know

Was there a heart murmur at birth? ____Yes ____ No ____ Don't Know
If Yes, specify the cardiac diagnosis_____

Were any other problems noted AT birth? ____ Yes ____ No ____ Don't Know
If Yes, please explain _____
_____

Were any other problems noted AFTER birth? ___ Yes ___ No ____ Don't Know
If Yes, please explain, and indicate the age of the child when the problem was noted _____
_____

A child whose parents are related by blood may have a higher chance of having health problems. For this reason, we need to know if there is any blood relationship between the birth parents. *If this child's parents are related by blood* please check off the relationship in the list below:

____ Father/daughter ____ Mother/son ____ Brother/sister ____ Half brother/sister
____ Uncle/niece ____ Aunt/nephew ____ Cousin ____ Other (please explain)

BIRTH AND MEDICAL INFORMATION FOR THIS CHILD

Sex of child: ____ Male ____ Female *Date of Birth:* _____ *Time of Birth:* _____

Hospital of birth: _____ *City:* _____ *State:* _____ *County:*_____

The baby was born: ____ At Term Premature at ____ weeks Postmature at ____weeks

Birth weight: _____ lbs. _____ oz. *Birth length:* _____ inches

APGAR score: _____ At one minute _____ At five minutes _____ Don't Know

Baby's blood type: __ A __ B __ AB __ O *Rh factor:* __ Positive __ Negative __ Don't Know

Were any of the following newborn screening tests positive?

	Yes	No	Don't Know
Cystic fibrosis	_____	_____	_____
Galactosemia	_____	_____	_____
Hypothyroidism	_____	_____	_____
PKU (phenylketonuria)	_____	_____	_____
Sickle cell disease	_____	_____	_____
Maple syrup urine disease	_____	_____	_____
Other (specify) _____	_____	_____	_____

Has the child had any genetic testing? ____ Yes ____ No ____Don't Know If Yes, please explain_____

Date: _____ Medical-Genetic Family Hx (circle): Birth Mother Birth Father Agency# _____ p. 1 of 8

Medical-Genetic Family History Questionnaire

Please supply the following information about yourself:

Your year of birth: _____ *Are you adopted?* ___Yes ___No ___Don't Know

Ethnic Background (circle all that apply): White Jewish African American Hispanic Origin Native American Asian Pacific Islander Other (Please list):
_____

Highest grade completed (circle): 1 2 3 4 5 6 7 8 9 10 11 12 13 14 15 16 17+

Were you ever in special classes to provide extra help in learning? ___ Yes ___No

Have you had any major illnesses? ___Yes ___No

If yes, please explain: _____

Do you have, or have you had, any mental illness? ___ Yes ___ No

If yes, please explain:_____

Have you ever been told that you have a genetic/inherited disease? ____ Yes ____No

If yes, please explain:_____

Have you ever been told that you are a carrier of a genetic/inherited disease? ___ Yes ___No

If yes, what disease? _____

Print the first names and descriptions of all of your children (i.e., the child's brothers and sisters). List in order of birth, including children who have died. If a child died, please indicate age at death and the cause of death.

First Name	Relationship to the present child (full, half, or step)	Date of Birth	Health Problems
1._____	_____	_____	_____
2._____	_____	_____	_____
3._____	_____	_____	_____
4._____	_____	_____	_____
5._____	_____	_____	_____
6._____	_____	_____	_____

Have you (or your partner) had any miscarriages? ____ Yes (How many?) _____ No_____

Date: _____   Medical-Genetic Family Hx (circle): Birth Mother Birth Father Agency# ___ p. 2 of 8

YOUR BROTHERS AND SISTERS

How many living brothers do you have? _____
Do you have any brothers who died? ___ Yes (list each below)   ___ No

Age at Death	Cause of Death	Medical Problem involved in the cause of death, if known
_____	_____	_____
_____	_____	_____
_____	_____	_____

Have any of your brothers had any serious health, physical, mental or learning problems?

_____ Yes   _____ No   _____ Don't Know
If yes, please explain:_____

How many living sisters do you have? _____
Do you have any sisters who died? ___ Yes (list each below)   ___ No

Age at Death	Cause of Death	Medical Problem involved in the cause of death, if known
_____	_____	_____
_____	_____	_____
_____	_____	_____

Have any of your sisters had any serious health, physical, mental or learning problems?

_____ Yes   _____ No   _____ Don't Know
If yes, please explain:_____

Do any of your brothers or sisters have a different father or mother? If yes, please indicate which brother or sister, and which parent was different from yours:

_____

YOUR PARENTS

In what year was your mother born? _____

Has she had any serious health, physical, mental or learning problems?

___Yes ___No ___Don't Know

If yes, please explain: _____

_____

If she has died, cause of death and age:_____

Highest grade she completed in school (circle): 1 2 3 4 5 6 7 8 9 10 11 12 13 14 15 16 17+

Did she receive special education? ___ Yes ___ No ___Don't Know

Date: _____ Medical-Genetic Family Hx (circle): Birth Mother Birth Father Agency# _____ p. 3 of 8

*In what year was your father born?*_____

Has he had any serious health, physical, mental or learning problems? ___Yes ___No ___Don't Know

If yes, please explain: _____

If he has died, cause of death and age: _____

Highest grade he completed in school (circle): 1 2 3 4 5 6 7 8 9 10 11 12 13 14 15 16 17+

Was he ever in special classes to provide extra help in learning? ___Yes ___ No ___Don't Know

YOUR GRANDPARENTS

Your Mother's Mother:

Has she had any serious health, physical, mental or learning problems? __Yes ___No ___Don't Know

*If yes, please explain:*_____

If she has died, cause of death and age: _____

Country of origin of her ancestors (for example, Italy, Scotland, etc.): _____

Ethnic Background (circle all that apply): White, Jewish, African American, Hispanic Origin, Native American, Asian, Pacific Islander, Other (Please list): _____

Your Mother's Father:

Has he had any serious health, physical, mental or learning problems? __Yes ___ No ___Don't Know

If yes, please explain: _____

If he has died, cause of death and age: _____

Country of origin of his ancestors (for example, Italy, Scotland, etc.): _____

Ethnic Background (circle all that apply): White, Jewish, African American, Hispanic Origin, Native American, Asian, Pacific Islander, Other (Please list): _____

Your Father's Mother:

Has she had any serious health, physical, mental or learning problems? ___Yes ___No ___Don't Know

If yes, please explain: _____

If she has died, cause of death and age: _____

Country of origin of her ancestors (for example, Italy, Scotland, etc.): _____

Ethnic Background (circle all that apply): White, Jewish, African American, Hispanic Origin, Native American, Asian, Pacific Islander, Other (Please list): _____

Your Father's Father:

Has he had any serious health, physical, mental, or learning problems? ___Yes ___No ___Don't Know

If yes, please explain: _____

If he has died, cause of death and age: _____

Country of origin of his ancestors (for example, Italy, Scotland, etc.): _____

Ethnic Background (circle all that apply): White, Jewish, African American, Hispanic Origin, Native American, Asian, Pacific Islander, Other (Please list): _____

Date: _____   Medical-Genetic Family Hx (circle): Birth Mother Birth Father Agency# ___ p. 4 of 8

Genetic-Medical History

Check "Yes" or "No" if you or any of your blood relatives (i.e., your parents, grand-parents, aunts, uncles, brothers, sisters, cousins, nieces and nephews) ever had, or now have, any of the medical conditions listed. Include only relatives who are your blood relatives (omit relatives related by marriage or adoption, but include half brothers and half sisters).

Specific Medical Conditions	Yourself Yes	No	Blood relative Yes	No	How related to you?
1. Blindness or other visual problems (note age affected)					
2. Cataracts (note age affected)					
3. Glaucoma (note age affected)					
4. Deafness, hearing difficulties (note age affected)					
5. Unusual shape or missing ear					
6. Speech problems					
8. Dental problems Example - extra or missing teeth					
9. Cleft lip (harelip)					
10. Cleft palate					
11. Learning disability (slow learner)					
12. Mental retardation (estimate severity)					
13. Attention deficit disorder and/or hyperactivity					
14. Down syndrome					
15. Other chromosome abnormality (please specify)					
16. Schizophrenia (note age affected)					
17. Bipolar depression (note age affected)					

If you answered yes to any of the above, please complete the following:

Number (from above)	Age when first affected	Relationship to the child	Comments (name of disorder if known)

Date: _____   Medical-Genetic Family Hx (circle): Birth Mother Birth Father Agency# ___ p. 5 of 8

Specific Medical Conditions	*Yourself*		*Blood relative*		*How related to you?*
	Yes	*No*	*Yes*	*No*	
18. *Other mental illness (please specify)*					
19. *Hydrocephalus (water on the brain)*					
20. *Microcephaly (small head)*					
21. *Birthmarks (please describe) Example - unusual shape, size, or number*					
22. *Patches of hair of different color*					
23. *Patches of skin of different color Example - white or brown spots*					
24. *Skin problems Severe eczema, acne, or other*					
25. *Bleeding problems or hemophilia*					
26. *Sickle cell disease*					
27. *Thalassemia*					
28. *High blood pressure (hyypertension) (specify age)*					
29. *Kidney problems (specify age)*					
30. *Stroke (specify age)*					
31. *Heart attack (specify age)*					
32. *Born with heart defect Example - hole in heart*					
33. *Born with open spine (spina bifida)*					
34. *Born with missing brain (anencephaly)*					
35. *Born with hip problems (dislocated hips)*					

If you answered yes to any of the above, please complete the following:

Number (from above)	Age when first affected	Relationship to the child	Comments (name of disorder if known)

Date: _____ Medical-Genetic Family Hx (circle): Birth Mother Birth Father Agency# ___ p. 6 of 8

Specific Medical Conditions	Yourself Yes	No	Blood relative Yes	No	How related to you?
36. *Dwarfism or short stature*					
37. *Spinal curvature (scoliosis)*					
38. *Unusually formed bones or many broken bones*					
39. *Unusually formed hands (please describe)* Example - extra/missing/webbed fingers					
40. *Unusually formed feet (please describe)* Example - extra/missing/webbed toes					
41. *Club foot*					
42. *Other birth defects (please specify)* (not listed above)					
43. *Arthritis, joint problems (specify age)*					
44. *Muscular dystrophy (age affected and type* *if known)*					
45. *Muscle weakness (note age affected)*					
46. *Loss of muscle control (note age affected)*					
47. *Pyloric stenosis (projectile vomiting)*					
48. *Breast cancer (age diagnosed)*					
49. *Colon cancer (age diagnosed)*					
50. *Ovarian cancer (age diagnosed)*					
51. *Other cancers (please specify type and age* *diagnosed)* (include childhood cancers)					
52. *Cystic fibrosis*					
53. *Alzheimer disease (note age affected)*					
54. *Dementia (note age affected)* (mental deterioration)					

If you answered yes to any of the above, please complete the following:

Number (from above)	Age when first affected	Relationship to the child	Comments (name of disorder if known)

Date: _____ Medical-Genetic Family Hx (circle): Birth Mother Birth Father Agency# ___ p. 7 of 8

Specific Medical Conditions	Yourself Yes	Yourself No	Blood relative Yes	Blood relative No	How related to you?
55. Huntington disease (chorea) (note age affected)					
56. Neurofibromatosis					
57. Multiple sclerosis (note age affected)					
58. Tay sachs disease					
59. Cerebral palsy					
60. Seizures, convulsions, epilepsy (note age affected and type if known)					
61. Adult diabetes (specify age) (insulin or non-insulin dependent)					
62. Childhood diabetes (specify age)					
63. Thyroid disorder (specify if under-active or over-active)					
64. Kidney problems (note age affected)					
65. Respiratory or breathing problems (specify age) Example - emphysema					
66. Asthma					
67. Allergies - hay fever (pollen)					
68. Allergies - food (please specify)					
69. Allergies - medicine (please specify)					
70. Chemical dependency (alcohol)					
71. Chemical dependency - other drugs (please specify)					
72. Weight problems (obesity or anorexia)					

If you answered yes to any of the above, please complete the following:

Number (from above)	Age when first affected	Relationship to the child	Comments (name of disorder if known)

Date: _____ Medical-Genetic Family Hx (circle): Birth Mother Birth Father Agency# ___ p. 8 of 8

Specific Medical Conditions	Yourself Yes	No	Blood relative Yes	No	How related to you?
73. *Infertility*					
74. *Miscarriages* If yes, how many?					
75. *Stillbirths* If yes, how many?					
76. *Neonatal deaths* (died before one month old)					
77. *Infant deaths* (died before one year of age)					
78. *Childhood deaths (specify age and cause)*					
79. *HIV (Human Immunodeficiency Virus)*					
80. *AIDS (Acquired Immunodeficiency Syndrome)*					
81. *Frequent Infections (Immune deficiency)*					

If you answered yes to any of the above, please complete the following:

Number (from above)	Age when first affected	Relationship to the child	Comments (name of disorder if known)

Has anyone in the family had any genetic testing? Please explain:

_____

_____

_____

_____

Is there anything else you think we should know about you or your family?

_____

_____

_____

_____

The development of this form was supported in part by the CORN Education Committee, Project #: NCJ-361011-03 and was revised with permission by Robin L. Bennett, MS, April 1998 and again in February 2009.

Joan Burns, MSW

Robin L. Bennett, MS

Barbara Bernhardt, MS

Kathleen Delp, MSW

Amy A Jarzebowicz, MS

Diane Plumridge, MSW

Cheryl Schroeder, EdD

Kerry Silvey, MA

Stephanie Smith, MS

The Genetics Library

The following is an annotated list of my recommendations for pedigree drawing programs and general Internet resources related to clinical genetics. It is not meant to be an exhaustive list and focuses mainly on resources in the United States and the European Union. All URLs were checked at the time of writing. All prices are in U.S. dollars. Resources for locating a genetics professional are available in Chapter 6.

PEDIGREE SOFTWARE DRAWING PROGRAMS

Resources for recording family history based on genealogy models can be found in Section 6.7. The U.S. Surgeon General's Internet tool for recording a family history is reviewed in Section 6.6.

Commercial Software Programs

PED 6.0.2 (www.medgen.de): Developed by Hansjoerg Plendl, *PED 6.0.2* is a Windows application for creating, drawing, and editing of pedigrees. The drawing features conform to the Pedigree Standardization Task Force recommendations. The program allows for uploading to the BOADICEA data file to estimate the risks of breast and ovarian cancer and the probability of being a carrier of *BRCA1* or *BRCA2* gene mutations. The costs varies from approximately $100 for a single user license, to $239 for up to 10 users. The costs are more for LINKAGE, CSV, and Boadicea format.

Pedigree-Draw: Genealogy Visualization for MacIntosh (www.pedigree-draw .com): A product of Jurek Software in San Antonio, Texas, this program is a native Macintosh OS X application that provides for creation, editing, and drawing of pedigrees. Pictures of relatives can be included. Output can be saved as a PDF for electronic distribution or posting on websites. The program can be purchased from the Kagi Online store with a single user license or as a CD-ROM. It is available in multiple languages. The price is approximately $60.

Progeny (www.progenygenetics.com): To date, *Progeny* is the only consistently available program for drawing a clinical pedigree. It is most useful for preparing pedigrees for publication, keeping track of evaluations of large families, or collecting pedigrees for research. Clinical and molecular data can be tracked and stored in relation to pedigree information. Progeny also incorporates several risk assessment tools such as the BRCAPRO model for predicting the likelihood of identifying a *BRCA1* or *BRCA2* mutation based on family history. Tools such as *Progeny* are likely to become more standard and useful as more medical records are stored and transferred electronically. The costs vary based on whether the program is for a single-user, networked model, or Web-based. Custom programs can be developed for patient populations (for example, a concentration on cancer or cardiovascular disease).

Cyrillic (www.exetersoftware.com/cat/cyrillic/cyrillic.html): Based in a Microsoft Access and Paradox file formats, this program allows for calculations using BRCAPRO and MENDEL. This version has not been updated in a while but there is still user support. The software is distributed by Exeter Software. The cost is approximately $800.

General Internet Resources

BayesMendel Lab (http://astor.som.jhmi.edu/BayesMendel/index.html): An essential resource for those doing cancer susceptibility counseling or research in this area. This workgroup has developed open source software to predict who may carry an inherited susceptibility to a variety of cancers (e.g., *BRCA1*) and *BRCA2* and BRCAPRO).

Centers for Disease Control, and Prevention, Office of Public Health Genomics (www.cdc.gov/genetics): This regularly updated website provides access to current information on the impact of human genetic research and the Human Genome Project on public health and disease prevention. You can register for their on-line newsletter, which includes headlines from the past week's news and highlights scientific publications, upcoming evens, and websites that are relevant to genetics and public health. There are several initiatives related to family history including Family Healthware.

European Directory of DNA Laboratories (www.eddnal.com): An extensive directory of DNA laboratories in EU countries, sponsored by the European Commission.

Family Village—A Global Community of Disability-Related Resources (www. familyvillage.wisc.edu): An easy to navigate site for parents of children with cognitive and other disabilities, providing medical information and resources for a variety of inherited disorders

Genetic Alliance (http://geneticalliance.org): This is not only an outstanding resource for locating support organizations for persons with various genetic disorders also is the premier advocacy group for persons and families affected by inherited disorders. The Genetic Alliance in partnership with the American Society of Human Genetics and the National Library of Medicine has developed a toolkit for collecting and recording family history.

Gene Reviews (www.genereviews.org): This is the best resource on the web for expert-authored clinical information related to genetic testing, diagnosis, management, and counseling of individuals and families with inherited disorders. If is funded by that National Library of Medicine and the National Human Genome Research Institute of Health and maintained by the University of Washington in Seattle. There are also educational modules related to medical genetics.

Gene Clinics (www.geneclinics.org): This is the linked database to GeneReviews, which lists the clinical and research laboratories providing genetic testing for various genetic conditions. Contact information is listed for the laboratories. Direct contact with the laboratories is then necessary to find out specifics about laboratory techniques used for diagnostics, costs of testing, and sample requirements. There is also a reference directory for finding genetics professional.

Genetics and Rare Disease Information Center (http://rarediseases.info.nih.gov): Sponsored by the National Institute of Health, Office of Rare Diseases Research, this site is a portal to rare disease information and research.

Genetics Education Center, University of Kansas Medical Center (Genetics and Rare Conditions Site, www.kumc.edu/gec/support; Genetic Professional Home Page, www.kumc.edu/gec/geneinfo.html; Genetics Education Center, www.kumc.edu/gec): This collective website is updated on a regular basis by genetic counselor Debra Collins, MS, at the University of Kansas Medical Center. Collins maintains an extremely comprehensive listing of clinical genetic resources, pedigree drawing programs, family support information, and on-line databases. There is a section on genetic education resources. The site has many useful links.

Genetics Home Reference (http://ghr.nlm.nih.gov/): A guide to understanding hundreds of genetic conditions. Sponsored by the National Institutes of Health and the National Library of Medicine.

GROW (Genetics Resources on the Web: www.geneticsresources.org): This is a search engine to optimize the use of the web to provide health professionals and the public with high-quality information related to human genetics, with a particular focus on genetic medicine and health.

HUGO Gene Nomenclature Committee (http://genenames.org): The resource for identifying human gene symbols and names, with links to other resources such as OMIM.

March of Dimes Homepage (http://modimes.org): General information about birth defects and their prevention, and a resource list of fact sheets on genetic disorders in various languages. There is also a genetics section for professionals and researchers, which includes a family history tool as part of the Genetics and Your Practice module for health professionals (www.marchofdimes .com/professionals/15829.asp).

National Cancer Institute (http://cancer.gov): This site is part of the NCI's main on-line information center for patients and physicians. It has several basic monographs on genetic testing and on testing by groups such as the American College of Medical Genetics, the American Society of Human Genetics, and the American Society of Clinical Oncologists. A valuable resource is the ability to query the database to locate a board-certified or eligible genetic counselor.

National Human Genome Research Institute (www.genome.gov): This is the website for the Human Genome Project. It includes information about the Center for Inherited Disease Research, ELSI (ethical, legal and social implications), a schedule of workshops and conferences, and timely topics in the news. My favorite section is the "talking glossary" of genetic terms that allows the user to download audio and video files; also available are genetic education modules for teachers. The NHGRI is a major partner with the U.S. Surgeon General's Office in relation to family history initiatives.

National Institutes of Health, Office of Rare Diseases Research (http://rarediseases .ino.nigh.gov): As noted on their website, a portal to rare disease information and research.

National Institute of Neurological Disorders and Stroke (www.ninds.nih.gov): Grouped by neurological conditions, this database provides a brief general description of the disease, its treatment, prognosis, research, and available support groups. In-depth references for health professionals are included.

NCHPEG (National Coalition for Health Professional Education in Genetics) (www.nchpeg.org): A resource for health professionals in genetics education. Includes a resource for learning and teaching core competencies in family history.

NORD (National Organization for Rare Disorders) (www.rarediseases.org): A network of organizations representing individuals with rare disorders and their families.

OMIM (On line Mendelian Inheritance in Man) (www.ncbi.nlm.nih.gov/sites/ entrez?db=omim): This site is a unique web resource and a common place to turn for information about a particular genetic issue. It is an extensive database of inherited disorders maintained by the Johns Hopkins University School of Medicine, providing information on genetic syndromes, clinical presentation, cytogenetics, genetic mapping, pathogenesis, and population genetics. There are links to the National Library of Medicine's MEDLINE database.

Rare Chromosome Disorder Support Group (Unique) (www.rarechromo.org/html/ByChromo.asp): Unique is a support organization based in the United Kingdom for families with rare chromosome disorders. There are many links to publications and opportunities for research regarding a range of structural and numerical chromosome disorders.

Wisconsin Stillbirth Services Program (WiSSP) (www.wisc.edu.wissp): A website containing the standard of care for the genetic evaluation of stillbirth (clinical evaluation, photographs, autopsy, chromosomes, radiographs, pre/perinatal history, and Kleihauaer-Betke testing). There are also links support of families who have experienced a stillbirth.

Appendix A.6

Genetics in Practice: Five Case Studies

Case 1: No News Is Good News–A Family History of Intellectual Disability

Nathan, aged 30 years, and his wife Natalie, aged 28 years, are planning a pregnancy in the next year. They are concerned because Nathan's 36-year-old brother, Billy, has mild intellectual disability.

The Medical-Family History

Records were obtained from Billy's evaluation for a seizure disorder at the Children's Hospital. He has an IQ of 60. He has no regression in his abilities. He lives with his parents. He is unable to make change or ride a bus independently. He is able to perform activities of daily living. Billy was the product of a full-term, no-stressed vaginal delivery. His mother did not take any medications during the pregnancy. She had an occasional glass of wine (perhaps five glasses total) during her pregnancy.

Billy is described as having an easygoing personality. He has no hearing or visual deficits. His speech is limited and repetitive. He is 5 feet 10 inches tall. Because Billy lives on the other side of the country, it was not possible to examine him. Natalie and Nathan brought some of their wedding pictures to their appointment. Billy does not seem to have anything unusual about the way he looks. His head appears normally shaped. His eyes and ears appear normally placed and shaped. He does not appear to have coarse facial features. His hair seems normal. His jaw appears somewhat prominent. Nathan does not recall any unusual birthmarks on his

The Practical Guide to the Genetic Family History, Second Edition, by Robin L. Bennett
Copyright © 2010 John Wiley & Sons, Inc.

brother. Billy reportedly does not have any skeletal anomalies or joint laxity. He had multiple seizures beginning at age 3 years until the age of 19 years. He still takes a seizure medication. His parents first noticed his delays soon after his seizures began. He does not appear to have any problems walking or with muscle weakness (several of the wedding pictures show him merrily joining in the dancing). He has no involuntary movements. Billy is not described as having symptoms suggestive of a metabolic problem (Table 4.12), such as severe childhood illnesses, episodic vomiting, hypoglycemia, unusual odors, or an unusual dietary pattern. Nathan does not recall if his brother has large testes.

Billy is Nathan's only sibling. Their father, Nate Sr. is 62 years old. He developed diabetes 3 years earlier. His diabetes is under good control with medication. Nate had three older full siblings. Nate's oldest brother, Norman, died at age 70 from a myocardial infarction. Norman and his wife had one miscarriage and two healthy daughters. Nate has two sisters—Edith, age 68, and Naomi, age 64. Edith has a son and a daughter who are both healthy. Naomi has a healthy son, Peter, from her first marriage, and a son, Carson, from her second marriage. Nate's father died of a heart attack at age 58. His mother is living at age 93. She has lost about 2 inches of height from osteoporosis, but is otherwise reasonably healthy.

Nathan and Billy's mother, JoAnne, age 63 years, had some knee surgery from a sports injury, but is otherwise healthy. She has two brothers—Roger, age 61 years, and her twin brother, Thomas. Roger has one daughter, and Thomas has three daughters and a son. They are all reportedly healthy. JoAnne's father died in a car accident at age 45, and her mother died at age 80 from pneumonia related to complications after a hip replacement.

JoAnne's father's family settled in the Ohio Valley more than 100 years ago; they were mostly of English and Irish ancestry. Her mother's father emigrated from Ireland in the early 1900s. Nathan laughs and states that his father's ancestry is "Heinz 57," although he is proud to say that his great-grandfather was a Native American from the Salish tribe.

Natalie is the youngest of eight siblings, having four full brothers and three full sisters. Her mother, Rosemary, is 76 years old and in good health. Natalie's father, Edward, came from a large family with three brothers and two sisters. They are all apparently healthy, as are their numerous children. Rosemary has a younger sister and a brother. Her sister never had children, and her brother has five healthy children. Rosemary's father and mother have lived in the United States for many years; and their ancestors were mostly from Germany, France, and Holland. Edward's parents were also of northern European ancestry.

Natalie and Nathan are not aware if their parents are related to each other either as cousins or more closely related. There is no other family history of intellectual disability, birth defects, or miscarriages.

Pedigree Analysis   The most through approach to providing a risk assessment for Natalie and Nathan is to have Billy evaluated by a medical geneticist because the etiology of his developmental delay has never been determined. Initially, Natalie and Nathan were reluctant to purse this option; they were concerned that Nathan's parents would feel guilty if they found out that Nathan and Natalie had a high chance to have a child with mental impairments. Nathan felt a conflict between his strong emotional attachment to Billy and his not wanting to have a child like Billy. Nathan decided to approach his parents because he felt that establishing a diagnosis for Billy might also benefit Billy's health and planning for his long-term care.

Nathan's parents agreed to have Billy evaluated by a medical geneticist near their home. A syndrome was not identified. He had a chromosome study and chromosome microarray analysis using a DNA chip and comparative genome hybridization for many known loci associated with intellectual delay. These studies were normal. He was also tested for fragile X syndrome.

The medical family history (Figure A.1) does not provide any obvious indicators to a possible hereditary etiology to Billy's problems. It is possible to provide Nathan and Natalie with empirical risk figures to have a child with intellectual delay based on their "normal" family history. The following risk possibilities were discussed with the couple:

- Autosomal dominant inheritance seems unlikely because Nathan and his parents are of normal intelligence, and they do not have any dysmorphic features. Billy could have a new dominant mutation but this would not affect his healthy adult brother.
- Autosomal recessive inheritance is a possibility. If Billy's parents are related as cousins (or more closely related), the likelihood of autosomal recessive inheritance would be greater. Many inborn errors of metabolism are inherited in an autosomal recessive pattern (Table 4.12), but Billy does not have features typical for these problems.
- If Billy's problems are a result of an autosomal recessive gene alteration, then Nathan's chance to be a heterozygous carrier is 66%. Because Nathan and Natalie are not consanguineous, the chance that she also carries this same gene alteration is probably less than 1%. An estimate of their chance to have an affected child is 0.66 (Nathan's chance to carry the gene alteration) times 0.50 (the chance he passes the gene alteration to his child) times 0.01 (an estimated risk that Natalie is a carrier for the same autosomal recessive gene alteration) times 0.5 (the chance Natalie passes the gene alteration to her child) = 1/300.
- Another possibility is that Billy's condition is X-linked. Fragile X syndrome is the most common form of intellectual disability in males. Billy had a normal fragile X DNA test. Billy could still have some other form of X-linked intellectual disability. Nathaniel's mother, JoAnne has two healthy brothers. This information does not rule out an X-linked syndrome, although it does slightly reduce the likelihood that Billy carries an X-linked gene mutation. Even if Billy does have an X-linked mutation, because Nathan is healthy and without intellectual disability, it is unlikely that Nathan is harboring the same gene alteration.
- A chromosme aberration such as a deletion, duplication, or unbalanced rearrangement should be considered in any individual with intellectual disability. Billy's chromosome study was normal; therefore, it is unlikely that Nathan

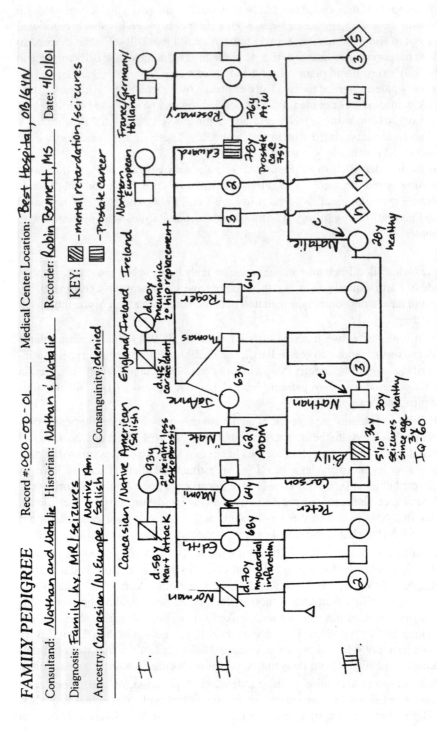

Figure A.1 Hypothetical pedigree of Nathan and Natalie. Nathan has a brother with an undiagnosed condition involving intellectual disability and a seizure disorder.

carries a chromosome rearrangement. Note that even if a person had a normal chromosome study several years ago, it is worth considering an additional chromosome study because of advances in the ability to detect subtle chromosome aberrations.

- Mitochondrial inheritance is an unlikely though remote possibility. Some mitochondrial disorders are associated with intellectual disability and seizures. Given that Billy's mother is apparently healthy, this is less likely. If this is a mitochondrial syndrome, Nathan does not appear to be affected, and Nathan's offspring would not be at risk because men do not pass mitochondria to their children.

In summary, the etiology of Billy's intellectual impairment remains unknown. His tests for the most likely causes of intellectual disability (chromosomal imbalances and fragile X mutations) were negative. Given both Nathan and Natalie's noncontributory family histories, they can be given risk figures from empirical tables. The chance that a healthy sibling of an individual with moderate intellectual disability will have a similarly affected child is about 1.8%. This compares to the approximately 1% chance that any couple has to have a child with intellectual disability.

Nathan and Natalie were reassured by this information. They have since gone on to have a healthy son and a healthy daughter.

Case 2: A Fresh Look at an Adolescent with Congenital Cataracts and Intellectual Disability

Bob Johnson is a 15-year-old moderately intellectually delayed youth who has found to have proteinuria when he was evaluated for his sports physical to participate in the Special Olympics. He was born blind, and he has had more than 20 surgeries for glaucoma and cataracts. His parents were told his congenital cataracts and intellectual delays were a result of congenital rubella syndrome. Given the combination of congenital cataracts, intellectual delay, and possible renal disease, it seemed wise to obtain a family history to see if there could be a genetic explanation for this combination of characteristics.

The Medical-Family History

Bob has proportionate short stature (height, 134 cm and weight, 29 kg, both below the 3rd percentile). His head circumference is 58.5 cm, which is above the 98th percentile. His blood pressure is 110/64. He has numerous sebaceous cysts on his face, hands neck, buttocks, legs, and ears. His eyes are deep set and hypoterloric. He has a broad nasal root and broad nasal tip. He has a large mouth with full lips. His ears are large. His palate is normal. He is hirsute. His lungs are clear to auscultation. His heart has regular rate and rhythm. His abdomen is normal. He has normal male genitalia with bilateral descended testes. He has broad and short hands and feet. He has decrease range of motion and difficulty with ambulation, given joint stiffness, particularly in his hips and knees. He does not have a history of diabetes or seizures.

Bob has quite a sense of humor and is very vocal. His mother, Ann, states he has some stereotypical behaviors such as head bumping and finger tapping. Ann is frustrated by Bob's disruptive temper tantrums. His development was delayed. Bob sat up at 2 years of age, walked at about age $2^1/_2$, developed his first words at 2, and was able to put a few words together by age $3^1/_2$. He can sign his name. Bob does not have regression of his learning.

Ann did have a fever and joint aches early in her pregnancy. She did not consume any alcohol or drugs during her pregnancy. Bob was delivered vaginally at 40 weeks of gestation. His cataracts were noted a few days after birth. Ann was told by Bob's pediatrician that the rubella she had while pregnant was the cause of Bob's problems.

Bob has a healthy sister, Julie age 19 years. Julie attends college in a premedical curriculum. Julie is five feet, 6 inches tall and has no health problems. Bob's mother, Ann, is 47 years old and is employed as an accountant. She has recently been diagnosed with cataracts. She is otherwise healthy. She had a brother, John, who died at age 37 years. Ann is not sure of the cause of her brother's death; he grew up in a home for the learning disabled. He had severe intellectual disability, glaucoma, and cataracts. Ann's mother, Sophie, died a year ago at age 77. She was recovering from a hip replacement and died of pneumonia. Sophie had one sister, Jasmine, who is reportedly healthy at age 75 years. She had one daughter, Georgia, who is healthy at age 45 years. Ann has little contact with this distant branch of the family, but apparently Georgia's youngest son, Sam, has cataracts, glaucoma, and some developmental disabilities. Ann believes Sam is about 12 years old and that he has two healthy sisters in middle school.

Bob's mother and father (Jim) divorced when Bob was 5 years old. Jim has not remained in contact with the family. Ann believes Jim has at least two other sons. Ann is not aware of any health problems in Jim or his sons. Jim came from a large family of three sisters and two brothers. Ann believes that they are all healthy as are their children. Ann knows that her ex-husband's parents are deceased but she is not sure of the causes. Jim is 48 years old and is 5 feet 11 inches tall.

Jim and Ann are both of African American ancestry. They are not known to be consanguineous.

Pedigree Analysis

It is unlikely that Bob, John, and Sam have glaucoma, cataracts, and varying degrees of intellectual disability by chance alone. The most likely explanation is an X-linked inheritance pattern because the affected males are related through an apparently healthy women. Ann's early cataracts are probably a manifestation of her being heterozygous for the gene alteration. It might be possible to obtain the prenatal records from Ann's pregnancy with Bob to document the occurrence of maternal rubella. Usually children with congenital rubella have a small head circumference (microcephaly), and Bob has a large head circumference. A syndrome with autosomal dominance with reduced penetrance is a possibility but less likely because predominantly males are affected in this family, and the only female who is possibly affected (Ann) has mild manifestations in comparison to the male relatives.

The family could have an inherited chromosome rearrangement where by chance only males have been affected. No one in the family is known to have had a miscarriage, which can be seen in carriers of a chromosome rearrangement.

Mitochondrial inheritance is another possibility because the males in this family are affected through females. However, you would expect to see females who are as severely as affected as males. Progression of the disease is often seen in mitochondrial disorders (owing to a continuing accumulation of mitochondrial mutations during cell division); there does not seem to be progression of the disease in Bob.

The collection of characteristics of congenital cataracts, intellectual disability, short stature, sebaceous cysts, dysmorphic features, joint problems, and probable renal disease (Figure A.2) suggests of the X-linked oculocerebrorenal (Lowe) syndrome (Table 4.9). A medical geneticist, using the appropriate diagnostic testing, confirmed this diagnosis in Bob. Because progressive tubular and glomerular renal disease is a major component of the syndrome, Bob was referred for a full assessment of his renal function. Treatment with phosphorus, calcium, carnitine, and/or vitamin D is usually beneficial for these individuals in managing their renal disease and bone degeneration.

Multiple family members were affected by a fresh look at Bob's medical-family history. Ann was pleased she finally had an explanation for her son's problems. She had always felt guilty that her son's problems were a result of something she had done in pregnancy. Knowledge that her son's temper outbursts were characteristic of boys with this condition was a relief because Ann had fretted that her parenting techniques were at fault. Ann was grateful to learn of the national support group for families with Lowe syndrome (the Lowe Foundation), and she could hardly wait to attend their next annual meeting to meet other parents who had children with similar problems. Ann planned to share information about Lowe syndrome with her daughter Julie who has a 50:50 chance to be a carrier of the oculocerebrorenal syndrome, so that Julie can make her own choices about childbearing and possible prenatal testing. Because Lowe syndrome is a multisystem disease, a final diagnosis in Bob is beneficial for his life-long health management. Sharing this information with Sam's parents and healthcare providers will also assist in his medical care.

Case 3: But I Thought That Was a Pediatric Disease

Rhonda Adams is a 40-year-old white woman seeking a new primary-care physician because she has recently moved to the area. She has been successful in her career as a software developer for the past 15 years. She has a significant history of chronic respiratory disease. She is a nonsmoker and nobody smokes in her household. As a child she had chronic sinusitis, and she has been hospitalized several times for pneumonia. She has constant postnasal drip. She has intermittent heartburn.

The Medical-Family History

Rhonda and her husband, Ron, have two healthy daughters—a Jane, age 20 and Angie, age 18. Rhonda had three full siblings. Her sister, Frieda, is 45 years old. She has nasal polyps and had one miscarriage at approximately 12 weeks of gestation.

FAMILY PEDIGREE

Consultand: Ms. Johnson Record #: 0-00-00-02 Medical Center Location: Best Hospital Pediatrics

Historian: Ann Johnson Recorder: Dr. Spock Date: 4/1/10

Proband: Bob Johnson
Diagnosis: MR/glaucoma/cataracts

KEY: ◼ – cataracts ◼ – mental retarda-
tion/learning
disabilities

Ancestry: African American

◼ – glaucoma

Consanguinity? denied

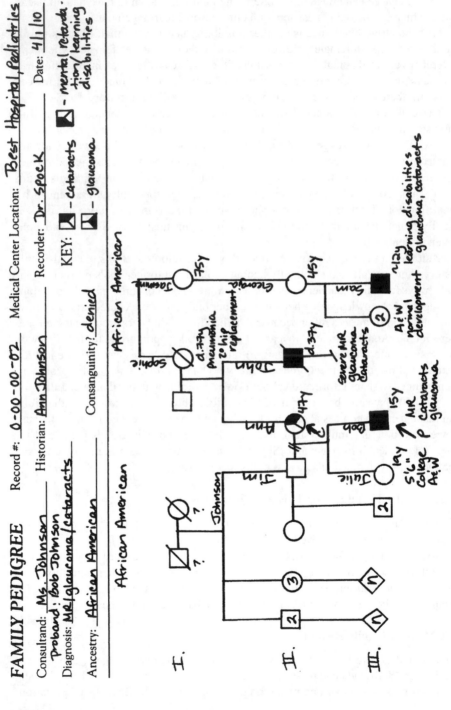

Figure A.2 Hypothetical pedigree of the Johnson family—a family with X-linked oculocerebrorenal (Lowe) syndrome.

A brother, Paul, is 36 years old. He and his wife have been trying to conceive a pregnancy for about 3 years. They have an appointment to see a fertility specialist.

Rhonda's mother, Joyce, died at age 65 from a myocardial infarction. She had one brother who died at age 24 in World War II. A sister is healthy at age 68 years, as are her three children and eight grandchildren. Joyce's mother died at age 85 of colon cancer, and Joyce's father died at age 77 of "old age." They are of Russian-German (Ashkenazi Jewish) ancestry.

Rhonda's father, Robert, has some arthritis at age 75 but is otherwise healthy. He has two older sisters, age 78 and 80 years, who are reportedly healthy, as are their children. A full sister died in infancy of unknown causes. Robert's father died of heart disease at age 90. Robert's mother had Parkinson disease and died in her 80s. They are of Polish (Ashkenazi Jewish) ancestry. The families are not known to be consanguineous.

There is no other history of miscarriages, infertility, or deaths in childhood. There is no family history of liver or pancreatic dysfunction or gastrointestinal disease. Rhonda does not report having foul smelling stools although she describes her stomach as always being a little "sensitive."

Pedigree Analysis

The family history suggests cystic fibrosis (Figure A.3). Paul's infertility could be due to congenital absence of the vas deferens. The report of nasal polyps in Stefanie and problem conceiving a pregnancy also suggests cystic fibrosis. The family history is compatible with autosomal recessive inheritance because there does not appear to be related health problems in more than one generation.

Rhonda was referred for a genetic evaluation, including a sweat-chloride test and DNA mutation analysis for mutations in the cystic fibrosis gene. Her sweat chloride was abnormal. She is a compound heterozygote for two of the more common mutations in the white, northern european population-delta F508 and R117H.

Rhonda's diagnosis of cystic fibrosis will now assist in the management of her pulmonary disease. Her siblings may have minor pulmonary manifestations of cystic fibrosis. Knowing whether they have cystic fibrosis can be important in their health-care. The diagnosis of affected or carrier status can be determined with DNA testing. Paul most likely has congenital absence of the vas deferens (see Section 4.18.3). At age 43, Stephanie may be considering future pregnancies. Decreased fertility in women is associated with cystic fibrosis. If Stephanie has inherited one or both mutations, her husband may want to have cystic fibrosis carrier testing. Rhonda's daughters are obligate carriers for a cystic fibrosis mutation. This information is important for their family planning.

Case 4: Life Isn't Always as It Seems

Jill is a successful 40-year-old costume designer for a local theater group. She is petrified of the cancer she describes as "running rampant" in her family. This clinic visit is prompted by the recent diagnosis of prostate cancer in her 76-year-old father, Thomas. Her mother, Evelyn, died 30 years earlier of ovarian cancer at age 44 years.

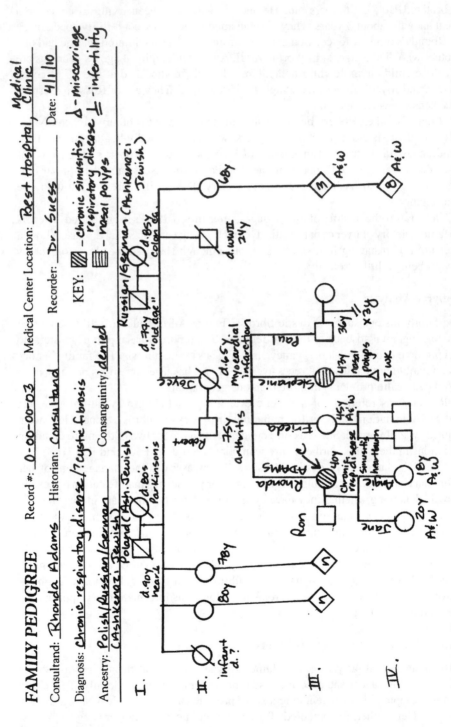

Figure A.3 Hypothetical pedigree of Rhonda Adams—a woman with chronic respiratory disease who has cystic fibrosis.

Jill has heard that breast and ovarian cancer can run in a family. She is considering having a prophylactic oophorectomy. She states, "Since I'm through having children, I would consider both having my breast and ovaries removed if this will allow me to live to watch my children grow old."

Medical-Family History

Jill and her partner, Dan, have two daughters, ages 6 years and 15 months. Jill is the oldest child of her mother and father, although she has two healthy half-brothers from her father's first marriage: Patrick, age 48 years, and Samuel, age 50 years. Samuel has two healthy step-daughters. Dan is of Mexican-American ancestry and he and Jill are not blood relatives.

Jill knows little about her mother's treatment for cancer. She knows her mother was diagnosed with cancer about a year before she died. Jill believes her mother was trying to "protect her." Jill is tearful as she recalls her mother's death. She regrets that her mother "enjoyed her vodka Collins" and "smoked like a chimney" until her death. Evelyn was estranged from her because her parents were apparently upset with her choice of a "life in the world of theater" and because Evelyn died when Jill was only 10 years old, Jill knows little of her mother's medical-family history. According to Jill, Evelyn left home at the age of 17 years because she found it difficult to live in a home where alcohol was abused, and her father was verbally abusive. Jill believes her mother's brother, Clark, died in his 50s from stomach cancer. He has no children. Jill is in contact with her mother's sister, Betty, who is apparently healthy at age 75 years. Betty has a son, Mark, age 45 years, and a daughter, Judy, age 48 years. Jill and Judy see each other socially quite often, and Judy recently confided to Jill that she had an abnormal Pap smear. Evelyn had another brother, Jack, who died of unknown kidney problems at age 67. He had at least three children, but Jill does not even know their names. Evelyn's mother, Janis, apparently died of brain cancer at the age of 78 years, and Evelyn's father, Bradley, committed suicide at the age of 60 years. He apparently was an alcoholic. Evelyn's parents met in their early 20s when they both were working in a textile factory in New York City. Both Evelyn's mother and father emigrated from England.

Jill's father, Thomas, is a retired attorney. He has one sister, Deidra, who is 70 years old and has one healthy daughter. Another sister, Janet, has heart disease at age 63, but is other wise healthy. Janet has a son and a daughter. Thomas grew up in Alaska and is of Native American (Tlingit tribe) ancestry. Thomas and Evelyn were divorced when Jill was only 2 years old, and Jill went to live with her father after her mother's death. His father died of "old age" at the age of 80 years, and his mother is alive at the age of 97 years.

Pedigree Analysis

On the surface there seems to be a lot of cancer in this family, which may represent a familial cancer syndrome (Figure A.4). To be absolutely certain, it is essential to obtain medical records and death certificates on the family members with cancer. With the help of Jill's aunt Betty, Jill is able to obtain the pathology reports on her mother's

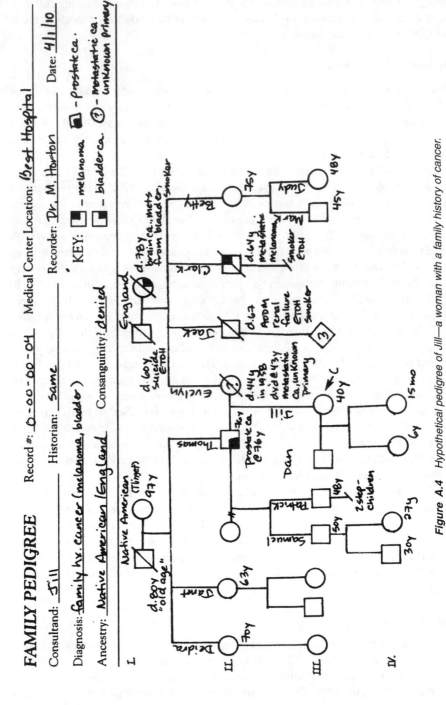

Figure A.4 Hypothetical pedigree of Jill—a woman with a family history of cancer.

cancer diagnosis, and death certificates on her uncle and maternal grandmother. Evelyn's medical records indicate that actually Evelyn had a metastatic abdominal cancer of unknown primary origin, but the surgical report indicates that the ovaries looked healthy. Jill and her aunt requested Clark's death certificate because they were unsure where he had his medical care. According to the death certificate, Clark died at age 64 years from metastatic melanoma. Jill's aunt Betty also adds that the whole family smoked tobacco heavily. Jack died of renal failure related to complications from diabetes and alcohol abuse. Evelyn's mother's death certificate states she died of metastatic brain cancer from the bladder.

Jill's family may have a single-gene mutation or mutations in more than one gene that predispose to cancer susceptibility (particularly if exposed to strong carcinogenic agents such as tobacco smoke). The occurrence of brain cancer in Jill's maternal grandmother Janis is probably explained by environmental factors, not heredity; bladder cancer is one of the most common cancers seen in heavy smokers, and brain cancer is a known metastatic site for bladder cancer (see Tables 5.5 and 5.6). Janis may have also been exposed to carcinogenic agents in the textile factory she was working at in the early 1900s. Aunt Betty also told Jill that Jill's uncles were notoriously noncompliant with their healthcare.

Given that Jill has multiple relatives with cancer, she should be judicious with her cancer screening, but her family history does not suggest that she needs to have screening at ages or intervals different from any other woman her age. Given her strong family history of alcohol addiction, she should be cautious in use of alcohol.

Jill was thrilled with this information. She thought her family history was a "cancer death sentence." As Jill approached the age that her mother had died, her fear of ovarian cancer was overwhelming; from her research, Jill felt the prognosis for anyone given a diagnosis of ovarian cancer was grim. She was greatly comforted that her mother's cancer was probably not ovarian in origin and indeed may have been related to her smoking and alcohol misuse. Jill was aware that she has no guarantees that she does not have an increased risk for cancer, but she does not need to be screened for cancer any differently from other women her age. Although obtaining information about Jill's family was time-consuming it helped Jill obtain peace of mind and saved her from further debate over the consideration of a prophylactic oophorectomy.

Case 5: A Pedigree Pickle

I like to use this song for a fun break in teaching (Figure A.5)

"I'm My Own Grandpaw": Words and music by Dwight Latham and Moe Jaffe © 1947. Renewed: Used by permission.

Many, many years ago when I was twenty-three
I was married to a widow who was pretty as could be.
The widow had a grown up daughter who had hair of red.
My father fell in love with her and soon, they too, were wed.

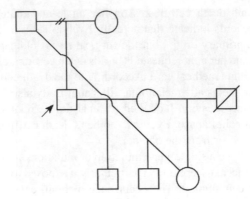

Figure A.5   *Teaching tool: pedigree of a man who is his own grandfather.*

Chorus
This made my dad my son-in-law, and changed my very life.
For my daughter was my mother cause she was my father's wife.
To complicated the matter even though it brought me joy,
I soon became the father of a bouncing baby boy

Chorus
My little baby then became a brother-in-law to Dad,
And so became my uncle, though it made me very sad.
For if he was my uncle then that also made him brother
Of the widow's grown-up daughter who, of course, was my stepmother.

Chorus
Father's wife then had a son who kept them on the run.
And he became my grandchild for he was my daughter's son.
My wife is now my mother's mother and it makes me blue
Because, although she is my wife, she's my grandmother too.

Chorus
Oh, if my wife is my grandmother, then I am her grandchild
And everytime I think of it it nearly drives me wild.
For now I have become the strangest case you ever saw;
As husband of my grandmother I am my own grandpaw.

Chorus
I'm my own grandpaw.
I'm my own grandpaw.
It sounds funny I know,
But it really is so;
I'm my own grandpaw.

List of Genetic Disorders, Gene Symbols and Names, and Patterns of Inheritance

Disorder and/or Locus[a]	Gene Symbol	Gene name	Inheritance Pattern
Aarskog (faciogenital dysplasia)	*FGD1*	FYVE, RhoGEF and PH domain containing 1	XL
Abetalipoproteinemia	*MTTP*	microsomally triglyceride transfer protein	AR
Aceruloplasminemia	*CP*	ceruloplasmin (ferroxidase)	AR
Achondroplasia	*FGFR3*	fibroblast growth factor receptor 3	AD
Acute intermittent porphyria	*HMPBS*	hydroxymethybilane synthase	AD
Adrenoleukodystrophy (aderenomyeloneuropahy)	*ABCD1*	ATP-binding cassette, sub-family D (ACD) member 1	XL
α-1 antitrypsin deficiency (AATD)	*SERPINA1*	serpin peptidase inhibitor, clade A(α-1 antiproteinase, antitrypsin), member 1	AR
α-thalassemia			AR
HBA1		hemoglobin, α 1	AR
HBA2		hemoglobin, α 2	AR
Alport syndrome	*COL4A5*	collagen, type IV, α 5	XL
COL4A3		collagen type IV, α 3	AR
COL4A4		collagen, type IV, α 4	AR

(Continued)

The Practical Guide to the Genetic Family History, Second Edition, by Robin L. Bennett
Copyright © 2010 John Wiley & Sons, Inc.

Disorder and/or Locus[a]	Gene Symbol	Gene name	Inheritance Pattern
Andersen-Tawil syndrome (Long QT7, atypical)	*KCNJ*	potassium inwardly rectifying channel, subfamily J, member 2	AD
Androgen insensitivity syndrome	AR	androgen receptor	XL
Angelman syndrome	*UBE3A*	ubiquitin-protein ligase E3A	Maternal inheritance
Arginase deficiency	ARG1	Arginase–1	AR
Arrhythmogenic right ventricular dysplasia			
	DSC2	Desmocollin 2	AD
	DSP	desmoplakin	AD
	PKP2	plakophilin 2	AD
	DSG2	desmoglein 2	AD
Aspartylglucosaminuria	*AGA*	aspartylglucosaminidase	AR
Ataxia-telangiectasia	*ATM*	ataxia telangiectasia mutated	AR
Barth syndrome	*TAZ*	tafazzin	XL
Biotinidase deficiency	*BTD*	biotinidase	AR
Birt-Hogg Dubé	*FLCN*	folliculin	AD
Blepharophimosis, ptosis, epicanthus inversus (BPES)	*FOXL2*	Foxhead box L2	AD
Bloom syndrome	*BLM*	Bloom syndrome, RecQ helicase–like	AR
Branchio-oto-renal spectrum disorders (BOR)	*EYA1*	eyes absent homolog 1	AD
	SIX1	SIX homebox 1	AD
	SIX5	SIX homeobox 5	AD
Breast-ovarian cancer syndrome			
	BRCA1	breast cancer 1, early onset	AD
	BRCA2	breast cancer 2, early onset	AD
Brugada syndrome	*SCN5A*	sodium channel, voltage–gated, type 5, alpha subunit	AD
CADASIL (cerebral autosomal dominant arteriopathy with subcortical infarcts and leukoencephalopathy)	*NOTCH3*	Notch homolog 3	AD
CARASIL (cerebral autosomal recessive arteriopathy with subcortical infarcts and leukoencephalopathy)	*HTRA1*	HtrA serine peptidase 1	AR
Canavan syndrome	*ASPA*	aspartoacylase	AR
Carney complex	*PKAR1A*	protein kinase, cAMP-dependent, regulatory, type 1, α (tissue specific extinguisher 1)	AD

Disorder and/or Locus[a]	Gene Symbol	Gene name	Inheritance Pattern
Carnitine palmitoyl transferase 1	CPT1	carnitine palmitoyltransferase 1A	AR
Carnitine palmitoyl transferase II	CPT2	carnitine palitoyltransferase II	AR
Catecholaminergic ventricular tachycardia			
	CASQ2	calsequestrin 2	AR
	RYR2	ryanodine receptor 2	AD
Cerebroreintal vasculopathy (CRV & HERNS)	TREX1	three prime repair exonuclease 1	AD
Cerebrotendinous xanthomatosis	CYP27A1	sterol 27-hydroxylase	AR
Charcot-Marie-Tooth type I (hereditary motor sensory neuropathy)	PMP22	peripheral myelin protein-22	AD
Chrondrodysplasia punctata (Conradi-Hunermann)	ARSE	arylsulfatase E	XL
Chondroectodermal dysplasia (Ellis van Creveld)	EVC	Ellis van Creveld	AR
	EVC2	Ellis van Creveld2	AR
Choreoacanthocytosis	VPS13A	vacuolar protein sorting 13 homolog A	AR
Cleft lip with/without cleft palate, non-syndromic	MSX1	msh homebox AD	AD
Cockayne syndrome			AR
	CSA	Cockayne syndrome A	
	CSB	Cockayne syndrome B	
Congenital adrenal hyperplasia	CYP21A2	cytochrome P450, family 21, subfamily A, polypeptide 2	AR
Congenital central hypoventilation syndrome	PHOX2B	paired-like homebox2b	AD
Congenital nephrotic syndrome (Pierson syndrome)	LAMB2	lamin beta-2	AR
Connexin 26 (DNB1), non-syndromic neurosensory deafness	GJB2/Cx26	gap junction protein β-2	
Coproporphyria	CPO	coproporphyrinogen oxidase	AD
Cowden syndrome	PTEN	phosphatase and tensin homologuo	AD
Creutzfeldt-Jacob diseases	PRNP	prion protein	AD, sporadic

(Continued)

Disorder and/or Locus[a]	Gene Symbol	Gene name	Inheritance Pattern
Cystic fibrosis	CFTR	cystic fibrosis transmembrane conductance regulator	AR
Cystinosis	CTNS	cystinosis, nephrotic	AR
Danon syndrome	LAMP2	lysosome-associated membrane protein 2	XL
DRPLA	ATN1	atrophin 1	AD
Duchenne-Becker muscular dystrophy	DMD	dystrophin	XL
Dysautonomia, familial	IKBKAP	inhibitor of kappa light polylpeptide gene enhancer in B-cells, kinase complex-associated protein	AR
Ehlers-Danlos type IV (vascular)	COL3A1	collagen, type III, α 1	AD
Emery-Dreifuss muscular dystrophy	LMNA	lamin A/C	AD
Exostoses, multiple	EXT1	exostoses, multiple 1	AD
	EXT2	exostoses, multiple 2	AD
	EXT3	exostoses, multiple 3	AD
	EMD	emerin	XL
Fabry disease	GLA	galactosidase α	XL
Familial adenomatous polyposis coli (FAP)	APC	adenomatous polyposis coli	AD
Familial amyloid angiopathy	CST3	cystatin C	AD
Familial atypical multiple mole-melanoma (FAMM)	CDKN2A	cyclin-dependent kinase inhibitor 2A	AD
	CDK4	cyclin-dependent kinase 4	AD
	CMM	cutaneous malignant melanoma/dysplastic nevus	AD
Familial fatal insomnia	PRNP	prion protein	AD
Familial hypercholesterolemia	LDLR	low density lipoprotein receptor	AD
Familial medullary thyroid cancer	RET	ret proto-oncogene	AD
Floating-Harbor syndrome	?		AD, sporadic
Fragile X syndrome	FMR1	fragile X mental retardation 1	XL
Friedreich ataxia	FXN	frataxin	AR
Frontotemporal dementia with parkinsonism (FTDP–17)	MAPT	microtubule-associated protein tau	AD
Frontotemporal dementia-CHMP2B-related	CHMP2	chromatin modifying protein 2B	AD
Frontotemporal dementia–GRN related	GRN	granulin	AD

Disorder and/or Locus[a]	Gene Symbol	Gene name	Inheritance Pattern
Galactosemia	*GALT*	galactose-1-phosphate uridyltransferase	AR
Galactokinase deficiency	GALK1	galactokinase 1	AR
Gaucher disease	*GBA*	glucosidase, β acid	AR
Glutaric aciduria	*GCDH1*	glutaryl-Coenzyme A dehydrogenase	AR
GM2 gangliosidosis (late-onset Tay-Sachs)	*HEXA*	hexosaminidase A (α polypeptide)	AR
Hallervorden-Spatz disease	*PANK2*	pantothenate kinase 2	AD
Hand-foot-genital syndrome	*HOXA13*	homeobox A13	AD
Hartnup disease	*SLC6A19*	solute carrier family 6 (neutral amino acid transporter), member 19	AR
Hemochromatosis (classic)	*HFE*	hemochromatosis	AR
Hemophilia A (factor VIII deficiency)	*F8*	coagulation factor VIII, procoagulant component	XL
Hemophilia B (factor IX deficiency)	*F9*	coagulation factor IX	XL
Hereditary diffuse gastric cancer (HDGC)	*CDH1*	cadherin 1, type 1, E-candherin (epithelial)	AD
Hereditary hemorrhagic telangiectasia (HHT or Osler-Weber-Rendu)	*ENG* *ACVRL1*	endoglin activin-A receptor type II-like 1	AD
Hereditary leiomyomatosis and renal cell carcinoma (HLRCC)	*FH*	fumarate hydratase	AD
Hereditary papillary renal cell	*MET*	met proto-oncogene (hepatocyte growth factor receptor)	AD
Hereditary parganglioma syndrome (PGL)			AD
PGL1	*SDHB*	succinate dehydrogenase complex, subunit B, iron sulfur	
PGL2	SDHAF2	succinate dehydrogenase complex assembly factor 2 (possible imprinting)	
PGL3	*SDHC*	succinate dehydrogenase complex, subunit C, integral membrane protein	
PGL4	SDHD	succinate dehydrogenase complex, subunit D, integral membrane protein (maternal imprinting)	

(Continued)

Disorder and/or Locus[a]	Gene Symbol	Gene name	Inheritance Pattern
Homocystinuria	*CBS*	cysthathionine beta-synthase	AR
Hunter syndrome (mucopolysaccharidosis type II)	IDS	iduronate 2-sulfatase	XL
Huntington disease	*HTT*	huntingtin	AD
Hypertrophic cardiomyopathy	*MYH7*	myosin, heavy chain 7, cardiac muscle beta	AD
	MYBPC3	myosin binding protein C, cardiac	AD
	TNNT2	troponin T type 2, cardiac	AD
Hypophosphatemia (vitamin D resistant rickets)	*PHEX*	phosphate regulating endopeptidase homolog, X-linked	XL
Hypohydrotic ectodermal dysplasia	*EDA*	ectrodysplain A	XL
Idiopathic pulmonary fibrosis (IPF)	*TERT*	telomerase reverse transcriptase	AD
	TERC	telomerase RNA component	AD
Incontinentia pigmenti	*IKBKG* (NEMO)	inhibitor of κ light polypeptide gene enhancer in B-cells kinase γ	XL
Inclusion body myopathy with early-onset Paget disease and frontotemporal dementia (IBMPFD)	*VCP*	valosin-containing protein	AD
Jervell-Lange Nielsen (JLNS1, JLNS2)			
	KCNQ1	potassium voltage-gated channel subfamily KQT member 1	AR
	KCNE1	Potassium voltage-gated channel subfamily E member (Isk-related) 1	AR
Juvenile polyposis	*BMPR1A*	bone morphogenetic protein receptor, type 1A	AD
	SMAD4	SMAD family member 4	AD
Kallmann syndrome (KS)			
KS1	*KAL1*	Kallman syndrome 1 sequence	XL
KS2	*FGFR1*	fibroblast growth factor receptor 1	AD
KS3	*PROKR2*	prokineticin receptor 2	AD
KS4	*PROK2*		AD

Disorder and/or Locus[a]	Gene Symbol	Gene name	Inheritance Pattern
Kartagener syndrome (see primary ciliary dyskinesia)			
Leri-Weill dyschondrosetosis (SHOX related haploinsufficiency disorders)	SHOX	short stature hemobox	del, point muta-tions of pseu-doauto-somal regions of X and Y
Lesch–Nyhan syndrome	HPRT1	hypoxanthine phosphoribosyl-transferase 1	XL
Loeys-Dietz syndrome	TGFBR1	transforming growth factor, β receptor 1	AD
	TGFBR2	transforming growth factor, β receptor 2	AD
Long QT (includes Romano-Ward)			
Long QT1	KCNQ1	potassium voltage gated-channel subfamily KQT member 1	AD
Long QT2	KCNH2	potassium voltage gated-channel subfamily H member 2	AD
Long QT3 (Brugada syndrome)	SCN5A	sodium channel protein type 5 subunit alpha	AD
Long QT4	ANK2	ankryin-B	AD
Long QT5	KCNE1	potassium voltage-gated subfamily E member 1	AD
Long QT6	KCNE2	potassium voltage-gated subfamily E member 2	AD
Long QT7 (Anderson-Tawil, atypical Long QT)	KCNJ2	potassium inwardly-rectifying channel, subfamily J, member 2	AD
Long QT8 (atypical, complex; Timothy syndrome)	CACNA1C		AD
Long QT9	CAV2	caveolin-3	AD
Long QT10	SCN4B	sodium channel subunit beta-4	AD
Li-Fraumeni syndrome	TP53	tumor protein p53	AD
Lowe syndrome (oculocerebrorenal)	OCRL1	oculocerebrorenal syndrome of Lowe	XL

(Continued)

Disorder and/or Locus[a]	Gene Symbol	Gene name	Inheritance Pattern
Lynch syndrome (HNPCC)			AD
	MLH1	mut homolog 1, colon cancer, nonpolyposis type 2	AD
	MSH2	mutS homolog2, colon cancer, nonpolyposis type	AD
	MSH6	mutS homlog 6	AD
	PMS2	PMS2 posmeiotic segregation increased 2	AD
	TACSTD1	tumor–associated calcium signal transducer 1	AD
Mandibulofacial dysostosis (Treacher-Collins syndrome)	TCOF1		AD
Maple syrup urine disease			AR
	BCKDHA	branched chain keto acid dehydrogenase E1, α polypeptide	
	BCKDHB	branched chain keto acid dehydrogenase E1, β polypeptide	
	DBT	dehydrolioamide branched chain transacyclase E2	
	DLD	dihydrolipoamide dehydrogenase	
Marfan syndrome	FBN1	fibrillin 1	AD
Marshall syndrome	COL11A1	collagen type XI, α	AD
Medium-chain-acyl-dehydrogenase	ACADM	acyl-coenzyme A dehydrogenase, C-4 to C-12 straight gene	AR
Metachromatic leukodystrophy	ARSA	arylsulfatase A	AR
MODY (maturity-onset diabetes of the young)			
MODY1	HNF4A	hepatocyte nuclear factor 4, α	AD
MODY2	GCK	glucokinase	AD
MODY3	HNF1A	hypatocyte nuclear factor-1, homeobox A	AD
MODY4	PDX1 or IPF1	pancreatic and duodenal homeobox 1	AD
MODY5	HNF1B	hepatocyte nuclear factor-1, homeobox B	AD
MODY6	NEUROD1 or BETA2	neurogenetic differentiation 1 or β cell E-box trans-activator 2	
Mohr-Tranebjaerb syndrome	TIMM8A	translocase of inner mitochondrial membrane homolog A	XL

Disorder and/or Locus[a]	Gene Symbol	Gene name	Inheritance Pattern
MTHF reductase (methylenetetrahydrofolate reductase)	*MTHFR*	5,10–methylene (NADPA)	AR
Multiple endocrine neoplasia 1 (MEN1)	*MEN1*	menin	AD
Multiple endocrine neoplasia 2 (MEN2)	*RET*	ret proto-oncogene	AD
MYH9-related disorders	*MYH9*	myosin, heavy chain 9, non-muscle	AD
MYH associated polyposis (MAP)	*MUTYH*	mutY homolog	AR
Myotonic muscular dystrophy	*DM1*	dystrophica myotonica 1	AD
Nail-patella syndrome (hereditary oncho-osteodysplasia)	LMX1	LIM homeobox transcription factor 1, β	AD
Nance-Horan	*NHS*	Nance-Horan syndrome	XL
Naxos disease	*JUP*	plakoglobin	AR
Nephrogenic diabetes insipidus	*AVPR2*	arginine vasopressin receptor 2	XL
Neurofibromatosis type 1	*NF1*	neurofibromin 1	AD
Neurofibromatosis type 2	*NF2*	neurofibromin 2 (merlin)	AD
Nevoid basal cell carcinoma syndrome (Gorlin syndrome)	*PTCH*	patched homolog 1	AD
Niemann-Pick Type C	*NPC1*	Niemann-Pick disease, type C1	AR
Non-syndromic neurosensory deafness (DFNB1)	*GJB2/Cx26*	gap junction protein β-2/connexin 26	AR
Non-syndromic neurosensory deafness (DFNA3)	*GJB6*	gap junction protein β-6/connexin 30	AD
Noonan syndrome			AD
NS1	*PRPN11*	protein tyrosine phosphtase, non-receptor type 11	
NS4	*SOS1*	son of sevenless homolog 1	
Norrie disease	*NDP*	Norride disease (pseudoglioma)	XL
Oculo-auriculo-vertebral spectrum	?	?	AD
Oculomandibulofacial syndrome (Hallerman Streiff)	?	Sporadic	
Opitz syndrome (spectrum of 22q deletion syndrome)			AD

(*Continued*)

Disorder and/or Locus[a]	Gene Symbol	Gene name	Inheritance Pattern
Ornithine transcarbamylase deficiency	*OTC*	ornithine transcarbamy-oltransferase	XL
Orofaciodigital syndrome 1	*OFD1*	oral-facial-digital syndrome 1	XL
Osteogenesis imperfecta			AD
	COLA1	collagen type 1, α 1	
Pancreatitis, hereditary	*PRSS1*	protease, serine 1 (trypsin 1)	AD
	SPINK1	serine peptidase inhibitor, Kazal type 1	AD
	COL1A2	collagen type 1, α 2	AD
Pendred syndrome (DFNB4)	*SLC26A4*	solute carrier family 26, member 4	AR
	FOXI1	forkhead box I1	AR
Peutz-Jeghers syndrome	*STK11*	serine/threonine kinase 11	AD
Phenylketonuria (PKU)	*PAH*	phenylalanine hydroxylase	AR
Polycystic kidney disease, adult			AD
	PKD1	polycystic kidney disease 1	AD
	PKD2	polycystic kidney disease 2	AD
	PKD3	polycystic kidney disease 3	AD
Polycystic kidney disease, infantile	*PKDH1*	polycystic kidney disease and hepatic disease 1	AR
Popliteal ptergium syndrome	*IRF6*	interferon regulatory factor 6	AD1
Porphyria variegate	*PPOX*	protoporphyrinogen oxidase	AD|
Primary ciliary dyskinesia (PCD; immotile cilia syndrome; Kartagener syndrome)			
	DNAI1	dynein axonemal, intermediate chain 1	AR
	DNAH5	dynein axonemal, heavy chain 5	AR
	DNAH11	dynein, axonemal, heavy chain 11	AR
	DNAI2	dynein, xonemal, intermediate chain 2	AR
	TXNDC3	thioredoxin domain-containing protein 3	AR
	RSPH9	radial spoke head 9 homolog	AR
	RSPH4A	radial spoke head 4 homolog A	AR

Disorder and/or Locus[a]	Gene Symbol	Gene name	Inheritance Pattern
Proprionic acidemia			AR
	PCCA	propionyl coenzyme A carboxylase α polypeptide	
	PCCB	propionyl coenzyme A carboxylase, β polypeptide	
Pseudohypoparathyroidism	*GNAS*	GNAS complex locus	AD
Pseudoxanthomas elasticum (PXE)	*ABCC6* (MRP6)	ATP-binding cassette, sub family X (CFTR/MRP) member 6	AR
Pyruvate carboxylase deficiency	*PC*	pyruvate carboxylase	AR
Refsum (adult) syndrome			AR
	PHYH	phytanoyl-CoA 2-hydroxylase	
	PEX7	perioxisomal biogenesis factor 7	
Retinoblastoma (RB)	*RB1*	retinoblastoma 1	
Rett syndrome	*MECP2*	methyl CpG binding protein 2	XL
Rhizomelic chondrodysplasia punctata	*PEX7*	peroxisomal biogenesis factor 7	AR
Romano Ward (see Long QT)			
Rothmund-Thompson	*RECAL4*	RECQ protein-like 4	AR
Saethre-Chotzen syndrome	*TWIST1*	twist homolog 1	AD
Sanfilippo syndrome (mucopolysaccharidosis III)			AR
MPS IIIA	*SGSH*	N-sulfoglucosamine sulfohydolase	
MPS IIIB	*NSGLU*	N-acetylglucosaminidase, α	
MPS IIIC	*HGSNAT*	heparin-α-glucoasminide-N-acetyltransferase	
MPS IIID	*GNS*	N-glucosamine 6 (N-acetyl)-sulfatase	
Short QT syndrome			
	KCNQ1 (*KVLQT*)	potassium voltage-gated channel subfamily KQT-like subfamily member 1	AD
	KCNH2 (*HERG*)	potassium voltage-gated channel subfamily H (eag-related) member 2	AD
	KCNJ2	potassium inwardly-rectifying, channel subfamily J member 2	AD

(*Continued*)

Disorder and/or Locus[a]	Gene Symbol	Gene name	Inheritance Pattern
Sickle cell anemia	HBB	hemoglobin, β	AR
Smith-Lemli-Opitz syndrome	DCHR7	7-dehydrocholesterol reductase	AR
Spinal muscular atrophy	SMN1	survival of motor neuron 1, telomeric	AR
Spinobulbar muscular atrophy	AR	androgen receptor	XL
Spinocerebellar ataxia 2 (SCA2)	ATXN2	ataxin 2	AD
Stickler syndrome (hereditary anthro-ophthalmopathy)			
STL1	COL2A1	collagen, type II, α 1	AD
STL2	COL11A1	collagen, type XI, α 1	AD
STL3	COL11A2	collagen type XI, α 2	AD
Tay-Sachs disease (GM2 gangliosidosis)	HEXA	hexosaminidase A (α polypeptide)	AR
Timothy syndrome (Long QT 8)	CACNA1C	calcium channel, voltage-dependent, L-type, α 1C subunit	AD
Treacher-Collins syndrome	TCOF1	Treacher Collins-Franceschetti syndrome 1	AD
Tricho-rhino-phalangeal syndrome	TRPS1	trichorhinophalangeal syndrome	AD
Tuberous sclerosis complex			AD
	TSC1	tuberous sclerosis 1	
	TSC2	tuberous sclerosis 2	
21-hydroxylase deficiency	CYP21A2	cytochrome P450, family 21, subfamily A, polypeptide 2	AR
Tyrosinemia type 1	FAH	fumarylacetacetate hydrolase (fumaryl acetoacetase)	AR
Usher syndrome (multiple loci, multiple types)			AR
Van der Woude syndrome	IRF6	interferon regulatory factor 6	AD
Vitamin D resistant rickets (see Hypophosphatemia)			XL
Von Hippel-Lindau syndrome	VHL	von Hippel-Lindau tumor suppressor	AD
Von Willebrand disease	VWF	von Willebrand factor	AD

Disorder and/or Locus[a]	Gene Symbol	Gene name	Inheritance Pattern
Waardenburg syndrome			
WS1	PAX3	paired box 3	AD
WS2	MITF	microophthalmia-associated transcription factor	AD
WS3	PAX3	paired box 3	AD
WS4	EDNRB	endothelin receptor type B	AD
	EDN3	endothelin 3	
	SOX10	SRY determining region Y box 10	
Werner syndrome	WRN	Werner syndrome	AR
Wilms tumor syndromes			AD
	WT1	Wilms tumor 1	
	WT2	Wilms tumor 2	
Wilson disease	ATP7B	ATPase, Cu++ transporting, β polypeptide	AR
Wolfram (DIDMOAD) syndrome	WFS1	Wolfran syndrome 1 (wolframin)	AR
	WFS2	Wolfran syndrome 2	AR
Young syndrome			
Xeroderma pigmentosum (XP) at least 9 loci			AR
Zellweger spectrum		multiple genes involved in peroxisome biogenesis	AR

[a]Many diseases are allelic and also have locus heterogeneity; therefore, this list is not intended to be exhaustive but a reference for many of the disorders mentioned throughout the book.

Source: HUGO Gene Nomcenclature Committee at the European Bioinformatics Institute. Available at http://genenames.org. Accessed November 28, 2009.

Index

The Practical Guide to the Genetic Family History, Second Edition, by Robin L. Bennett
Copyright © 2010 John Wiley & Sons, Inc.